AF712024

SMALL-ANIMAL SPECT IMAGING

Matthew A. Kupinski
Harrison H. Barrett
(Eds.)

Small-Animal SPECT Imaging

With 123 Figures

Springer

Matthew A. Kupinski
Optical Science Center
The University of Arizona
Tucson, AZ 85721
USA

Harrison H. Barrett
Department of Radiology
The University of Arizona
Tucson, AZ 85721
USA

Library of Congress Control Number: 2005923844

ISBN-10: 0-387-25143-X eISBN: 0-387-25294-0 Printed on acid-free paper.
ISBN-13: 978-0387-25143-1

© 2005 Springer Science+Business Media, Inc.
All rights reserved. This work may not be translated or copied in whole or in part without the written permission of the publisher (Springer Science+Business Media, Inc., 233 Spring Street, New York, NY 10013, USA), except for brief excerpts in connection with reviews or scholarly analysis. Use in connection with any form of information storage and retrieval, electronic adaptation, computer software, or by similar or dissimilar methodology now known or hereafter developed is forbidden.
The use in this publication of trade names, trademarks, service marks and similar terms, even if they are not identified as such, is not to be taken as an expression of opinion as to whether or not they are subject to proprietary rights.

Printed in the United States of America. (EB)

9 8 7 6 5 4 3 2 1

springeronline.com

Contents

List of Figures

List of Tables

About the Editors

Matthew A. Kupinski is an Assistant Professor of Optical Sciences and Radiology at the University of Arizona. He earned his Ph.D. degree from the University of Chicago in 2000 and joined the faculty at the University of Arizona in 2002.

Harrison H. Barrett is a Regents Professor of Radiology and Optical Sciences at the University of Arizona in Tucson, Arizona. Professor Barrett joined the University of Arizona in 1974, he is the former editor of the *Journal of the Optical Society of America A*, and is the recipient of the IEEE Medical Imaging Scientist Award in 2000. He is the coauthor of two books on image science.

Preface

In January 2004, the Center for Gamma-Ray Imaging (CGRI), a research resource funded by the National Institute of Biomedical Imaging and Bioengineering (NIBIB), hosted "The Workshop on Small-Animal SPECT" in Tucson, Arizona. Over 80 people from around the world attended this workshop, which included numerous short courses and contributed papers. The primary objective of the workshop was to provide education in some of the key technologies and applications that have been going on in the Center. Topics presented at this workshop included scintillation and semiconductor detector technologies, digital signal processing techniques, system modeling and reconstruction algorithms, animal monitoring and handling, and applications of small-animal imaging. The workshop presented an opportunity for free interchange of ideas among the researchers, faculty, and attendees through presentations, panel discussions, lab tours, and question and answer sessions. The members of the Center for Gamma-Ray Imaging thought it important that the many interesting results and ideas presented at this workshop be written down to, hopefully, benefit other researchers. This volume is the result of that endeavor. Most short courses and contributed presentations are included in chapter form. The first seven chapters were contributed by faculty members in the Center, followed by chapters from our colleagues around the world.

MATTHEW A. KUPINSKI

Acknowledgments

This book would not have been possible without the help of Jane Lockwood, Lisa Gelia, and Nancy Preble. Dr. Georgios Kastis deserves much of the credit for the initial planning of the workshop and for obtaining the funding necessary to organize the conference and publish this volume. We are especially thankful to Corrie Thies for her careful editing of this entire volume. Finally, we thank the over 80 attendees of the Workshop of Small-Animal SPECT Imaging.

Chapter 1

Biomedical Significance of Small-Animal Imaging

James M. Woolfenden and Zhonglin Liu*

1. Introduction

Small animals are used widely in biomedical research. Mice in particular are favorite animal subjects: they are economical, reproduce rapidly, and can provide models of human disease. Mice with compromised immune systems have been used for many years in studies of human tumor xenografts. The sequence of the mouse genome has been determined, and knockout mice (in which expression of a particular gene has been disabled) are available as models of various metabolic abnormalities.

Most studies in mice and other small animals are translational studies of human disease. Such studies are supported by government and private-sector research grants and by major pharmaceutical corporations. Other research studies are directed at cellular and subcellular processes that do not necessarily have immediate applications in human disease. Small animals are also used for some studies of animal diseases that do not have direct human analogues, but these studies are confined largely to centers of veterinary medicine.

In all of these biomedical studies of small animals, imaging can play a key role. Imaging studies can determine whether a new drug reaches the intended target tissue or organ and whether it also reaches other sites that may result in toxic effects. More-detailed studies of biodistribution and pharmacokinetics are possible, provided the spatial resolution and dynamic capabilities of the imaging systems are adequate. In the case of new radiopharmaceuticals for imaging and therapy, radiation-dose estimates can be made from the biodistribution data.

Imaging studies have significant advantages over postmortem tissue distribution studies. Although a few animals may need to be sacrificed to validate the imaging data, far fewer must be sacrificed than with conventional tissue biodistribution studies. Radiolabeled compounds that have unfavorable biodistribution or pharmacokinetics can be identified rapidly and either modified or discarded. Longitudinal studies in the same animals are possible, and the effects of interventions such as drug treatment can be assessed.

*The University of Arizona, Department of Radiology, Tucson, Arizona

Imaging of internal biodistribution of molecules in small animals generally means gamma-ray imaging, although imaging of superficial structures may be possible using other methods. The remainder of this discussion will assume that the objective is gamma-ray imaging and that the gamma-emitting radionuclides serve as reporters of physiologic functions of interest. (Imaging of characteristic x-ray emissions is technically not gamma-ray imaging, but no distinction will be made between the two.)

2. Selection of radiopharmaceuticals

2.1 Choice of radiolabeled molecule

There are several categories of molecules that are commonly radiolabeled for use in small-animal imaging:

1. Receptor-directed molecules are useful for imaging organs or tissues that have elevated expression of the receptor compared to other tissues. For example, somatostatin receptors have increased expression in various neuroendocrine tumors, and radiolabeled somatostatin-receptor ligands such as In-111 pentetreotide are used in both human and animal imaging.

2. Molecules may serve as substrates for metabolic processes. Examples include F-18-fluorodeoxyglucose as a marker of glucose metabolism. Most malignant tumors have increased glucose utilization compared to normal tissues, although some increase in glucose metabolism may also occur at inflammatory sites.

3. A molecule may serve as a reporter for a physiologic function such as perfusion or excretion. For example, myocardial imaging agents such as Tc-99m tetrofosmin and sestamibi are reporters of regional myocardial perfusion.

4. Occasionally the radionuclide itself is the molecule of interest, usually in ionic form. Examples include any of the radioisotopes of iodine, administered as sodium iodide for studies of the thyroid.

2.2 Choice of radionuclide

Several factors affect the choice of radionuclide. First, the goals of imaging should be considered. If a radiopharmaceutical is being developed with the objective of human use, then the radionuclide that is intended for human use should be used in the animal studies if at all possible. This will simplify submission of preclinical data to the U.S. Food and Drug Administration. In some cases, however, the use of a different radionuclide for some of the preclinical studies is unavoidable. For example, if therapy is planned using a pure beta-emitter such as Y-90, then a surrogate such as In-111 will be needed for imaging. If no translational uses are anticipated, and only a quick screen of biodistribution is needed, then ease of radiolabeling may dictate the choice of radionuclide. If autoradiography is planned, then selecting a radionuclide with a reasonable abundance of particle emissions (including conversion and Auger electrons) is better than attempting autoradiography with photons.

The physical properties of the radionuclide are likely to affect the choice. The gamma energy should be appropriate for the imaging system and the animal being imaged. Detector thickness and photon-detection efficiency should be considered. Silicon detectors are nearly transparent to the gamma-ray energies used in clinical nuclear-medicine imaging, but they can be used for low-energy photons (as well as particle emissions). I-125 should work well with a silicon imaging array, but I-123, I-131, and Tc-99m would not. Animal thickness is also relevant. I-125 has a tissue half-value layer of approximately 1.7 cm, which precludes its use for most human imaging studies. This attenuation is only a minor problem in mice, although it becomes more of a problem in larger animals. If the animal being imaged is a small submammalian species such as C. elegans, then very low-energy photons or even direct particle detection can be used.

Chemical properties of the radionuclide may influence its choice. For example, there are several standard methods of radioiodination, and radiolabeling is often relatively easy. If rapid assessment of biodistribution is the goal, then one of the iodine radioisotopes may be a good choice. If Tc-99m is desired as the radiolabel, then a linking chelator may be needed, and the chemistry becomes somewhat more complex. If large molecular complexes are used for radiolabeling, the biodistribution of the radiolabeled molecule may be changed. It may be necessary to validate such radiolabeled molecules by comparing their biodistribution to that of the molecule without the labeling complex, using an incorporated radiolabel such as H-3 or C-14, along with liquid scintillation counting of tissue samples.

Disposal issues may affect the choice of radionuclide. As a general rule, most radionuclides in reasonable quantities can be stored for approximately 10 half-lives, surveyed for any residual radioactivity, and if none is present then they can be disposed of as ordinary waste. If a radionuclide with a long half-life is selected, such as I-125 (60 days) or Co-57 (270 days), then waste management is likely to be an issue.

2.3 Other issues in small-animal imaging

The anticipated biological fate of the radionuclide may need to be considered. If the radionuclide is separated from the molecule it was labeling, it may be recycled or excreted. For example, deiodinases cleave radioiodine from tyrosyl and phenolic rings, and the radioiodine is then available for thyroid uptake and incorporation into thyroid hormone.

The radiation dose to the animal from imaging studies should be considered, particularly when serial studies are planned, in order to prevent unwanted biological effects. The administered radionuclide doses per unit weight for small-animal imaging are typically quite large, in comparison to human studies, in order to obtain sufficient photons for imaging. If CT imaging is also used, this further increases the radiation dose.

Good spatial resolution is necessary in small-animal imaging studies, particularly when quantitative measurements are desired, but it may not be sufficient. Even in human imaging studies using radionuclides, organ boundaries are frequently indistinct, and localization of sites of uptake can be problematic. A major benefit of hybrid PET-CT systems is the definition of anatomy on CT so that the site of F-18 fluorodeoxyglucose uptake can be identified. Similarly, micro-CT units as part of multimodality small-animal imaging systems are very helpful for defining anatomy. MRI can play a similar role, although care must be taken to ensure accurate image fusion, because the gamma-ray and MR images are acquired on different systems.

3. Applications: Ischemic heart disease

3.1 Clinical imaging studies

Heart disease is the leading cause of death in the United States. In 2001, the last year for which complete data are available, heart disease was responsible for 29.0% of deaths, and cancer, the second-leading cause, resulted in 22.9% of deaths [Centers for Disease Control and Prevention]. Most of the cardiac deaths are from ischemic heart disease.

Myocardial infarction typically causes electrocardiographic changes and elevation of blood markers such as troponin-I and the myocardial fraction of creatine kinase. Clinical imaging has not played a large role in diagnosis of acute myocardial infarction, although several nuclear-medicine imaging studies are available. Tc-99m-pyrophosphate, a bone-imaging agent, was noted about 30 years ago to accumulate in acute myocardial infarcts; the uptake is probably associated with calcium deposition in the irreversibly damaged tissue. The In-111 antimyosin antibody also has been used for imaging acutely infarcted myocardium; myosin is normally sequestered inside cardiac myocytes, but following infarction, it is available for antibody binding.

Myocardial imaging agents that are widely used in diagnostic imaging of stress-induced myocardial ischemia can also be used to screen for perfusion defects associated with acute myocardial infarction. A normal imaging study has a high predictive value for the absence of infarction and can obviate the need for hospital admission and monitoring while results of other tests to exclude infarction are pending. If a perfusion defect is present, however, the imaging study cannot distinguish between acute infarction, prior infarction, chronically ischemic (hibernating) myocardium, and acutely ischemic but viable (stunned) myocardium.

Myocardial stunning is a reversible form of a category of myocardial dysfunction known as ischemia-reperfusion injury. This injury typically accompanies restoration of myocardial perfusion by angioplasty or thrombolysis following acute coronary-artery occlusion. There is evidence that development and severity of ischemia-reperfusion injury can be modulated by drugs and ischemic preconditioning. Small-animal imaging studies provide a means to evaluate the effects of such modulation.

3.2 Imaging of ischemia-reperfusion injury

We have implemented a model for studies of ischemia-reperfusion injury using Sprague-Dawley rats. A left thoracotomy incision is made, and a ligature is placed around the left coronary artery and a small amount of myocardium. The ligature can be tightened and released for desired periods of ischemia and reperfusion. Animals are maintained under isoflurane anesthesia and ventilated using a mixture of oxygen and room air during surgery and imaging.

Tc-99m sestamibi is a standard agent for imaging the distribution of myocardial perfusion; it remains within the myocardial cells for at least several hours after injection. If subsequent imaging studies with another Tc-99m-labeled compound are planned, then perfusion can be assessed using Tc-99m-teboroxime, which rapidly washes out of myocardial cells. We have validated the distribution of the perfusion agents by comparing the tomographic images to corresponding post-mortem myocardial slices. In order to define the myocardium at risk, the ligature is tightened, and Evans blue dye is injected prior to sacrifice; the area at risk remains unstained. Viable myocardium is demonstrated on the post-mortem sections by staining with triphenyltetrazolium chloride (TTC); nonviable myocardium remains unstained.

We have used Tc-99m glucarate to demonstrate areas of acute myocardial infarction following ischemia. Glucarate is a 6-carbon dicarboxylic acid sugar that is a natural catabolite of glucuronic acid metabolism in mammals. It is taken up in acutely necrotic myocytes, mainly by binding to nuclear histones [Khaw et al., 1997]. It has little uptake in ischemic, but viable, cells or in apoptotic cells. We have also used Tc-99m annexin-V to demonstrate apoptosis in the ischemic-reperfused myocardium.

The ischemia-reperfusion model permits assessment of interventions such as ischemic preconditioning and use of various chemicals and drugs to decrease the area of myocardial damage that results from the ischemic episode.

4. Applications in oncology

4.1 Problems in clinical oncology

A major problem in clinical oncology is predicting response to therapy. Most cancer chemotherapy drugs have significant toxicity to tissues other than the targeted tumor, particularly bone marrow and intestinal mucosa. Many chemotherapy drugs are expensive, and treatment of drug side effects is another expense. If drug efficacy could be predicted prior to treatment, then ineffective or marginally effective drugs could be discarded, needless side effects avoided, and costs minimized.

An example of predicting response to therapy is found in breast cancer, where the expression of estrogen receptors is highly predictive of response to estrogen-receptor ligands. Another example in a variety of tumors is expression of multidrug resistance (MDR), in which the multidrug-resistance gene encodes p-glycoprotein, a transmembrane protein that exports a variety of xenobiotics from the cell, including various chemotherapy drugs.

Assessing response to chemotherapy after initial exposure to the drug would be desirable if the prediction cannot be made in advance. Imaging studies using Ga-67 citrate and F-18 fluorodeoxyglucose in lymphoma have shown predictive value for subsequent clinical response to chemotherapy [Front et al., 2000; Kostakoglu et al., 2002]. Preliminary data suggest that Tc-99m annexin-V may have similar value by demonstrating apoptosis in tumors after initial exposure to chemotherapy [Mochizuki et al., 2003].

Another problem in clinical oncology is documenting response to therapy. A standard method for assessing response is measuring change in tumor size, using either bidimensional measurements or volume estimates. Size is a lagging indicator, however, and the size of some tumors with fibrotic or necrotic portions may not decrease significantly after the cancer cells have been eradicated. Metabolic activity should be a much earlier and more accurate marker for tumor response than size alone.

4.2 Small-animal imaging to predict tumor response to therapy

We have implemented several small-animal models to address the problem of predicting response to therapy. We have used MCF7 human breast cancer xenografts in SCID mice to assess modulation of expression of multidrug resistance (MDR). A sensitive cell line, MCF7/S, responds to doxorubicin chemotherapy, but a resistant line, MCF7/D40, does not; the resistance results from increased p-glycoprotein expression. Modulation of MDR can be assessed by uptake of radiolabeled substrates for MDR; Tc-99m sestamibi is such a substrate. Dynamic imaging is useful, because the level of MDR expression affects the rate of substrate export from the cell.

We have used another tumor model for early assessment of tumor response to chemotherapy. We have implanted A549 human lung cancer in SCID mice and evaluated response to taxotere therapy. The imaging reporter is Tc-99m annexin-V, which binds to phosphatidylserine in the membrane of cells undergoing apoptosis. Phosphatidylserine is normally not expressed on the cell surface, but the energy-dependent regulation of cell-membrane structure is disrupted in early apoptosis, and phosphatidylserine becomes exposed. Preliminary studies suggest that Tc-99m annexin-V uptake correlates with tumor response to therapy.

4.3 Small-animal imaging of reporter genes

Successful gene therapy requires that a transfected gene be expressed in the targeted tissue. Gene expression may not be immediately apparent, however, and use of a reporter gene that is transfected along with the therapeutic gene may be useful to confirm successful delivery. Several different strategies for reporter genes have been used. One type of reporter gene encodes a membrane receptor, such as the human somatostatin receptor, to which a radiolabeled ligand will bind [Zinn et al., 2002]. A similar concept is cell-membrane expression of the sodium/iodide symporter (NIS), for which iodide and other monovalent anions such as pertechnetate are substrates [Chung, 2002].

The DNA sequences encoding NIS have been identified and cloned for both rats and humans. Cell-membrane expression of NIS results in uptake of radiolabels such as radioiodine, pertechnetate or perrhenate in the targeted cells. Because the radiolabels are not retained in cells other than thyroid (and radiolabels other than iodide are not retained in thyroid), additional strategies may be needed to promote cellular retention. Thyroid peroxidase is involved in organification of iodide, and co-transfection of the thyroid peroxidase gene with NIS may aid in retention of radioiodine.

In collaboration with Drs. Frederick Domann, Michael Graham, and others from the University of Iowa, we have imaged a line of human head-and-neck squamous-carcinoma cells (HEK) implanted in the thighs of nude mice. A replication-incompetent adenovirus that expresses NIS is injected into the tumor. A control adenovirus that expresses BgIII instead of NIS is injected into the tumor in the contralateral thigh. Images are obtained at 48-72 hours using Tc-99m pertechnetate. Preliminary images have shown pertechnetate localization in the NIS-containing tumors but little uptake in the control tumors.

5. Summary

Small-animal gamma-ray imaging studies provide valuable data in translational studies of human disease. Because serial studies in the same animals are possible, progression of disease and effects of intervention can be monitored. Radiolabeled molecular probes can be used to image gene expression, and reporter genes can be used to monitor gene therapy. Imaging systems with high spatial resolution and dynamic capability greatly increase the range of biological studies that can be undertaken. High-resolution tomographic imaging systems can in effect provide *in vivo* autoradiography.

References

[Centers for Disease Control and Prevention] Centers for Disease Control and Prevention, National Center for Injury Prevention and Control, Web-based Injury Statistics Query and Reporting System. Accessed January 2004 at: http://www.cdc.gov/ncipc/wisqars

[Chung, 2002] J.-K. Chung. "Sodium iodide symporter: its role in nuclear medicine," *J. Nucl Med.*, vol. 43, pp. 1188-1200, 2002.

[Front, 2000] D. Front, R. Bar-Shalom, M. Mor, N. Haim, R. Epelbaum, A. Frenkel, D. Gaitini, G.M. Kolodny, O. Israel. "Aggressive non-Hodgkin lymphoma: early prediction of outcome with 67Ga scintigraphy," *Radiology*, vol. 214, pp. 253-257, 2000.

[Khaw, 1997] B.-A. Khaw, A. Nakazawa, S.M. O'Donnell, K.-Y. Pak, and J. Narula. "Avidity of Technetium-99m glucarate for the necrotic myocardium: *in vivo* and *in vitro* assessment," *J. Nucl. Cardiol.*, vol. 4, pp. 283-290, 1997.

[Kostakoglu, 2002] L. Kostakoglu, M. Coleman, J.P. Leonard, I. Kuji, H. Zoe, and S.J. Goldsmith. "PET predicts prognosis after 1 cycle of chemotherapy in aggressive lymphoma and Hodgkin's disease," *J. Nucl. Med.*, vol. 43, pp. 1018-1027, 2002.

[Mochizuki, 2003] T. Mochizuki, Y. Kuge, S. Zhao, E. Tsukamoto, M. Hosokawa, H.W. Strauss, F.G. Blankenberg, J.F. Tait, and N. Tamaki. "Detection of apoptotic tumor response *in vivo* after a single dose of chemotherapy with 99m-Tc-annexin V," *J. Nucl. Med.*, vol. 44, pp. 92-97, 2003.

[Zinn, 2002] K.R. Zinn and T.R. Chaudhuri. "The type 2 human somatostatin receptor as a platform for reporter gene imaging," *Eur. J. Nucl. Med.*, vol. 29, pp. 388-399, 2002.

Chapter 2

Detectors for Small-Animal SPECT I

Overview of Technologies

Harrison H. Barrett and William C. J. Hunter*
barrett@radiology.arizona.edu

1. Introduction

Indirect imaging systems such as SPECT have three essential components: an image-forming element, an image detector, and a reconstruction algorithm. These components act together to transfer information about the object to the end user or *observer*, which can be a human or a computer algorithm. As we shall see in Chapter 5, the efficacy of this information transfer can be quantified and used as a figure or merit for the overall imaging system or for any component of it. Fundamentally, image quality is defined by the ability of some observer to perform some task of medical or scientific interest.

In many cases, the limiting factor in task performance is the image detector. Only when the detector is capable of recording finer spatial or temporal detail can more information be transferred to the observer. Conversely, any improvement in detector capability can be translated into improved task performance by careful design of the image-forming element and the reconstruction algorithm.

In the case of nuclear medicine with single-photon isotopes, however, it has long been the conventional wisdom that there is no need for improved detectors because the limiting factor is always the image-forming element. This view stems from consideration of the usual imaging configuration in which a parallel-bore collimator is placed in front of an image detector such as an Anger camera. To a reasonable approximation, the resolutions of the detector and collimator add in quadrature and, when the detector resolution is much better than that of the collimator, the latter dominates. Continuing the argument, many authors conclude that improvements in collimator resolution are obtainable only at the expense of photon-collection efficiency; thus there is little hope of any improvement in single-photon gamma-ray imaging.

*The University of Arizona, Department of Radiology, Tucson, Arizona

This chapter has two goals. The first is to show that the conventional wisdom is wrong, that improvements in detector capability can indeed be translated to measurable benefits in system performance in SPECT. The second goal is to survey the available technologies for improving detector performance, especially for small-animal applications.

Because detector requirements depend on the image-forming element, we begin in Section 2 by looking broadly at methods of image formation in gamma-ray emission imaging. As we shall see, pinhole imaging is an attractive alternative to parallel-hole collimators, with some perhaps unexpected advantages. In Section 3, we look more specifically at small-animal SPECT and assess the requirements on the gamma-ray detectors to be used there.

In Section 4, we examine the various physical mechanisms that might be used for gamma-ray detection. The unsurprising conclusion will be that semiconductor and scintillation detectors in various forms are the most promising; these two technologies will be examined in more detail in Sections 5 and 6, respectively.

2. Image formation

This section is a catalog of methods of forming images of emissive gamma-ray sources, with a few comments on applicability to small-animal SPECT. The reader is presumed to be familiar with the elementary properties of collimators and pinholes, but a review can be found in Barrett and Swindell [1981, 1996b].

2.1 Multi-bore collimators

Parallel-hole collimators made of lead are the image-forming elements of choice in clinical SPECT. Typically, for that application, the bore length is 2–3 cm, the bore diameter is 1–3 mm, and the septal thickness is of order 1 mm. These parameters are chosen to give a collimator resolution of 1 cm or so at a distance of about 15 cm from the collimator face. The resulting collimator efficiency (fraction of the emitted photons passed by the collimator) is around 3×10^{-4}.

Parallel-hole collimators also can be used for small-animal SPECT, but quite different parameters are needed. At the Center for Gamma-ray Imaging (CGRI), we use a laminated tungsten collimator with 7 mm bore length, 260 μm square bores, and 120 μm septa, yielding an efficiency of 5×10^{-5} and submillimeter resolution out to about 2.5 cm from the collimator face. Further improvement could be achieved by fabricating the collimator from gold, which is economically feasible for small animals but not for clinical applications.

Focusing collimators with nonparallel bores are sometimes used clinically to magnify or minify the object onto the camera face, but to the authors' knowledge, they have not been used for small animals.

For a thorough discussion of collimator design and optimization, see Gunter [1996].

2.2 Pinholes

2.2.1 Simple pinhole imaging. Most small-animal SPECT imaging today is done with pinholes. Pinholes are very flexible, with the main free parameters being the pinhole diameter d_{ph}, the perpendicular distance s_1 from the pinhole plane to an object plane of interest, and the perpendicular distance s_2 from the pinhole to the detector plane. The collection efficiency is controlled by the ratio $[d_{ph}/s_1]^2$, while the magnification is given by s_2/s_1. The spatial resolution depends on all three parameters and on the spatial resolution of the detector. As a general rule, the magnification should be adjusted so that the contribution of the detector to the overall spatial resolution is equal to or less than the contribution of the pinhole; with low-resolution detectors, a large magnification is very useful.

Other design considerations in pinhole imaging concern penetration of the radiation through the edges of the pinhole and vignetting in the imaging of off-axis points. For good discussions of these points, see Jaszczak et al. [1993] and Smith and Jaszczak [1998].

2.2.2 Multiple pinholes and coded apertures. With pinholes or collimators and a fixed imaging geometry, there is an inevitable tradeoff between photon-collection efficiency and spatial resolution; a smaller pinhole or collimator bore improves resolution but degrades efficiency. In practice, however, there is no reason for the imaging geometry to remain fixed. A simple way of avoiding the tradeoff in pinhole imaging is to use more pinholes; a system with N pinholes has N times the collection efficiency of a single pinhole of the same size. As long as the pinhole images do not overlap on the detector surface, the overall gain in sensitivity is also a factor of N.

As N increases, however, overlapping, or *multiplexing*, of the pinhole images occurs, and we refer to the multiple-pinhole system as a *coded aperture*. In that case, the system performance is no longer simply related to the collection efficiency. While it is true that the total number of detected photons increases by a factor of N, each photon conveys less information about the object because of the uncertainty about which pinhole it came through.

The effect of multiplexing on the noise properties of the images has been studied thoroughly for nontomographic imaging of planar objects; see Barrett and Swindell [1981, 1996b] for a discussion in terms of signal-to-noise ratio in the image and Myers et al. [1990] for a treatment in terms of detection tasks. In brief, for an object of finite size, the system performance increases linearly with N until the images overlap, after which the rate of improvement drops.

For tomographic (SPECT) imaging, it is important to realize that multiplexing *always* occurs, even for a single pinhole. One pinhole and one detector element define a tube-like region or *ray* through a 3D object, and emissions from all points along the ray contribute to the photon noise in that one detector reading. For detection of a nonrandom lesion in a uniform object, the effective degree of multiplexing for a single pinhole is of order L/δ, where L is the average length of the intersection of the ray with the object, and δ is the size of the lesion. If there are N pinholes, and

M rays through the object strike one detector element, the degree of multiplexing increases to ML/δ. Because the total number of counts is proportional to N, the detectability scales as $N\delta/ML$ (i.e., N divided by the degree of multiplexing). If there is no overlap of the pinhole images, then $M = 1$, and we gain the full benefit of N pinholes, just as in the planar case, but there is the additional loss of detectability (by a factor of δ/L) in any tomographic system due to multiplexing along the ray.

The degree of multiplexing is not the whole story, however, because performance on a task of clinical interest might be limited by object nonuniformity (anatomical noise) as well as by photon noise. As discussed more fully in Barrett and Myers [2004] and in Chapter 5 of this volume, the performance limitations arising from anatomical noise are related to the deterministic properties of the system rather than the stochastic properties such as Poisson noise. Discrimination against anatomical noise is best accomplished if the system collects sufficient data that an artifact-free reconstruction can be formed.

Early work in coded-aperture imaging did not satisfy this condition because projections were collected over a relatively small range of angles. As with any limited-angle tomography system, there were significant null functions which resulted in artifacts and loss of task performance in the presence of anatomical noise. More recent work has recognized that multiplexing and limited-angle imaging are two different problems, the main connection being that they both lead to null functions.

An example of a small-animal SPECT system that separates these two problems is the work of Schramm and co-workers at Jülich [Schramm et al., 2002]. In their work, a multiple-pinhole aperture is rotated around an animal so that a full range of view angles is sampled; excellent images are obtained despite multiplexing.

Meikle et al. [2002, 2003] are also developing coded-aperture systems for small-animal applications, using both multiple-pinhole apertures and Fresnel zone plates [Barrett, 1972]. By using up to four detector heads, the limited-angle problems are avoided, and generally artifact-free image are obtained in simulation.

Another recent project applying coded apertures to small-animal SPECT is the work at MIT using uniformly redundant arrays [Accorsi, 2001a, 2001b]. Originally developed for x-ray and gamma-ray astronomy, these arrays produce images that can be decoded to yield a sharp point spread function for an object that consists of a single plane. For 3D objects, they provide a form of longitudinal tomography or laminography in which one plane is in focus while other planes are blurred in some way, but the location of the in-focus plane can be varied in the reconstruction step. Promising results have been obtained despite the limited-angle nature of the data.

2.2.3 Pinholes and high-resolution detectors. A little-recognized aspect of multiple-pinhole imaging is that it allows us to gain sensitivity without sacrificing final image resolution, provided we can improve the detector performance. If we develop a detector with improved resolution, we can use it with a smaller pinhole or finer collimator and improve the final image resolution at the expense of sensitivity, but we can also use it to improve sensitivity. To do so, we move the detector closer to the pinhole, thereby reducing the magnification and leaving room for more pinholes

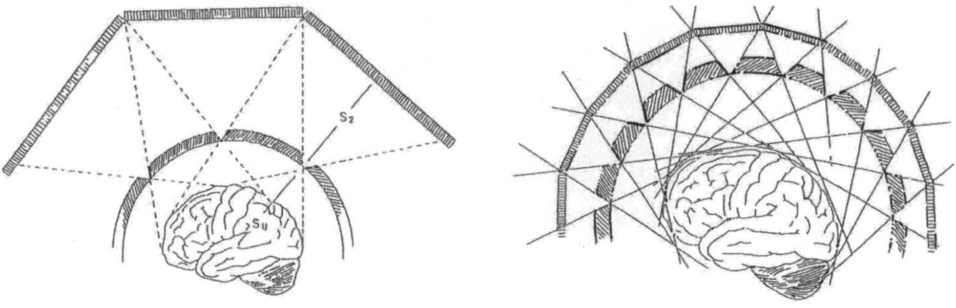

Figure 2.1. (Left) Illustration of a multi-pinhole imager used with low-resolution detectors. (Right) Illustration of a multi-pinhole used with high-resolution detectors. With the same final resolution and field of view as in the Left figure, the system illustrated to the Right can have much higher sensitivity.

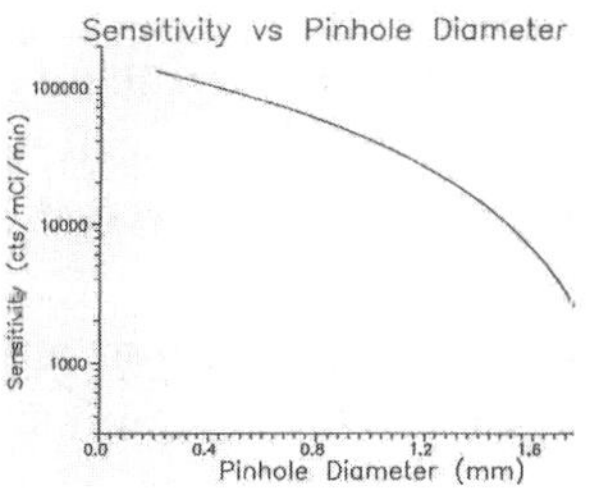

Figure 2.2. Sensitivity of an optimally designed system vs. pinhole diameter.

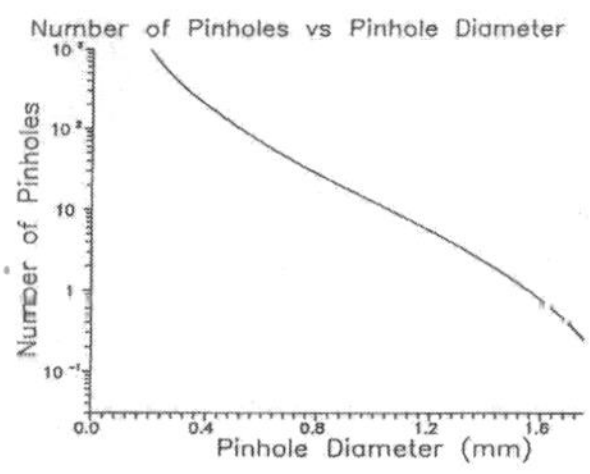

Figure 2.3. Allowed number of pinholes for no image overlap.

without encountering problems from overlapping or multiplexed images (see Fig. 2.1). Even though smaller pinholes are then needed for the same final resolution, the number of pinholes increases faster than the area of each decreases; thus, the overall sensitivity is actually increased [Rogulski, 1993]. The effect can be seen quantitatively in Figs. 2.2–2.4, taken from the Rogulski paper for the case of clinical brain imaging. Fig. 2.2 shows the paradoxical end result: the photon-collection efficiency *increases* as *smaller* pinholes are used. The explanation of the paradox is shown in Fig. 2.3; because the smaller pinholes are used with lower magnification, many more of them can be placed around the brain. The technological price one has to pay is shown in Fig. 2.4; the detector resolution must be much greater with the smaller pinholes and lower magnification if the same final resolution is to be maintained. Turning the argument around, if one has a certain detector resolution, Fig. 2.4 can be used to select a pinhole size which, with optimal choice of magnification, will lead to the specified resolution (2 mm for the graphs shown). Then Fig. 2.3 shows the number of pinholes that can be used without multiplexing, and Fig. 2.2 shows the resultant sensitivity.

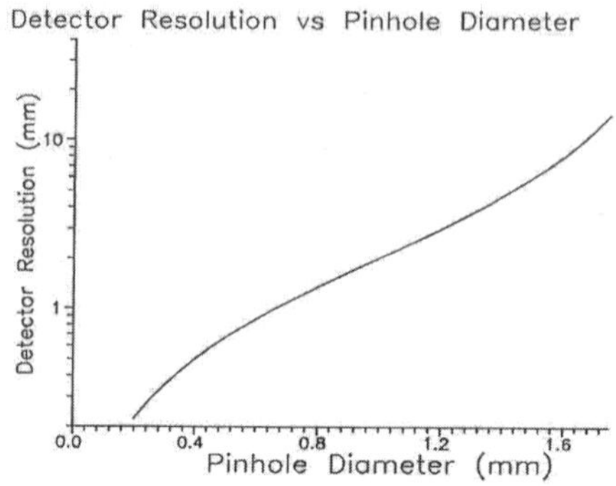

Figure 2.4. Required detector resolution in order to use a given pinhole diameter and the number of pinholes shown in Fig. 2.3 with constant final resolution (2 mm).

2.3 Synthetic collimators

There is still another way of using multiple pinholes, in a system that can be regarded as a hybrid between coded apertures and unmultiplexed pinholes. Referred to in our group as the *synthetic collimator*, this approach is designed to overcome the limitations of real collimators [Clarkson, 1999; Wilson, 2000].

To understand the objective of the synthetic collimator, let us first define an ideal parallel-hole collimator. This physically unrealizable device would acquire a two-dimensional (2D) projection of a 3D object with a spatial resolution and sensitivity independent of position in the object. More precisely, a detector element placed behind one bore of the ideal collimator would be uniformly sensitive to radiation emanating from anywhere in a tube-like region of space formed by mathematically extending the bore into the object, and it would be totally insensitive to radiation originating outside this tube. This detector would therefore measure the integral of the object activity over this tube region, and other detector elements would do the same for other tubes. The collection of tube integrals is the ideal planar projection. In a synthetic collimator, we attempt to collect a data set from which these tube integrals can be estimated by mathematical operations on actual data.

A suitable data set for this purpose can be collected by a simple multiple-pinhole aperture. A plate of gamma-ray-absorbing material is placed in the plane $z = 0$, and the object is contained in the halfspace $z > 0$. The plate is essentially opaque except for K small pinholes, and the image detector is placed in the plane $z = -s$. In the absence of noise, the mth detector element records a measurement given by

$$g_m = \int_S d^3\mathfrak{r}\, f(\mathfrak{r}) h_m(\mathfrak{r}). \tag{2.1}$$

where $\mathfrak{r}$ is a 3D vector, $f(\mathfrak{r})$ is the object activity, S is the region of support of the object, and $h_m(\mathfrak{r})$ is the sensitivity function that specifies the response of the detector to radiation emanating from point $\mathfrak{r}$. If the detector can "see" the object through all K pinholes, then $h_m(\mathbf{r})$ is appreciable over K cone-like regions through the object.

The parameters we would like to estimate are the ideal tube integrals, given by

$$\theta_j = \int_S d^3\mathbf{r}\, f(\mathbf{r}) t_j(\mathbf{r}). \tag{2.2}$$

where $t_j(\mathbf{r})$ is the tube function, defined to be unity in the region of the jth tube and zero elsewhere. The key question is whether we can recover the values of θ_j from the measured data, at least in the absence of noise. The answer is yes if we can write the tube functions themselves as a linear superposition of the sensitivity functions, so that

$$t_j(\mathbf{r}) = \sum_{m=1}^{M} B_{jm} h_m(\mathbf{r}). \tag{2.3}$$

If this condition can be satisfied, then we can find all of the tube integrals by

$$\theta_j = \sum_{m=1}^{M} B_{jm} g_m. \tag{2.4}$$

When noise is taken into account, it is advantageous to estimate the tube integrals by maximum-likelihood (ML) methods such as the expectation-maximization (EM) algorithm, but the success of the synthesis still depends on being able to represent the tube functions as a linear superposition of sensitivity functions as in equation 2.3.

We have performed a large number of simulation studies to determine the circumstances under which this synthesis can be performed. In brief, we find that a single multiple-pinhole image is not sufficient. It is necessary to collect additional information, for example by varying the aperture-to-detector distance s, possibly with different pinhole patterns at each s. When we do this, the simulations and theoretical analysis show that an excellent approximation to the ideal collimator can be synthesized and that the results are quite robust to noise.

There are several ways to implement the synthetic-collimator concept in practice. One is to fix a multiple-pinhole plate relative to the object and to take data with several (3–4) spacings between the plate and the detector. The synthesis then gives a single 2D projection of the 3D object, and the object or the pinhole-detector assembly can be rotated to obtain multiple projections for 3D reconstruction. Alternatively, the data acquired with multiple detector distances but no rotation can be processed by ML methods to yield 3D images directly; the results with this approach are surprisingly good in practice, even though it is limited-angle tomography. A third approach combines the first two, acquiring data with 3 or 4 detector spacings and a few rotations, for example rotating the object in $45°$ steps. Finally, the requirement for mechanically moving the detector relative to the pinhole plate can be avoided by using several (say four) separate detectors, each with its own spacing s, and again rotating the object or the detector assembly to gather sufficient data for 3D reconstruction.

2.4 Other methods of image formation

At 140 keV, pinholes or collimators appear to be the only viable option for forming gamma-ray images. Approaches based on grazing-incidence reflective optics are of interest at much lower energies; they deserve attention for small-animal imaging, especially below 30 keV, but the grazing angles are quite small and probably impractical at higher energies. Similarly, multilayer thin films operated near normal incidence show promise at low energies but have very low efficiency at 30 keV and above. Approaches based on diffraction from crystals have shown good efficiency at high energies, but the requirement for matching the Bragg condition leads to systems with very long focal lengths and/or small fields of view.

At higher energies, an interesting approach to image formation in nuclear medicine is the Compton camera. In this method, there is no collimator; instead, the photons impinge on a semiconductor detector (usually germanium) where they undergo Compton scattering and are redirected to a second detector (often a scintillation camera). If the first detector can measure the energy of the Compton event, the scattering angle can be estimated. If both detectors also have 2D spatial resolution, then for each photon we can estimate the angular deviation at the first detector and the line of propagation between the two detectors. This has the effect of localizing the source of the photon to a fuzzy conical shell in the object space. By comparison, a pinhole and one 2D detector localizes the source to a fuzzy ray through the object; therefore, the Compton camera suffers from additional multiplexing around the periphery of the conical shell. This deficiency is compensated to a degree by the improved collection efficiency resulting from omission of the pinhole.

Compton cameras are most suited for high-energy isotopes because the energy loss on scattering increases as the square of the incident energy, and also because the detectors have better relative energy resolution at higher energy. If high-energy isotopes become of interest in small-animal SPECT, Compton cameras should be reconsidered, but for 140 keV and lower, they do not appear to be practical.

3. Detector requirements

Gamma-ray detectors are characterized by their spatial resolution, area, energy resolution, count-rate capability, and sensitivity. We shall discuss each of these performance characteristics in the context of small-animal SPECT, with regard to the different methods of image formation discussed in Section 2.

3.1 Clinical SPECT versus small-animal SPECT

Before getting into specifics on the detector requirements for small-animal SPECT, it is useful to contrast that application with conventional clinical SPECT.

As seen in Table 2.1, the most obvious difference is in the required field of view and spatial resolution; roughly speaking, the field of view for small animals is ten times smaller (in linear dimension), but the resolution must be about ten times finer than for human imaging. When clinical detectors are adapted to animal studies, it is common to use pinholes in order to magnify the image $\sim 10\times$ onto the detector

Table 2.1. Comparison of clinical and small-animal SPECT.

Clinical SPECT	Small-animal SPECT
~ 1 cm resolution	mm or sub-mm resolution
FOV ~ 50 cm	FOV ~ 5 cm
Collimators used to cover FOV	Pinholes used to get magnification
Body dimensions >> $1/\mu$	Body dimensions << $1/\mu$
Strong scatter and attenuation	Weaker scatter and attenuation
Multiple scatter likely	Single-scatter approx. more useful
Need E $\gtrsim$100 keV	Can use E ~ 30 keV
Radiation dose critical	Volume of tracer critical
Want half-life ~ hours (e.g., ^{99m}Tc)	Can use longer half-life (e.g., ^{125}I)
General-purpose instruments strongly preferred (commercially)	Adaptable, special-purpose instruments more attractive
Quantitative accuracy desirable (Detection tasks common clinically)	Quantitative accuracy crucial (Estimation tasks needed for research)

face. For more discussion on the use of clinical detectors in small-animal SPECT, see Section 4.2.

Another distinction is that the object being imaged is typically much less scattering and absorbing in small-animal applications than clinically. Of course, the attenuation and scattering coefficients are the same in the two cases, but the body dimensions are different. At 140 keV, for example, the attenuation in soft tissue is almost entirely due to Compton scatter, and the total attenuation coefficient μ is about 0.14 cm^{-1}. Thus, the attenuation length μ^{-1} is about 7 cm, which is large compared to a mouse but small compared to a human. The most probable event in mouse SPECT imaging at 140 keV is that the emitted photon will escape the body with no scattering at all, and multiple scattering is very rare.

The small body dimensions also open up the possibility of using lower-energy isotopes. In particular, ^{125}I is very attractive because many biologically important molecules are available pre-tagged with this tracer. The 60-day half-life makes it possible to order these radiopharmaceuticals ahead of the planned study and to follow the biodistribution over weeks.

Radiation dose is, of course, a critical concern in clinical imaging. It is less important in animal studies so long as it can be established that there are no radiation-induced physiological changes over the period of the study. The more pressing concern is the physical volume of the injection, which must be restricted to about 0.2 ml for mice. Thus, there is a need for high specific activity, mCi/ml.

In terms of commercial instrumentation, it appears to be the conclusion of most companies in the field that there is no market for specialized instruments that are dedicated to one or a few clinical studies. It is the premise of CGRI, however, that great progress can be made in animal studies by using flexible, modular imaging systems that can be adapted to the needs of specific animal studies.

In terms of task-based performance criteria, there is no difference in principle between clinical and animal systems, but in practice clinical SPECT studies are largely nonquantitative. Great effort has been expended on correcting for scatter, attenuation, and other effects that degrade quantitative accuracy; in most cases, however, the desired clinical outcome is accurate detection or classification rather than quantitation. In research, however, quantitative accuracy is more important, and fortunately the lower attenuation and scatter with small animals facilitates its achievement.

3.2 Spatial resolution

It follows from the considerations in the previous section that excellent resolution is needed for small animals because of the small scale of the details to be imaged. More precisely, as we shall see, high resolution is needed for both detection and estimation tasks.

In addition, certain image-acquisition geometries place great demands on the detector resolution. In particular, the use of multiple pinholes with significant minification, as discussed in Section 2.2.3, requires that the detector resolution be much better than would be needed with 1 : 1 imaging or magnification.

3.2.1 Spatial resolution and lesion detection. Tsui et al. [1978, 1983] were the first to study the effects of spatial resolution on lesion detection in nuclear medicine. They considered detection of a lesion of known size and location superimposed on a uniform but unknown background. They found that the optimum aperture size was approximately equal to the size of the lesion to be detected and that increasing the aperture size beyond this point resulted in reduced detectability despite increased counts.

Numerical and psychophysical studies by Rolland [1990] demonstrated clearly that random inhomogeneities in the background were an important determinant of image quality and of the tradeoff between sensitivity and resolution. Barrett [1990] published a detailed study of the effects of these inhomogeneities on image quality, and Myers et al. [1990] published a study on aperture optimization for planar emission imaging. The conclusion of this latter study was qualitatively similar to that of Tsui et al. [1978]: the optimum aperture resolution is approximately equal to the size of the lesion to be detected. For small, poorly resolved lesions in inhomogeneous backgrounds, however, the improvement in detectability with improvements in aperture resolution could be dramatic. In some cases, a reduction by a factor of two in aperture size could increase the detectability index (SNR^2) by two orders of magnitude despite the four-fold reduction in counts. These theoretical predictions were verified to a high degree in psychophysical studies [Rolland, 1990; Rolland and Barrett, 1992].

Similar dramatic effects have been noted in PET. Muehllehner [1985] published a series of PET simulations showing that far fewer photons are required for detection of small details if the spatial resolution of the imaging system can be improved. He arrived at the rule of thumb that, for every 2 mm improvement in detector spatial resolution (in the range 4 – 14 mm), the total number of counts can be reduced by a factor of three to four for equal subjective image quality.

These studies all show that small improvements in spatial resolution can result in a large improvement in objective performance measures. Theoretical studies such as Wagner and Brown [1985] and Barrett [1990] make it clear that aperture and detector resolution are much more important than post-detection image reconstruction or processing. Resolution improvements achieved algorithmically are irrelevant to an ideal observer. For the human observer, algorithmic resolution variations have a small effect [Abbey and Barrett, 1995; Abbey, 1996], but the real leverage is in the design of the detection system.

3.2.2 Spatial resolution and estimation tasks. Similar conclusions hold for estimation tasks. Consider the common task of estimating the activity of a tracer in some region of interest (ROI). This task is usually performed simply by manually outlining the region on a reconstructed image and then adding up the grey values in the region defined this way. Many factors, including scatter and attenuation, contribute to the errors in the resulting estimate, but even if these factors are controlled, there is still the effect of the finite spatial resolution. A bright source outside the region of interest can contribute to the sum of grey values within the region because of tails on the point spread function. In fact, the bias in the estimate is a strong function of the object distribution *outside* the region, and it is impossible even to define an estimator that is unbiased for all true values of the parameter [Barrett and Myers, 2004, Chapter 13].

There are two ways of ameliorating this effect. The first is to use an estimator that explicitly takes into account the detector resolution as well as the noise statistics [Barrett, 1990]. The second, and much better, approach is to improve the system resolution.

Other estimation tasks also benefit from improved resolution. For example, in a careful study of optimal collimator selection for estimation of tumor volume and location, Müller et al. [1986] found that collimators designed for high resolution, even at substantial cost in sensitivity, would lead to significant improvements for brain SPECT.

3.2.3 Specifying the resolution. For both detection and classification tasks, the fundamental limitation is the resolution associated with the hardware — the collimator and detector. The resolution contribution from the algorithm has no effect at all on task performance if the task is performed optimally. For suboptimal observers, such as a human reading the image or a simple ROI estimator, the algorithm indeed plays a role, but that may point to the need for better observers rather than better reconstruction algorithms. For example, a computer-assisted diagnosis algorithm can in principle be designed to overcome the limitations of the human in detection tasks, and optimal estimators can be designed to extract the desired quantitative parameters.

Thus, at a fundamental level, the best way of specifying system resolution is in terms of the hardware only, without reference to any particular reconstruction algorithm. One way of doing this is to use the Fourier cross-talk matrix [Barrett and Gifford, 1994; Barrett, 1995a, 1996] which makes it possible to define a kind of modulation transfer function for systems that are not even approximately shift-invariant. The Fourier cross-talk matrix is an exact description of the deterministic properties of any linear digital imaging system. It is independent of the task the system must perform, but methods developed in Barrett et al. [1995a] can be used to compute task performance from the cross-talk matrix and information about the measurement noise.

Another reason not to include the algorithm in specifications of resolution is that the final point spread function (PSF) in a reconstructed image can be varied over a wide range by setting reconstruction parameters such as smoothing factors, number of iterations and voxel size. With accurate modeling and iterative reconstruction, one can obtain almost arbitrary reconstructed resolution, generally at the expense of noise although not necessarily at the expense of task performance. Thus, it is highly misleading to state "the resolution" of a system that includes a reconstruction step.

Moreover, when resolution is specified in tomographic imaging, it is necessary to distinguish volumetric and linear resolution. A linear resolution of about 1 mm is obtainable these days in both animal PET and animal SPECT; if this resolution is obtained isotropically, it corresponds to a volume resolution of about 1 μL, legitimizing the terms microPET and microSPECT. It is really the volumetric resolution, mainly of the hardware, that determines the limitation on task-based image quality for either detection or estimation tasks.

3.2.4 Pixellated versus continuous detectors. As we shall see below, two distinct kinds of scintillation detectors are used in SPECT (and also in PET, although we shall have very little to say about PET detectors). One kind uses a monolithic detector like the large NaI crystal used in clinical Anger cameras. The other kind of detector, favored in small-animal systems based on position-sensitive photomultipliers (PSPM Ts), uses a segmented or pixellated crystal. In decision-theoretic terms, the data-processing task with monolithic crystals is to estimate the position of the scintillation event on a continuous scale, binning the estimate into discrete pixels for storage and display only. With the segmented crystals, the data processing must decide in which segment the event occurred, thus performing a classification task rather than an estimation task.

A similar situation arises with semiconductor detectors. Discrete arrays of individual elements are a quick way of constructing imaging detectors, but the complexity and cost of the systems increase rapidly with the number of elements. To avoid these problems, monolithic semiconductor crystals are used with discrete electrodes (see Section 5.2).

The question then arises as to how to specify and compare the resolutions of these two distinct kinds of detectors. The common approach is to use the segment size as the resolution measure in pixellated detectors and the full width at half maximum (FWHM) of the detector PSF as the measure for monolithic detectors.

This approach is unsatisfactory for two reasons. First, it takes no account of the task the system is expected to perform. Second, the distinction between the two kinds of detector is really a false dichotomy. Consider a monolithic semiconductor crystal with a discrete array of small electrodes. Is this a pixellated detector? It is if the location of the event is estimated, as it commonly is, by the address of the electrode that receives the largest amount of charge. On the other hand, the discrete electrodes are no different in principle from the discrete PMTs in an Anger camera, and one event gives a signal in multiple electrodes, therefore position estimation on a continuous scale can be performed as well. The size of the electrode is no more a resolution limitation than is the size of a PMT in an Anger camera.

These points will be discussed in more detail in the next chapter where we cover optimal approaches to position estimation with both semiconductor and scintillation detectors.

3.2.5 3D detectors. So far, we have discussed detector resolution as if it were associated with the 2D response of the detector. For many purposes, however, the detector is required to sense the position of the gamma-ray event in 3D. Consider, for example, a simple pinhole imaging system where the pinhole is placed close to an extended object. Then some of the photons from the object pass through the pinhole at oblique angles, up to 45° or more, and hence impinge on the detector at the same angle. Because gamma-ray detectors necessarily have a finite thickness in order to absorb the photons, the 3D location of the interaction event must be determined in order to accurately estimate the path of the photon. In other words, the detector must provide information about the depth of the interaction as well as its lateral position.

Many schemes are found in the literature for increasing the sensitivity of a gamma-ray detector to depth of interaction. Whatever scheme is used, the maximum-likelihood methods to be presented in Chapter 3 can be used to estimate the 3D coordinates of the interaction.

3.3 Detector area and space-bandwidth product

Another key parameter of a detector is its physical area. With a parallel-bore collimator, the area of the detector directly determines the field of view. With pinhole imaging, however, area alone is not what matters. A large-area, low-resolution detector can be used at large magnification to achieve the same field of view and final resolution as a small-area, high-resolution detector used at lower magnification (see Fig. 2.1).

The total number of independent measurements that the detector can make is what really matters. For a discrete detector array, that number is the number of individual elements in the array. For a continuous detector such as an Anger camera, the maximum number of independent measurements that can be made can be approximated by the area of the detector divided by the area associated with the PSF after position estimation. Because the reciprocal of the width of the PSF is a measure of width of the modulation transfer function (for a shift-invariant system), we can say that the important quantity in detector performance is the *space-bandwidth product*, defined by

$$\begin{aligned} \text{Sp-BW} &= (\text{Area of detector}) \,/\, (\text{Area of PSF}) \\ &= (\text{Area of detector}) \times (\text{2D bandwidth}). \end{aligned} \tag{2.5}$$

A larger detector is of no use if the image does not fill the detector area. In a statement probably attributable to W. L. Rogers, pinholes and coded apertures are simply ways of taking advantage of the available detector space-bandwidth product. The arguments presented in Section 2.2.3 show how an increase in either the resolution or the area of the detector can be used to increase the performance of a multiple-pinhole system without multiplexing; if the object has a sparse structure, so that relatively few detector elements receive significant radiation, then further advancement can be achieved with multiplexing.

3.4 Energy resolution

Most gamma-ray detectors have the ability to estimate the energy deposited in an interaction event as well as the position of the interaction. Note the wording: The detector does not estimate the energy of the *photon*, and in any case it provides only an *estimate* rather than an unambiguous determination of the energy it senses.

This energy estimate has two main uses. First, if two separate isotopes are used in a study, the energy information provides data needed to reconstruct two separate images; accuracy of the energy estimate determines the degree of influence one isotope distribution has on the reconstructed image of the other distribution.

The energy estimate also is used to discriminate against photons that have undergone Compton scatter in the patient's body, on the assumption that scattered photons carry little spatial information and hence degrade system performance. Whether this assumption is valid is an interesting question, discussed briefly in Section 3.4.2 after we look at scatter discrimination in small-animal imaging.

3.4.1 Energy resolution and scatter discrimination. As noted in Section 3.1, Compton scattering is not as strong in small-animal studies as it is clinically because the body dimensions are so much smaller. How important the residual scatter is depends, of course, on the task and observer. For now, let us assume that the scatter is undesirable and see what can be done about it.

The effectiveness of energy discrimination in rejecting scatter depends on the energy of source, on the energy resolution of detector, and on a choice the user makes in setting the tradeoff between rejecting scattered photons and rejecting the presumably desirable unscattered photons.

As a numerical example, the resolution of typical scintillation detectors at 140 keV, as measured by the FWHM of the distribution of energy estimates, is about 15 keV. High-atomic-number, room-temperature semiconductor detectors such as cadmium zinc telluride (CZT) can have energy resolutions of order 2–3 keV as single elements and 6–8 keV as imaging arrays. For comparison, a 45° Compton scatter at 140 keV produces an energy loss $\Delta E = 10$ keV. Thus a CZT detector is superior to a scintillation camera for scatter rejection with ^{99m}Tc, but neither is perfect.

There also is considerable interest in small-animal imaging with ^{125}I, which has several emission lines in the vicinity of 30 keV. At that energy, a 45° scatter yields an energy loss $\Delta E = 0.5$ keV. Neither scintillation detectors nor CZT detectors offer much chance of scatter discrimination in this case.

Silicon detectors are attractive at 30 keV, and the best single-element silicon devices can give resolutions less than 1 keV. Even this is not really good enough, however, because the gamma-ray emission of ^{125}I is not monoenergetic to start with, and silicon imaging arrays have much poorer energy resolution than single-element detectors in any case.

Whatever the energy resolution of the detector, the user must employ some algorithm to discriminate scattered from unscattered radiation. If that decision is to be made for each event in isolation, as it usually is, then the only information for making the decision is the energy estimate. The conventional — though scarcely optimal — approach is simply to compare the energy estimate to a threshold and make the decision to accept the event if the estimate exceeds the threshold. (An upper threshold can also be used but it isn't relevant to scatter rejection because Compton processes always result in energy loss.) Setting the threshold too high results in rejecting too many unscattered photons, while setting it too low results in accepting too many scattered photons.

To study this tradeoff, Jyh-Cheng Chen [1997] used a kind of receiver operating characteristic (ROC) curve in which the probability of accepting an unscattered photon (true positive) is plotted vs. the probability of accepting a scattered photon (false positive). He used this kind of plot to compare different methods of energy estimation and to choose a setting of the threshold.

We shall return to issues of energy estimation and scatter rejection in Chapter 3.

3.4.2 Energy information and task performance. The importance of scattered radiation in SPECT imaging depends on the task and observer and on the reconstruction algorithm, as well as on any scatter-discrimination method used.

For simple detection tasks in uniform backgrounds, White [1994] found that best ideal-observer performance was obtained with a wide-open energy window; the increased acceptance of unscattered photons outweighed the degradation due to scatter. For a similar task, Rolland et al. [1989, 1991] showed that the long tails of the scatter PSF degraded human performance but that much of the effect could be recovered by simple linear deconvolution. Unpublished work by White and Gallas indicates that the similar conclusions may hold for detection in a more complicated background: there might not be much of a penalty in detection task performance when a wide energy window is used.

There may even be some benefit to collecting scattered radiation, estimating the energies, and using this augmented data set for detection. Kwo et al. [1991] studied this possibility for intraoperative tumor detection, a setting similar to small-animal imaging in that the lesion can be rather close to the detector. They found that detection performance for an ideal linear (Hotelling) observer increased when the scattered photons were used optimally. They also showed that HgI_2 and CdTe semiconductor detectors offered some advantage over NaI(Tl), not for scatter rejection but for providing more accurate energy information to the observer. For more on optimal use of scattered radiation, see Barrett et al. [1998].

3.5 Count-rate capability

Traditionally, one of the main limitations of gamma cameras has been the count-rate capability. Depending on the technology, modern cameras show a loss in sensitivity or degradation of resolution when the count rate exceeds 100,000 – 200,000 cps. The problems only become more serious for small-animal imaging where the desire for high spatial resolution and reasonable imaging times often leads to injection of large amounts of activity, all of which can end up in the field of view of the detectors. Moreover, the high collection efficiency of coded apertures and multiple-pinhole systems leads to still higher count rates.

3.5.1 Modularity. Although improvements in electronics are always desirable, the best way to deal with high total count rates is with multiple independent camera modules. Although this approach is used clinically, with 2, 3, or even 4 camera heads, it is possible to use many more in small-animal SPECT. Of the systems being developed at CGRI (see Chapter 6), FastSPECT uses 24 modules, FastSPECT II uses 16, and SemiSPECT currently uses 8 modules but can be upgraded to 16. A system with N independent modules automatically has N times the count-rate capability (not to mention N times the sensitivity) of an otherwise identical system with a single module.

Other practical advantages of modular systems include the low cost of individual modules, the ease of troubleshooting and repair, and the flexibility in rearranging the modules for different applications.

3.5.2 Rationale for counting. Another way to deal with the demands of high count rates is to just say no – to use an integrating detector instead of a photon-counting one. Integrating detectors are the standard in digital radiography, where it is very difficult to build counting arrays that will have adequate speed. Why not just use these same detectors for nuclear medicine? We shall have more to say about this question in Section 4.2.2, but for now we simply enumerate the reasons for doing counting in the first place.

One reason for photon counting is so we can do energy discrimination and hence scatter rejection. We argued above, however, that scatter was not all that important in degrading small-animal SPECT images, so this reason for counting is not compelling.

The second reason for counting is that different absorbed gamma rays produce different pulse heights, because of Compton scatter in the body or detector, escape of K x-rays from the detector, or absorption or scattering in the detector material itself. With a photon-counting detector, these pulses are analyzed individually and accepted or rejected for inclusion in the image. No matter what the acceptance criterion is, the resulting image will obey Poisson statistics [Barrett and Myers, 2004]. With integrating detectors, however, each pulse makes a contribution to the image proportional to the pulse height, and the random variation in pulse height produces an additional noise often called Swank noise, after the person who first analyzed it. We shall discuss Swank noise in more detail in Chapter 3, but for now we merely note that it is seldom more than a 20% increase in noise variance above the Poisson level.

The final reason for counting is that integrating detectors have additional noise contributions arising from dark current and thermal noise in the readout electronics. For more on these noise sources and ways of controlling them, see Section 4.2.2.

3.5.3 Counting with an integrating detector. The distinction between photon-counting and integrating detectors is another false dichotomy. Depending on the rate of arrival of photons and the frame rate, it may well be possible to identify the effects of individual photons in each frame from an integrating detector. Furenlid et al. [2000] analyzed the statistics of this process and determined the allowable count rate as a function of the frame rate, the number of detector pixels affected by each gamma-ray photon, and the allowable degree of overlap.

We shall return to this question several times below, in the context of integrating arrays of semiconductor detectors and of lens-coupled CCD cameras.

3.6 Sensitivity

For a photon-counting device, the detector efficiency is defined as the fraction of incident photons that are counted; in other words, it is the fraction absorbed multiplied by the probability of being counted through the energy window or other thresholding means. Often the term *photopeak efficiency* is used. This quantity is to be contrasted with the overall system efficiency which also includes the probability that an emitted photon will pass through the imaging aperture.

In system design, we may trade absorption efficiency for spatial resolution (e.g., by using thinner crystals), but then obtain the overall sensitivity back, say by use of multiple pinholes. When this possibility is considered, a useful figure of merit for the detector is the space-bandwidth-efficiency product, defined as

$$\text{FOM} = \frac{\text{Area of Detector}}{\text{Area of resolution cell}} \times \text{Detector efficiency}. \tag{2.6}$$

4. Approaches to gamma-ray detection

Having established the general characteristics, we wish to achieve in detectors for small-animal SPECT, we now look broadly at how we might go about achieving them. In this section, we consider the nature of the initial interaction between the gamma ray and the detector material and ways of sensing the effect of that interaction, possibilities for adapting existing clinical detectors to small-animal SPECT, and some of the advantages of dedicated small-animal detectors.

4.1 The initial interaction

The inelastic interaction of sub-MeV gamma rays with matter takes place by the photoelectric effect or Compton scattering. In both cases, the result is that a high-energy electron is produced in the material. Different detector technologies are distinguished by how they sense this initial interaction. To see what the options are, we examine the events that occur in any nonmetallic material after the interaction.

4.1.1 Cascades. After production of a high-energy electron, there is a complicated cascade of events. The high-energy electron can excite lattice vibrations (mainly optical phonons), and it can also produce hole-electron pairs by exciting electrons across the band gap. The holes and electrons can be very energetic; that is, the electron energy might be far above the bottom of the conduction band and the hole might be far below the top of the valence band. The holes and electrons lose energy either by producing phonons or by exciting other hole-electron pairs.

After they have lost most of their energy, the holes and electrons can bind together to form excitons, and they eventually recombine, often through the intermediary of impurities. The recombination can be *radiative*, meaning that low-energy optical photons are produced, or *nonradiative*, meaning that the energy is dissipated through phonons.

In addition to the high-energy electron, the initial gamma-ray interaction also produces one or more high-energy photons. If the initial event is Compton scattering, the scattered gamma ray may escape from the crystal, or it can be absorbed or scattered at a second location, producing another high-energy electron and starting a similar cascade of hole-electron production at that location. Similarly, if the initial event is photoelectric, it leaves a vacancy in an inner shell of the atom it interacts with, and this vacancy is filled by production of a characteristic x ray. Like the Compton-scattered photon, this x ray can escape the crystal, or it can interact and start another cascade.

The cascades of events produce charge (holes and electrons), light (optical photons) and heat (phonons); any of these products can be used to transduce the initial interaction into a signal in an external circuit. Semiconductor detectors sense the charge, scintillation detectors sense the light, and microbolometers or superconductors sense the heat.

4.1.2 Nonlocality. As the spatial resolution of gamma-ray detectors improves, it becomes relevant to inquire about the spatial scale of the events described in Section 4.1.1. For numerical illustration, we consider a CZT detector and a 140 keV gamma ray, but the scales will be similar for other detectors.

For this material and gamma-ray energy, the attenuation length is about 2.5 mm; hence, the detector thickness must also be near this value to obtain reasonable absorption efficiency. If the 140 keV gamma ray interacts photoelectrically with the K shell of one of the constituents of CZT, it produces a photoelectron of energy around 100–120 keV, depending on whether the interaction is with cadmium, tellurium, or zinc. The range of this photoelectron is of order 20 μm, and this dimension specifies the size of the distribution of the hole-electron pairs, and hence also that of the light distribution for the radiative recombination. The range of the K x ray is around 100 μm, again depending on which constituent it comes from; because this number is small compared to typical detector thicknesses, it is highly likely that the x ray will be reabsorbed.

The ranges of the photoelectron and K x ray are comparable to the detector resolution we would like to achieve. At CGRI, we have built CZT detectors with pixels as small as 125 μm and silicon detectors with 50 μm pixels.

4.2 Clinical detectors

Next we investigate the prospects for using available clinical detectors for small animal SPECT. Both clinical scintillation cameras and detectors developed for digital radiography will be discussed.

4.2.1 Clinical scintillation cameras. Clinical scintillation cameras are bulky and expensive, and they do not provide the flexibility needed for optimal small-animal SPECT. The spatial resolution is typically around 3 mm at 140 keV, but they do have respectable space-bandwidth products, around 20,000 per detector head, because of their large area.

In practice, there may be some difficulty in utilizing the available detector area. If we attempt to use the edges of the camera with pinholes at large magnification, we encounter an additional problem: rays arriving at the edges do so at an oblique angle, and clinical cameras do not have depth resolution; therefore, the effective spatial resolution is degraded.

As noted above, there is considerable interest in small-animal SPECT with the 30 keV radiation from ^{125}I, and commercial cameras do not work well at this energy. Some of them do not even permit setting the energy window this low. Those that do will inevitably have poor spatial resolution because the light output in any scintillator is proportional to the photon energy; 30 keV gamma-ray photons produce less than one quarter the light of 140 keV photons, and thus have a point spread function that is over twice as wide.

Nevertheless, numerous groups are making very good use of commercial scintillation cameras with small pinholes placed very close to a mouse or rat. Several of the contributed papers in this volume describe the state-of-the-art in this endeavor.

4.2.2 Digital-radiography detectors. X-ray detectors for digital radiography (DR) are an active area of research, and several viable technologies have appeared. The most promising at this writing appear to be amorphous selenium layers and CsI scintillators with photodiode readouts, but detectors based on polycrystalline PbI_2 and HgI_2 layers also are getting serious attention.

For our purposes, DR detectors are attractive because of their high space-bandwidth product. Digital mammography detectors, in particular, must have high spatial resolution (50–100 μm), and they have a convenient size for imaging mice and rats.

The active layers in these detectors are usually rather thin (100–200 μm), which is good for pinhole SPECT because it minimizes blurring for photons arriving at oblique angles, but bad for higher-energy applications because the efficiency is reduced. As argued in Section 3.6, however, it is often advantageous to trade efficiency for space-bandwidth product.

The most salient property of DR detectors, however, is that they operate in an integrating mode instead of photon counting. As noted above, this means that there is excess noise arising from the readout electronics, dark current, and pulse-height variations. In SPECT applications, dark current and electronic noise can be minimized if the frames are read out rapidly and if an individual threshold is applied to each frame. The idea is that an individual gamma ray produces high-amplitude signals confined to a few detector pixels, while electronic noise and dark current give low-amplitude signals in all pixels. Depending on the signal levels, it may be possible to choose a threshold such that the excess noise is effectively eliminated, provided that only a few photons are detected in each frame. It must be noted, however, that because rapid frame rates require higher electronic bandwidths and hence yield higher read noise, the success of this strategy will depend on the characteristics of the particular DR detector as well as on the arrival rates and energies of the gamma rays.

As we shall see in Chapter 3, Swank noise is probably not a serious limitation in using DR detectors for small-animal SPECT, but if it is, it can be eliminated by a similar frame-by-frame analysis. Each frame can be analyzed to determine the locations of gamma-ray events, and the random pulse amplitudes can be replaced by constant signals at those locations. The resulting image statistics will be purely Poisson, with no remaining excess noise.

4.3 Dedicated small-animal detectors

4.3.1 Objectives. Even though clinical gamma cameras and digital-radiography detectors are applicable to small-animal SPECT, there is still considerable motivation for developing dedicated gamma-ray detectors for this application. The goals of this endeavor are to produce inexpensive, high-resolution modules that are well suited to small animals. Such modules would allow considerable flexibility in system design and optimization. If each module has a high resolution and many modules can be placed in close proximity to the animal, a large effective space-bandwidth product can be achieved.

Moreover, with many modules and many pinholes, all of the projection data needed for tomographic reconstruction can be obtained in parallel, with no motion of the animal or the imaging system. As with the FastSPECT systems developed at CGRI, this opens up the possibility of true 4D imaging, i.e., 3D tomography with no inherent limitation in temporal resolution.

4.3.2 Current technologies. In addition to CGRI, several other laboratories are developing gamma-ray detectors, especially for small-animal SPECT. The devices receiving the most attention at this writing are based on either scintillation crystals or semiconductors. Scintillation devices under investigation include modular scintillation cameras, scintillation cameras based on multi-anode photomultiplier tubes, and discrete arrays of small photodiodes. Semiconductor detectors of current interest are either arrays of discrete elements or integrated ("hybrid") devices in which a slab of semiconductor material is bonded in some way to one or more application-specific integrated circuits (ASICs) for readout.

More details on semiconductor and scintillation detectors will be given in Sections 5 and 6, respectively.

4.3.3 Other potential detector technologies.

Proportional counters. In a gas, constant-gain ion multiplication can be achieved within a range of electric field strengths denoted by the proportionality region, see Knoll [1999]. Ion multiplication (termed Townsend Avalanche) results from the large mean free path of the electrons. Above a critical field strength, the free electrons gain enough energy to ionize additional gas molecules before they collide. The heavier ions have a larger interaction cross section and do not gain enough energy between collisions to ionize other molecules.

Proportional counters are useful in detection and spectroscopy of low-energy x-radiation (2–60 keV). Energy resolution is typically about 15%, and time resolution is about 1 μsec, which is comparable to the performance of lithium-drifted silicon detectors for these energies. However, energy resolution can be very sensitive to nonuniformities of the ionization chamber and of the anode wire. In addition, instabilities in the gas can result in spurious pulses. Finally, conventional proportional counter chambers are relatively large for use in small-animal imaging.

Gas-electron multiplication (GEM) device. Building on the concept of gas-ionizing detectors, a number of groups have developed alternative methods to generate position- and energy-sensitive devices capable of single-photon detection and imaging. One of the more recent of these gas-ionizing detectors is the GEM. A GEM detector consists of metal-insulator-metal foil with an array of double conical, hourglass holes drilled through the foil. The foil is suspended in a gas-filled chamber between two electrodes with an applied potential, divided across the electrodes and the GEM metal layers. Ionized electrons accelerate and converge on the holes, where the electric field intensifies, causing charge multiplication. The amplified charge pulse then passes out of the foil, where it transfers to either another GEM layer or to collection electrodes. Most ions generated in the avalanche region drift along field lines away from the holes, mitigating the charge buildup on the insulating layer.

GEM devices can be built in large or small areas and with a fine pitch between holes ($\sim 100\mu$m pitch with $\sim 50\mu$m diameter holes). However, as with all gas detectors, the sensitivity to noncharged radiation such as x-ray or gamma-ray sources is small unless a thick gas layer is used, reducing the spatial resolution. One alternative that has recently been pursued is to hybridize this technology with a photocathode and a scintillator to improve the sensitivity of the device to gamma rays and x rays; see Breskin et al. [2002] and Mörmann et al. [2002]. This technique is now in competition with flat-panel, multi-anode photomultipliers that have recently been developed.

Micro-arrays of Superconducting Tunnel Junctions (STJ). Interaction of radiation with the superconducting electrodes of an STJ produces excited states of the superconducting Cooper pairs, referred to as quasiparticles. The energy gap for the quasiparticle excitations in a superconductor is small ($\sim$ 1 meV), which results in three orders of magnitude more charge carriers per incident photon than with conventional semiconductor detectors. Consequently, an STJ is very sensitive to variations of energy of the incident radiation. With a bias applied, these quasiparticles tunnel through the insulating barrier, generating a current pulse with amplitude proportional to the absorbed energy. With excellent energy resolution ($5eV$ for radiation for energies below $1keV$) and good temporal resolution ($10\mu sec$), these compact devices are capable of simultaneous imaging and spectroscopy. However, STJ sensitivity falls off at higher energies ($> 10keV$), and cryogenic cooling is required.

Photostimulable phosphors (PSPs). PSPs store energy from absorbed x rays by trapping generated electron-hole pairs in impurity levels deep within the bandgap of the crystal. The depth of the trap makes thermal detrapping unlikely. The distribution of the deposited energy can later be read out and digitized by scanning a focused laser over a PSP. Trapped charge carriers are re-excited and can recombine with some probability. In this way, the stored energy is read out, one pixel at a time. Resolution is typically limited by the spot size of the laser and by diffusion of laser

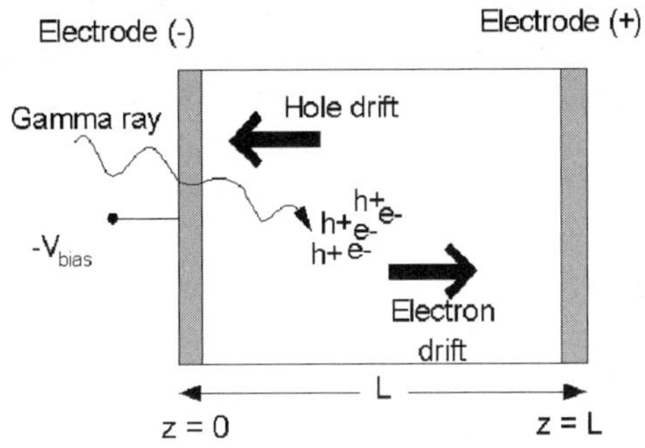

Figure 2.5. Basic principle of a single-element semiconductor detector.

light into the PSP. Because radiation fluence is integrated in the PSP, identification and counting of individual events is not possible. Limits in sensitivity (or resolution for thicker phosphor plates), and the requirement to scan the plate after each projection, make this method a slow and generally noncompetitive technology for use in SPECT.

5. Semiconductor detectors

A brief introduction to semiconductor detectors is provided in this section. Topics discussed include the basic physics of charge generation and transport, device configurations for imaging, and the considerations in the choice of materials.

5.1 Charge generation and transport

The operation of a simple single-element (nonimaging) semiconductor detector is illustrated in Fig. 2.5. As discussed in Section 4.1, the gamma ray undergoes a photoelectric or Compton interaction and produces a high-energy electron, which subsequently dissipates its energy by generating lattice vibrations (phonons) and charge (holes and electrons). Semiconductor detectors operate by sensing the presence of the charge.

5.1.1 Mobility and trapping. When a bias voltage is applied to the semiconductor detector shown in Fig. 2.5, it creates an electric field in the interior of the material. The field distribution depends on the nature of the electrode contacts and the bias voltage. If blocking (diode-like) electrodes are used, and the bias is high enough, then any free carriers that might arise from thermal excitation are swept out and the device is said to be *fully depleted*. It is also useful to assume that the transverse dimensions of the crystal are large compared to its thickness and that the material is homogeneous. If all of these assumptions are valid, the electric field in the device is uniform, just as it would be in a dielectric-filled plane-parallel capacitor.

The electrons in this uniform field move toward the anode, while the positively charged holes move toward the cathode. Because of interactions with phonons and impurities, however, the holes and electrons do not accelerate indefinitely but quickly reach a terminal velocity related to the field. For sufficiently small fields, the terminal velocity v is simply proportional to the field E. We call the constant of proportionality the mobility and denote it as μ, so $v = \mu E$. Practical units of μ are (cm/sec)/(Volts/cm) or cm^2/Volt-sec. As an example, in CZT, μ for electrons is around 1000 cm^2/Volt-sec and for holes it is about 100 cm^2/Volt-sec.

When they are free, the electrons and holes move at their respective drift velocities μE, but they can also be trapped at sites of impurities or lattice defects. If they remain free for a mean time τ, they move a mean distance $\nu\tau$ or $\mu\tau E$. After trapping, the carriers can be detrapped by thermal excitation or they can recombine. It is often assumed that, if detrapping occurs, it does so on a long time scale when compared to the measurement time of the electronics and can hence be neglected.

5.1.2 Charge induction. One might think that the carriers would need to drift to the electrodes to be observable, but in fact any motion of the carriers within the material induces a time-varying charge on the electrodes and hence an observable current in the external circuit. One way to see why this is so is to recognize that the bias circuit holds the potentials on the electrodes at constant values; for example, as shown in Fig. 2.5, the anode is held at 0 V. Thus, a negative point charge within the interior must be balanced by a fictitious positive image charge an equal distance on the other side of the anode, and it is the movement of this image charge that is sensed as a current. More physically, the actual negative charge draws charge from the circuit in such a way that a net positive distribution of surface charge on the anode is induced, maintaining the anode at ground potential.

5.2 Imaging arrays

5.2.1 Types of arrays. The simplest way to make an imaging semiconductor detector is to produce N individual detectors, of the type shown in Fig. 2.5, and mount them in a regular array to yield a discrete image detector with N pixels. For large N, this approach is costly because it requires N separate detectors and N sets of electronics.

Another approach is to start with a monolithic slab of semiconductor material, deposit electrodes on both sides, and use photolithography to partition one or both of the electrodes into separate channels. If, say, the cathode is left unpartitioned but the anode is divided into a regular array of N pixels, then electrically the system is similar to an array of N individual detectors, but mechanically it is much easier to construct. This type of device still requires N sets of electronics.

An alternative to pixel arrays is to use a semiconductor detector with orthogonal strip electrodes on opposite faces and synthesize pixels by detecting coincident signals on the row and column strips [McCready, 1971]. This approach has been used with CZT by a number of gamma-ray astrophysics research groups [Ryan, 1995; Stahle, 1996; Matteson, 1997]. The largest of these devices, the BASIS array built at NASA Goddard Space Flight Center [Stahle, 1997], has more than 5×10^5 defined pixels.

Many other clever electrode schemes have been suggested. Some have as their objective overcoming the effects of charge trapping, while others are intended to give more information about the depth of interaction.

5.2.2 Application-specific integrated circuits. Modern semiconductor detector arrays almost always use application-specific integrated integrated circuits (ASICs) for the readout electronics, thereby greatly reducing the cost per channel.

There is considerable variability in the specific circuitry implemented on each channel, but two general categories can be identified. The first is *event-driven electronics*, in which the presence of a gamma-ray interaction is recognized, and some characteristics of the resulting pulse are measured. The second is *integrating electronics*, in which the signal from each electrode is integrated over a fixed period, whether or not an event occurs.

In Section 3.5.3 we briefly mentioned the use of an integrator to detect individual gamma rays and measure their energy, and this approach can work very well with pixellated semiconductor arrays. With readout times of order one millisecond, a pixel rarely contains more than one gamma-ray hit, and individual events are easily identified and segmented.

A drawback to integrating detectors is that they integrate not only the current resulting from gamma-ray events but also the leakage current inherent in semiconductors. This current, which adds noise to the signals and degrades the energy resolution, can be reduced by using higher-resistivity material, cooling the device, or reducing the electric field; the latter is undesirable because it also reduces the drift lengths ($\mu \tau E$) for holes and electrons.

5.2.3 Charge spreading and induction in arrays. As we have emphasized above, it is highly desirable to have imaging detectors with high spatial resolution and large space-bandwidth product, but small pixels lead to interesting problems with semiconductor arrays.

Consider again a CZT detector for 140 keV photons. As noted in Section 4.1.2, the detector thickness t must be around 2–3 mm to obtain good absorption efficiency; yet, we would like to have detector resolutions of 0.5 mm or less for small-animal SPECT. At CGRI, we have built CZT arrays with pixels as small as 0.125 mm, and our standard semiconductor detector uses 0.380 mm pixels. The aspect ratio (material thickness t divided by pixel width w) is in the range 5–20.

It would make little sense to use such aspect ratios for photodetectors in conventional scintillation cameras because the light would spread by an amount comparable to the thickness as it propagated to the photodetector plane. In semiconductors, however, the charge carriers tend to follow the field lines; ideally, all carriers generated by a gamma ray would be drawn to the electrodes along paths perpendicular to the electrode planes, and charge would be collected in only one detector pixel for each interaction.

In reality, there are several mechanisms for sharing charge among multiple pixels. The initial interaction produces a compact cloud of holes and electrons, and there is charge diffusion driven by the concentration gradients that causes the cloud diameter to grow with time. Moreover, once the holes and electrons have separated, there is a Coulomb repulsion that tends to spread the clouds further. When this cloud of charge arrives at an electrode plane segmented into small pixels or small strips, each event can produce signals in several output channels.

Another effect that can cause charge sharing is trapping. Suppose there is no diffusion or Coulomb repulsion, so that each carrier is drawn in a straight line toward the electrode plane, but that many of the carriers are trapped before reaching the plane. The effect of the trapped charge on different pixels is described by something called the *weighting potential* associated with that pixel, but the net effect is that one event can give signals in several pixels. See Eskin et al. [1999] and references cited there for details on calculating the weighting potential and analyzing its effect. Additional discussion can also be found in Barrett and Myers [2004, Chapter 12].

5.2.4 Small-pixel effect. The weighting potential associated with small pixels can be put to good use with CZT and other materials in which electron transport is much better than hole transport. Often the drift length for electrons is large compared to the detector thickness, $\mu_e \tau_e E \gg t$; hence, the electrons readily propagate all the way across the detector. For holes, however, it is often the case that $\mu_h \tau_h E \ll t$; thus, holes have a high probability of being trapped before traversing the detector.

The impact of hole trapping depends on the size of the pixel and the detector thickness. For a pixel of width w, the weighting potential extends to a distance of order w into the material. If $w \gg t$, as it is in typical single-element detectors, then the pixel is equally sensitive to carriers at all distances from the pixel, and the total effect of any carrier depends on how far it moves. If the interaction occurs near the cathode, holes can make it to their collecting electrode and give their full contribution to the output signal. For interactions nearer the anode, however, the holes make a smaller contribution; therefore, the overall signal is strongly dependent on depth of interaction, with severe degradation in the pulse-height spectrum.

With small pixels ($w \ll t$), this effect can be greatly ameliorated simply by making the pixels the anodes. The pixels are sensitive mainly to carriers that move to within w of the anode plane. Because electrons are unlikely to be trapped, they move into this sensitive region no matter where they are produced, but holes move away from the anode pixel, thus, hole trapping is almost irrelevant.

This so-called *small-pixel effect* [Barrett, 1995b] can have a dramatic impact on the pulse-height spectrum, with many more of the events concentrated in the photopeak. If the pixel width w is made too small, however, diffusion and Coulomb repulsion come into play, and the pulse-height spectrum is again degraded. For CZT, the optimal pixel size for a single-pixel spectrum is around 0.5 mm [Eskin, 1999], which is very convenient for small-animal SPECT.

On the other hand, Marks et al. [1999] showed that significant improvements in energy resolution can be obtained for much smaller pixels if multiple pixel signals are used in the energy estimation. Integrating detectors are particularly convenient if this kind of processing is anticipated, because it is straightforward to read out the signals on several contiguous pixels.

5.3 Materials

5.3.1 Desirable material properties. From the above discussions, we can readily compile a list of the properties we would like to have in an ideal semiconductor material for use in small-animal SPECT.

The material also should have high gamma-ray absorption, which means it should have high density and high atomic number. Compounds of Pb, Hg, and Tl are particularly attractive in this regard.

The material should have high resistivity at room temperature, which necessitates both high bandgap and low impurity density. High resistivity is especially important if the material is to be used with an integrating detector. The resistivity requirement is reduced with event-driven electronics which do not integrate the leakage current or with system designs that permit modest cooling.

The material should exhibit good charge transport, with high mobility and low trapping, which in turn requires homogeneous, defect-free crystals. Because mobility and trapping time are only weak functions of temperature in most materials of interest, cooling does not help the charge transport appreciably.

Of course, low cost is always of interest, but especially so when large-space-bandwidth products are desired. If the cost per unit area of the material is high, or large crystals are simply not available, it may be economically prohibitive to fabricate large-area detectors. Small-animal SPECT has an advantage over clinical SPECT because the required field of view is less, and an increased space-bandwidth product can be achieved with smaller pixels rather than a larger detector area.

5.3.2 Candidate materials. A few of the materials that have been investigated as gamma-ray detectors are listed in Table 2.2, along with qualitative ratings (by number of gammas rather than stars) of their absorption, resistivity, charge transport and crystal quality.

Silicon and germanium have been widely developed in the semiconductor device industry. High-quality crystals with low trapping are readily available, but neither material has the gamma-ray absorption that would be desired at higher gamma-ray energies. Silicon is restricted to 30 keV or below, while thick germanium detectors are marginally useful at 140 keV. However, germanium is expensive and requires complex cryogenics, typically operating at around 100 K.

Mercuric iodide and thallium bromide have excellent gamma-ray absorption and high resistivity, but unfortunately the resistivity is obtained in part by low mobility. Crystal quality is still lacking, and HgI_2 is soft and difficult to work with.

Cadmium telluride and cadmium zinc telluride appear to be the best compromise at this writing, rating 2–3 gammas in each key characteristic.

Table 2.2. Comparison of some common semiconductor materials.

	Gamma-ray absorption	Resistivity	Charge Transport	Crystal quality
Si	γ	γγ	γγγγγ	γγγγγ
Ge	γγ	γ	γγγγγ	γγγγγ
CdTe	γγγ	γγ	γγγ	γγγ
CZT	γγγ	γγγ	γγγ	γγ
HgI_2	γγγγ	γγγγγ	γγ	γγ
TlBr	γγγγ	γγγγ	γ	γγ

5.3.3 Typical length scales. In Section 4.1.2, we examined the size of the region of energy deposition for a 140 keV gamma ray interacting in CZT; in Section 5.2.4, we presented some considerations on pixel size. To see how these pieces fit together and what they imply for small-animal SPECT with semiconductor detectors, we now summarize the typical length scales for a CZT detector operating at 1000 V/cm bias and used with 140 keV gamma rays. The relevant lengths are given approximately by:

Attenuation length:	2.5 mm
Detector thickness:	1-2 mm
Range of photoelectron:	20
Range of K x ray:	100 μm
Pixel pitch (Arizona Hybrid):	380 μm
Feasible pixel pitch:	50-100 μm
Diameter of "diffusion ball":	100 μm
Electron drift length:	2 cm
Hole drift length:	200 μm

As noted, the effect of the small hole drift length can be mitigated by using small pixels, although then the charge sharing due to the range of the K x ray and carrier diffusion can become appreciable. However, neither of these effects should be regarded as a fundamental limit on resolution. As we shall discuss in more detail in the next chapter, much finer resolution can be obtained with accurate statistical models and optimal position estimation.

6. Scintillation detectors

The use of scintillation detectors in gamma-ray imaging, and especially in small-animal SPECT, is surveyed in this section. The organization is similar to that of Section 5; topics include the physics of light production, materials considerations, optical detectors, and camera configurations.

6.1 Physics of light production

6.1.1 Scintillation processes. The interaction of ionizing radiation with a scintillator creates an inner shell vacancy and an excited primary electron. Subsequently, a cascade of excited electrons is generated by radiative decay, auger processes, and inelastic electron-electron scattering. However, much of the energy dissipates as thermal energy, and the efficiency for generating ionized electrons can be quite low (15–50%). When the electron energies decrease below the ionization threshold, further nonradiative processes (thermalization, lattice relaxation, and charge trapping) can result, lowering the scintillation efficiency yet further. Processes resulting in the production of light can be divided into four categories:

Self-trapped, excitonic, and recombination luminescence. Unbound electrons and holes or bound e-h pairs (excitons) move mostly unperturbed in a perfect crystal, and spontaneous recombination is relatively slow. However, the probability for recombination is enhanced through localization of one or both charge carriers (trapping) as a result of lattice discontinuities or by a shared charge affinity of a group of atoms (self-trapping). Lattice discontinuities may be a result of atomic impurities, boundary conditions, or lattice defects that formed during crystallization. Furthermore, single charge carriers that have been trapped serve as Coulomb defects that can trap charge carriers of the opposite charge. Examples of materials that exhibit these scintillation processes are BaF_2 and pure NaI.

Intrinsic ion-activated luminescence. For some materials, an intrinsic ionic component of the crystal can luminesce by undergoing an intra-ionic transition or by a charge-transfer transition. Such ions are termed activation ions or luminescent species. Examples of such ions are Bi^{2+} in $Bi_4Ge_3O_{12}$ (BGO) and $[WO_4]^{2-}$ in $CdWO_4$, respectively.

Dopant ion-activated luminescence. Some materials can be doped with impurity ions that serve to activate luminescence (see intrinsic ion-activation above). If the dopant activation ions are sparse, electron-hole pairs may be trapped and recombined by relatively few activation ions. This process could be inhibitive, slowing the scintillation response. However, the dopant-induced lattice defect results in an increased rate of electron-hole trapping. Examples of scintillators with dopant activators are $LaBr_3$:Ce, CsI:Na, and Lu_2SiO_5:Ce (LSO).

Cross-luminescence or core-valence luminescence (CVL). When a vacancy forms in the top core band of a crystal, a valence electron transitions to fill the vacancy [Rodnyi, 1992]. If the energy generated in this process is less than the fundamental bandgap, then the process is Auger free, and CVL may occur. Although this de-excitation process is fast ($\sim$ 1 ns), initial ionization of core electrons is an inefficient process, yielding at most a few photons per keV. Examples of CVL scintillation occur in BaF_2, CsCl, RbF, and $BaLu_2F_8$.

6.1.2 Nonproportionality. The amount of light produced by a scintillator depends on the likelihood of the radiative and nonradiative processes dissipating the deposited energy. These likelihoods will depend on the conditions in the scintillator, including the scintillator composition, structure, temperature, and even the amount of deposited energy. Generally, we would like process likelihoods to be independent of the deposited energy and for the light production to be a constant gain process. However, the deposited energy often does affect conditions in the scintillator, resulting in nonlinearities in the response. Nonlinear deviations of the scintillator response are termed nonproportionalities. Much work has been done to better understand and measure nonproportionalities, see Dorenbos et al. [1995], and Moses [2002].

6.2 Materials

Scintillators commonly used in SPECT include thallium-doped NaI (NaI:Tl) and either thallium- or sodium-doped CsI. However, over the past several decades, there has been an intense search for brighter, faster, more reliable, and cost-effective alternatives; see Derenzo and Moses [1993], van Eijk [2002], and Weber [2002]. This research has resulted in a wealth of new scintillators and a significant advancement in performance and fundamental knowledge of scintillation processes.

Table 2.3 gives a list of many viable scintillators for use in small-animal SPECT. A more complete compilation with detailed references is posted on the CGRI webpage: http://www.gamma.radiology.arizona.edu.

Interestingly, NaI:Tl, which was developed a few years after the photomultiplier was invented (mid-1940s), remains a viable contender for use in SPECT. In addition to new scintillators, many new fabrication methods have been developed, including columnar growth of CsI:Tl (parallel columns grown by vapor deposition with length $\sim$ 1 mm and diameter $\sim$ 3 μm).

Criteria for material selection for small-animal SPECT include absorption lengths, light yield, decay times, energy resolution, mechanical and radiological durability, chemical stability, and price. Light yield is especially important for Anger-type scintillation cameras where the interaction position is to be estimated from the relative signal on different photodetectors; low light yield means poor signal-to-noise ratio and hence poor spatial resolution in such devices. Light yield also is important in energy resolution and hence scatter rejection, but this factor is less critical for small-animal imaging, where there is significantly less scatter from the object than in clinical imaging.

Table 2.3. Properties of some useful scintillation materials.

	Hygro-scopic	Max.Emis. Wavelng. (nm)	30KeV Att.Coeff (cm^{-1})	140KeV Att.Coeff (cm^{-1})	Decay Times (ns)	Light Yield (ph/KeV)
$CeCl_3$	Yes	360	28.89	2.89	4.4(6%), 23(70%), 70(8%), >10000(16%)	28
Cs_2LiYCl_6:Ce	Yes	380	29.48	2.02	2(3%), 6500(97%)	22
CsI:Na	Yes	420	40.76	4.46	460(90%), 4180(10%)	39
CsI:Tl	Slightly	540	41.58	4.53	680(63%), 3340(37%)	65
Gd_2O_2S:Tb (GOS)	No	547	91.62	9.30	>4000	78
$Gd_3Ga_5O_{12}$:Cr,Ce	No	730	49.65	5.16	140000	40
K_2LaI_5:Ce	Yes	409	36.68	3.94	65(90%)	52
$LaBr_3$:Ce	Yes	358	79.09	3.42	35 (90%),	61
$LaCl_3$:Ce	Yes	350	27.93	2.82	20(70%), 213(30%)	49
$Lu_{1.8}Y_{0.2}SiO_5$:Ce (LYSO)	No	430	52.75	4.08	48	32-34
Lu_2O_3:Eu,Tb	No	611	167.37	16.28	>10,000	20
Lu_2S_3:Ce	No	592	101.91	9.78	32	28
$Lu_2Si_2O_7$:Ce (LPS)	No	385	86.55	8.51	38	26
Lu_2SiO_5:Ce (LSO)	No	430	115.41	11.28	47	27
LuI_3:Ce	Yes	465	68.50	7.07	34(79%), 630(21%)	47
NaI:Tl	Yes	415	28.19	3.12	230	38
$RbGd_2Br_7$:Ce	Yes	420	80.44	3.60	45(53%), 400(47%)	56
$Y_{1.34}Gd_{0.60}O_3$:$(Eu,Pr)_{0.06}$ (YGO)	No	610	116.88	5.72	1000000	42
Y_2SiO_5.Ce (YSO)	No	420	39.74	0.95	70	45
$YAlO_3$.Ce (YAP)	No	350	71.71	1.81	25-31	20-21
ZnS:Ag	No	450	37.34	1.03	110	49

6.3 Segmented versus monolithic crystals

As mentioned in Section 3.2.4, scintillation crystals can be used as segmented or monolithic detectors. Many recently developed gamma imaging systems use arrays of segmented scintillation crystals coupled to position-sensitive optical detectors (e.g., MAPMT, APD, etc.). The multichannel outputs of the position-sensitive devices are then combined by using external resistive networks implementing Anger arithmetic into X and Y signals that are then used to identify the segment in which a gamma ray interacted; see Dhanasopon et al. [2003], Inadama et al. [2003] and Pani et al. [2003, 2004].

The advantage of this approach is that the final detector has a reasonable spatial resolution (essentially the size of the crystal segments, which have been as small as 1 mm^2) in a compact, modular package. Disadvantages are that the crystal is fairly costly because of the segmentation, the sensitivity becomes smaller as the segment size is reduced (packing fraction decreases), the energy resolution is degraded because not all of the light gets out of the crystal segment, and there is no way to estimate depth of interaction (DOI) within the scintillator without auxiliary optical detectors or further segmentation.

In addition to lateral segmentation of the crystal, the crystal can be segmented to give DOI information. Segmentation in DOI is accomplished by encoding a change of the properties of the segments at different depths. This encoding can be done by changing the scintillation properties (wavelength, pulse decay time, etc.) or even by changing the reflectivity of the septa between segments at different depths; see Orita et al. [2003] and Chung et al. [2003].

An alternative approach, under investigation at CGRI, is to use a monolithic (nonsegmented) scintillation crystal with a position-sensitive optical detector (e.g., Hamamatsu H8500 MAPMT). Instead of using Anger arithmetic as the first step, we propose to acquire all signal outputs for each event, either storing them individually for later processing or combining them on the fly into a smaller set of signals that preserve the pertinent information. A discussion of maximum-likelihood estimation methods for processing these data is given in Chapter 3.

6.4 Seeing the light

6.4.1 Photomultipliers tubes (PMTs). Since their conception in the mid-1940s, PMTs have been the workhorse in amplification of low-intensity optical signals. PMTs provide large gain, on the order of 10^6 or more, and amplification noise is typically small. For scintillation cameras, the most important PMT characteristics are the *spectral response* and the *quantum efficiency* (QE) of the photocathode.

The spectral response must be chosen to match the emission spectrum of the scintillator used. Because the most important scintillators emit in the blue or near UV, it is possible to use a photocathode with no response in the green or red. Such photocathodes have a large photoelectric work function and hence a large thermal work function; thus, dark current is almost nonexistent, even at room temperature.

As discussed in much more detail in the next chapter, the QE is critical in scintillation cameras because spatial and energy resolution are fundamentally limited by the Poisson statistics of the photoelectrons liberated at the photocathode. QE in the range of 15–50% is common, but for limited spectral ranges. For a bi-alkali photocathode (e.g., Sb-Rb-Cs, Sb-K-Cs), QE is about 20% in the visible range. Hydrogenated, polycrystalline diamond has a QE of about 35% in the UV range. For solid-state III-V photocathodes, such as GaAs(Cs) and GaAsP(Cs), a QE of nearly 50% for visible and 15% for near-infrared is possible.

6.4.2 Multi-anode PMTs. A number of groups have developed small gamma cameras based on position-sensitive photomultiplier tubes (PSPMTs). A PSPMT typically consists of four signal outputs at the corners of a resistive anode plane of a PMT (combinations of these outputs give the equivalent of the computed Anger signals of a modular Anger camera). Interest in this area has been boosted recently by the introduction of the flat-paneled multi-anode photomultiplier tube (MAPMT), which is essentially an array of PMTs in a single glass envelope.

Currently available devices such as the Hamamatsu H8500 now have 8×8 anodes in a 5 cm $\times$ 5 cm area. Devices with even more anodes will soon be available. Keeping the same packaging size, Hamamatsu is in the final pre-production stages of a 16×16 anode device [Inadama, 2003], and Burle has a 32×32 MCP flip-chip device under development.

Electron multiplication in these flat-paneled devices is accomplished either by layers of dynode gratings (e.g., Hamamatsu H8500) or microchannel plates (Burle 85011). Due to their size and geometry, these devices have a large percent active area, minimal anode cross talk, and excellent pulse resolution. For example, the H8500 has 89% active area, <3% crosstalk, and 300psec pulse resolution [Hadig, 2002].

6.4.3 Photodiodes. Because silicon photodiodes are highly developed and have high quantum efficiency, it is natural to inquire into their usefulness as photodetectors in scintillation cameras. The main drawback of photodiodes is that they have no internal gain mechanism; thus, the noise associated with the detector and the external electronics will be much more serious than for PMTs.

The major noise components to be considered are the thermal noise of the photodiode, shot noise from leakage current through the diode, and thermal and 1/f noise in the amplifier that follows the photodiode and integrates the current to obtain a measure of the charge associated with each gamma-ray event. These different noise sources have different effects depending on the response characteristics of the amplifier and pulse-shaping network; for a detailed discussion, see Radeka [1988].

The analysis by Radeka shows that there are several terms in the variance of the noise charge, but the one of interest in this discussion is proportional to the mean-square amplifier noise multiplied by the square of the total capacitance seen at the amplifier input. The total capacitance includes the photodiode capacitance as well as that of the integrating capacitor and any cables used. Large-area photodiodes have large capacitance as well as large leakage current; therefore, in practice, the use of photodiodes with scintillators is limited to devices only a few millimeters across [Bird, 1993; Moses, 1994, 1995].

An interesting variant on simple planar photodiodes is the silicon drift detector [Gatti and Rehak, 1984]. These devices have small, point-like anodes so they can have large optical collection area but small capacitance.

Materials other than silicon also have been used for photodiodes in scintillation-counting applications. For example, HgI_2 photodiodes have been used with CsI(Tl) scintillators by Wang et al. [1995].

6.4.4 Avalanche photodiodes. Avalanche photodiodes (APDs) are silicon diodes operated at large reverse bias so that the carriers gain enough energy to excite new electron-hole pairs, in a manner similar to the gas proportional counters discussed in Section 4.3.3. Thus they function like PMTs, as photodetectors with internal gain. Because the gain can occur at any point in the depletion region, rather than at discrete dynodes as in PMTs, however, the gain noise tends to be larger in APDs.

It is also possible to construct APDs with resistive anodes in such a way as to obtain signals related to the position where a photon is absorbed. Hence, these so-called position-sensitive APDs function like miniature Anger cameras.

6.4.5 Video detectors. Because optical cameras have much better spatial resolution than gamma-ray cameras, it is natural to inquire whether it is possible to obtain high intrinsic resolution for gamma rays simply by imaging a scintillation crystal onto an optical camera. This idea has been evaluated by numerous groups in the past, but usually it has been rejected on statistical grounds. If the required field of view (size of the scintillation crystal) is $L \times L$ and the area of the optical camera is $w \times w$, with $w \ll L$, then the crystal must be demagnified by a factor of w/L, and the optical collection efficiency of the lens is reduced by the square of this quantity. As a result, the number of photoelectrons produced in one pixel of the optical camera for a single gamma-ray interaction may drop below one, or at least below the noise floor set by dark current and read noise. Under these conditions, the detective quantum efficiency of the system can be considerably less than the absorption efficiency of the scintillator. Moreover, even if an adequate number of photoelectrons per gamma ray can be produced, the system still operates as an integrating detector rather than a photon-counting one; therefore, energy discrimination is not possible, and the noise properties of the image suffer further, as discussed in Section 4.2.2.

Several developments over the last two years suggest that we should reconsider these conclusions. First, optical detector arrays are now much larger and have much lower noise than before; 6 cm $\times$ 6 cm CCDs (charge-coupled devices) are now available at reasonable cost and, when cooled modestly, they have essentially no dark current. Noise in the readout electronics also is being reduced by built-in electron multiplication or parallel readout. Moreover, these new devices have very high quantum efficiency for incident optical photons, over 90% in some cases; for comparison, conventional PMTs have a quantum efficiency around 25–30%.

Most important, for application to small-animal imaging, the field of view can be much smaller, and it is even possible to use $1:1$ magnification for imaging the scintillator onto the CCD. With this magnification and well-corrected lenses of large numerical aperture, the optical-photon collection efficiency can be excellent.

Another motivation for lens-coupled gamma cameras is the current strong interest in bioluminescence and fluorescence studies in small animals. Many laboratories already have a low-noise CCD camera, and it should be possible to add a scintillator and suitable optics to convert it into a dual-modality SPECT/optical imager.

7. Summary and future directions

Progress in small-animal SPECT requires better temporal and spatial resolution in the final images, and this in turn requires better detectors. Improvements can be measured broadly in terms of the usable space-bandwidth product of the detector system which, as discussed in Sec. 2.2.3, can be used to improve either the final image resolution, the system sensitivity, or both. It is also important that detectors to be used with pinholes be able to resolve the depth of interaction and, when multiple pinholes are used, the detectors must have high count-rate capability. Of the conventional detector characteristics, perhaps the least important in small-animal SPECT is energy resolution.

Although new technologies such as superconducting tunnel junctions and gas ionization devices may hold promise in the long run, significant improvements in detector performance are still possible with relatively conventional scintillation cameras and semiconductor detector arrays.

As with any engineering effort, performance of the final system is closely tied to characteristics of the materials used. For scintillation detectors, there is a continuing need for brighter, faster scintillation crystals; for semiconductor arrays, the need is for better charge transport and material homogeneity. In both cases, high density and high atomic number are very desirable.

Improved system performance can often be achieved by use of modular detectors, with each unit mechanically, optically, and electronically independent of all others. The modular approach allows flexibility in system design, high count-rate capability, and easy interchangeability for maintenance and design modification.

A less-obvious route to improved imaging systems is through the use of rigorous methods from statistical decision theory. The performance of all gamma-ray imaging systems is limited by the random fluctuations of the object, the Poisson statistics of the gamma-ray flux, and the signals produced by each photon; it is crucial to understand these limitations if one is to analyze and systematically optimize system performance. Specifically for gamma-ray detectors, it is important to catalog all of the noise sources that influence our ability to detect and localize individual gamma-ray events, to develop rigorous statistical characterizations of each noise source, and to use this statistical knowledge in optimal signal processing. These issues will be dealt with in the next chapter.

The future for small-animal SPECT is bright. As we noted in Section 3.2.3, the linear resolution of current small-animal PET and SPECT systems is about 1 mm isotropically, corresponding to a volume resolution of about 1 μL and making it reasonable to characterize the systems as microPET or microSPECT. It follows from the discussion of detector technologies presented in this chapter that a resolution of 100 μm is currently within reach for small-animal SPECT (although probably not for small-animal PET), and this linear resolution corresponds to a volume resolution of 1 nL. True NanoSPECT is probably achievable within two years of this publication. True picoSPECT (10 μm linear, 1 pL volumetric resolution) is not out of the question, at least for ^{125}I imaging.

References

[Abbey, 1995] C. K. Abbey, H. H. Barrett, "Linear iterative reconstruction algorithms: Study of observer performance," *XIVth International Conference on Information Processing in Medical Imaging* (IPMI), Ile de Berder, France, pp. 65-76, June 26-30, 1995.

[Abbey, 1996] C. K. Abbey, H. H. Barrett, D. W. Wilson, "Observer signal-to-noise ratios for the ML-EM algorithm," *Proc SPIE*, vol. 2708, 1996.

[Accorsi, 2001a] R. Accorsi, F. Gasparini, R. C. Lanza, "A Coded Aperture for High-Resolution Nuclear Medicine Planar Imaging with a Conventional Anger

Camera: experimental results," *IEEE Trans Nucl Sci*, vol. 48, no. 6, pp. 2411-2417, December 2001a.

[Accorsi, 2001b] R. Accorsi, F. Gasparini, R. C. Lanza, "Optimal Coded Patterns for Improved SNR in Nuclear Medicine Imaging," *Nucl Instr Meth Phys Res A*, vol. 474 , pp. 273-284, 2001b.

[Barrett, 1972] H. H. Barrett, "Fresnel zone plate imaging in nuclear medicine," *J. Nucl Med*, vol. 13, no. 6, pp. 382-385, 1972.

[Barrett, 1981] H. H. Barrett, W. Swindell, *Radiological Imaging: Theory of Image Formation, Detection, and Processing*, vols. I and II, New York, Academic Press, 1981.

[Barrett, 1990] H. H. Barrett, "Objective assessment of image quality: effects of quantum noise and object variability," *J. Opt Soc Am A*, vol. 7, pp. 1266-1278, 1990.

[Barrett, 1994] H. H. Barrett, H. C. Gifford, "Cone-beam tomography with discrete data sets," *Phys Med Biol*, vol. 39, pp. 451-476, 1994.

[Barrett, 1995a] H. H. Barrett, J. L. Denny, R. F. Wagner, K. J. Myers, "Objective assessment of image quality. II Fisher information, Fourier crosstalk, and figures of merit for task performance," *J. Opt Soc Am A*, vol. 12, no. 5, pp. 834-852, 1995a.

[Barrett, 1995b] H. H. Barrett, J. D. Eskin, H. B. Barber, "Charge transport in arrays of semiconductor gamma-ray detectors," *Phys Rev Lett*, vol. 5, no. 1, pp. 156-159, 1995b.

[Barrett, 1996a] H. H. Barrett, J. L. Denny, H. C. Gifford, C. K. Abbey, "Generalized NEQ: Fourier analysis where you would least expect to find it," *Proc SPIE*, vol. 2708, pp. 41-52, 1996a.

[Barrett, 1996b] H. H. Barrett, W. Swindell, *Radiological Imaging: Theory of Image Formation, Detection, and Processing*, Paperback edition, New York, Academic Press, 1996b.

[Barrett, 1998] H. H. Barrett, B. Gallas, E. Clarkson, A. Clough, "Scattered radiation in nuclear medicine: A case study in the Boltzmann transport equation," *Computational Radiology and Imaging: Therapy and Diagnosis*, Borgers, C., Natterer, F. eds., Springer Verlag, 1998.

[Barrett, 2004] H. H. Barrett, K. J. Myers, *Foundations of Image Science*, New York, John Wiley and Sons, 2004.

[Bird, 1993] A. J. Bird, T. Carter, A. J. Dean, D. Ramsden, B. M. Swinyard, "The optimisation of small CsI(Tl) gamma-ray detectors," *IEEE Trans Nucl Sci*, vol. 40, no. 4, pp. 395-399, 1993.

[Breskin, 2002] A. Breskin, A. Buzulutskov, R. Chechik, B. K. Singh, A. Bondar, L. Shekhtman, "Sealed GEM photomultiplier with a CsI photocathode," *Nucl Instr Meth Phys Res A*, vol. 478, pp. 225-229, 2002.

[Chen, 1997] J. C. Chen, "Scatter Rejection in Gamma Cameras for Use in Nuclear Medicine," *Biomed Eng Appl Basis Comm*, vol. 9, pp. 20-26, 1997.

[Chung, 2003] Y. H. Chung, Y. Choi, G. Cho, Y. S. Choe, K.-H. Lee, B.-T. Kim, "Optimization of Dual Layer Phoswich Detector Consisting of LSO and LuYAP for Small Animal PET," *Proc IEEE Med Imag Conf*, 2003.

[Clarkson, 1999] E. Clarkson, D. W. Wilson, H. H. Barrett, "The synthetic collimator for 2D and 3D imaging," *Proc SPIE Med Imag*, vol. 3659, pp. 107-117, 1999.

[Derenzo, 1993] S. E. Derenzo, W. W. Moses, "Experimental efforts and results in finding new heavy scintillators," *Heavy Scint for Sci and Indust Apps*, De Notaristefani, F., LeCoq, P., Schneegans, M. eds., Gif-sur-Yvette, France, Editions Frontieres, pp. 125-135, 1993.

[Dhanasopon, 2003] A. P. Dhanasopon, C. S. Levin, A. M. K. Foudray, P. D. Olcott, J. A. Talcott, F. Habte, "Scintillation Crystal Design Features for a Miniature Gamma Ray Camera," *Proc IEEE Med Imag Conf*, 2003.

[Dorenbos, 1995] P. Dorenbos, J. T. M. de Haas, C. W. E. van Eijk, "Non-proportinoality in Scintillator Response and Energy Resolution Obtainable with Scintillator Crystals," *IEEE Trans Nucl Sci*, vol. 42, pp. 2190-2202, 1995.

[Eskin, 1999] J. D. Eskin, H. H. Barrett, H. B. Barber, "Signals induced in semiconductor gamma-ray imaging detectors," *J. Appl Phys*, vol. 85, pp. 647-659, 1999.

[Furenlid, 2000] L. R. Furenlid, E. Clarkson, D. G. Marks, H. H. Barrett, "Spatial pileup considerations for pixellated gamma-ray detectors," *IEEE Trans Nucl Sci*, vol. 47, pp. 1399-1402, 2000.

[Gatti, 1984] E. Gatti, P. Rehak, "Semiconductor drift chamber – an application of a novel charge transport scheme," *Nucl Instr Meth*, vol. 225, pp. 608-614, 1984.

[Gunter, 1996] D. L. Gunter, "Collimator Characteristics and Design." In *Nuclear Medicine*, Henken, R. E., ed., Mosby Year Book, St. Louis, Chap. 8., 1996.

[Hadig, 2002] T. Hadig, J. Schwiening, C. Field, G. Mazaheri, M. Jain, D. G. W. S. Leith, B. Ratcliff, J. Va'vra, "Study of Timing and Efficiency Properties of the Hamamatsu H-8500 Photomultiplier," *Proc IEEE Nucl Sci Symp*, 2002.

[Inadama, 2003] N. Inadama, H. Murayama, M. Watanabe, T. Omura, T. Yamashita, H. Kawai, N. Orita, T. Tsuda, "Performance of 256ch flat panel PS-PMT with small crystals for a DOI PET detector," *Proc IEEE Med Imag Conf*, 2003.

[Jaszczak, 1994] R. J. Jaszczak, J. Li, H. Wang, M. R. Zallutsky, R. E. Coleman, "Pinhole collimation for ultra-high resolution, small-field-of-view SPECT studies," *Phys Med Biol*, vol. 39, pp. 425-437, 1994.

[Knoll, 1999] G. F. Knoll, *Radiation Detection and Measurement*, 3rd ed., New York, Wiley, 1999.

[Kwo, 1991] D. P. Kwo, H. B. Barber, H. H. Barrett, T. S. Hickernell, J. M. Woolfenden, "Comparison of NaI(Tl), HgI2 and CdTe surgical probes II: Effect of scatter compensation on probe performance," *Med Phys*, vol. 18, pp. 382-389, 1991.

[Marks, 1999] D. G. Marks, H. B. Barber, H. H. Barrett, J. Tueller, J. M. Woolfenden, "Improving performance of a CdZnTe imaging array by mapping the detector with gamma rays," *Nucl Instr Meth Phys Res A*, vol. 428, pp. 102-112, 1999.

[Matteson, 1997] J. L. Matteson, W. Coburn, F. Duttweiler, W. A. Heindl, G. L. Huszar, P. C. LeBlanc, M. R. Pelling, L. E. Peterson, R. E. Rothschild, R. T. Skelton, P. L. Hink, C. Crabtree, "CdZnTe arrays for astrophysics applications," *Proc SPIE*, vol. 3115, pp. 160-175, 1997.

[McCready, 1971] V. R. McCready, R. P. Parker, E. M. Gunnersen, R. Ellis, E. Moss, W. G. Gore, "Clinical tests with a prototype semiconductor gamma camera," *Brit J. Radiology*, vol. 44, pp. 58, 1971.

[Meikle, 2003a] S. R. Meikle, R. Wojcik, A. G. Weisenberger, M. F. Smith, S. Majewski, P. Kench, S. Eberl, R. R. Fulton, M. Lerch, A. B. Rosenfeld, "CoALA-SPECT: A coded aperture laboratory animal SPECT system for preclinical imaging," *2002 IEEE Nucl Sci Symp Conference Record*, Scott Metzler, ed., Norfolk, Virginia, ISBN 0-7803-7637-4, November 10-16, 2002a.

[Meikle, 2003b] S. R. Meikle, P. Kench, A. G. Weisenberger, R. Wojcik, M. F. Smith, S. Majewski, S. Eberl, R. R. Fulton, A. B. Rosenfeld, M. J. Fulham, "A prototype coded aperture detector for small animal SPECT," *IEEE Trans Nucl Sci*, vol. 49, pp. 2167-2171, 2003b.

[Mörmann, 2002] D. Mörmann, A. Breskin, R. Chechik, P. Cwetanski, B. K. Singh, "Gas avalanche photomultiplier with a CsI- coated GEM," *Nucl Instr Meth Phys Res A*, vol. 478, pp. 230-234, 2002.

[Moses, 1994] W. W. Moses, S. E. Derenzo, "Design studies for a PET detector module using a pin photodiode to measure depth of interaction," *IEEE Trans Nucl Sci*, vol. 41, no. 4, pp. 1441-1445, August 1994.

[Moses, 1995] W. W. Moses, S. E. Derenzo, C. L. Melcher, R. A. Manente, "A room temperature LSO/pin photodiode PET detector module that measures depth of interaction," *IEEE Trans Nucl Sci*, vol. 42, no. 4, pp. 1085-1089, August 1995.

[Moses, 2002] W. W. Moses, "Current trends in scintillator detectors and materials," *Nucl Instr Meth Phys Res A*, vol. 487, pp. 123-128, 2002.

[Muehllehner, 1985] G. Muehllehner, "Effect of resolution improvement on required count density in ECT imaging: a computer simulation," *Phys Med Biol*, vol. 30, no. 2, pp. 163-173, 1985.

[Müller, 1986] S. P. Müller, J. F. Polak, M. F. Kijewski, B. L. Holman, "Collimator Selection for SPECT Brain Imaging: The Advantage of High Resolution," *J. Nucl Med*, vol. 27, pp. 1729-1738, 1986.

[Myers, 1990] K. J. Myers, J. P. Rolland, H. H. Barrett, R. F. Wagner, "Aperture optimization for emission imaging: Effect of a spatially varying background," *J. Opt Soc Am A*, vol. 7, pp. 1279-1293, 1990.

[Orita, 2003] N. Orita, H. Murayama, H. Kawai, N. Inadama, T. Tsuda, "Three Dimensional Array of Scintillation Crystals with Proper Reflector Arrangement for a DOI detector," *Proc IEEE Med Imag Conf*, 2003.

[Pani, 2003] R. Pani, R. Pellegrini, M. N. Cinti, C. Trotta, G. Trotta, R. Scafe, M. Betti, F. Cusanno, L. Montani, G. Iurlaro, F. Garibaldi, Del A. Guerra, "A novel compact gamma camera based on flat panel PMT," *Nucl Instr Meth Phys Res A*, vol. 513, no. 1, pp. 36-41, 2003.

[Pani, 2004] R. Pani, R. Pellegrini, M. N. Cinti, M. Mattioli, C. Trotta, L. Montani, G. Iurlaro, G. Trotta, D'L. Addio, S. Ridolfi, De G. Vincentis, I. N. Weinberg, "Recent advances and future perspectives of position sensitive PMT," *Nucl Instr Meth Phys Res B*, vol. 213, pp. 197-205, 2004.

[Radeka, 1988] V. Radeka, "Low-noise techniques in detectors," *Ann Rev Nucl Part Sci*, vol. 38, pp. 217-277, 1988.

[Rodnyi, 1992] P. A. Rodnyi, "Core-valence band transitions in wide-gap ionic crystals," *Sov Phys Solid State*, vol. 34, pp. 1053-1066, 1992

[Rogulski, 1993] M. M. Rogulski, H. B. Barber, H. H. Barrett, R. L. Shoemaker, J. M. Woolfenden, "Ultra-high-resolution brain SPECT: simulation results," *IEEE Trans Nucl Sci*, vol. 40, pp. 1123-1129, 1993.

[Rolland, 1989] J. P. Rolland, H. H. Barrett, G. W. Seeley, "Quantitative study of deconvolution and display mappings for long-tailed point-spread functions," *Proc SPIE*, vol. 1092, pp. 17-21, 1989.

[Rolland, 1990] J. P. Rolland, *Factors influencing lesion detection in medical imaging*, Ph.D. Dissertation, University of Arizona, Tucson, Arizona, 1990.

[Rolland, 1991] J. P. Rolland, H. H. Barrett, G. W. Seeley, "Ideal versus human observer for long-tailed point spread functions: Does deconvolution help?" *Phys Med Biol*, vol. 36, no. 8, pp. 1091-1109, 1991.

[Rolland, 1992] J. P. Rolland, H. H. Barrett, "Effect of random background inhomogeneity on observer detection performance," *J. Opt Soc Am A*, vol. 9, no. 5, pp. 649-658, 1992.

[Ryan, 1995] J. M. Ryan, J. R. Macri, M. L. McConnell, B. K. Dann, M. L. Cherry, T. G. Guzik, F. P. Doty, B. A. Apotovsky, J. F. Butler, "Large area sub-millimeter resolution CdZnTe strip detector for astronomy," *Proc SPIE*, vol. 301, pp. 2518:292, 1995.

[Schramm, 2002] N. Schramm, G. Ebel, U. Engeland, M. Behe, T. Schurrat, T. M. Behr, "Multi-pinhole SPECT for small animal research," *J. Nucl Med*, vol. 43, no. 5, pp. S.913, 2002.

[Smith, 1998] M. F. Smith, R. Jaszczak, "An analytic model of pinhole aperture penetration for 3D pinhole SPECT image reconstruction," *Phys Med Biol*, vol. 43, pp. 761-775, 1998.

[Stahle, 1996] C. M. Stahle, A. Parsons, L. M. Bartlett, P. Kurczynski, J. F. Krizmanic, L. M. Barbier, S. D. Barthelmy, F. Birsa, N. Gehrels, J. Odom, D. Palmer, C. Sappington, P. Shu, Teegarden B. J., J. Tueller, "CdZnTe strip detector for arc second imaging and spectroscopy," *Proc Society Photo-Optical and Instr Eng*, vol. 2859, pp. 74-84, 1996.

[Tsui, 1978] B. M. W. Tsui, C. E. Metz, F. B. Atkins, S. J. Starr, R. N. Beck, "A Comparison of Optimum Detector Spatial Resolution in Nuclear Imaging based on Statistical Theory and on Observer Performance," *Phys Med Biol*, vol. 23, no. 4, pp. 654-676, 1978.

[Tsui, 1983] B. M. W. Tsui, C. E. Metz, Beck, R. N. "Optimum detector spatial resolution for discriminating between tumour uptake distributions scintigraphy," *Phys Med Biol*, vol. 28, no. 7, pp. 775-788, 1983.

[Wagner, 1985] R. F. Wagner, D. G. Brown, "Unified SNR analysis of medical imaging systems," *Phys Med Biol*, vol. 30, no. 6, pp. 489-518, 1985.

[Wang, 1995] Y. J. Wang, B. E. Patt, J. S. Iwanczyk, S. R. Cherry, Y. Shao, "High efficiency CsI(Tl)/HgI2 2 gamma ray spectrometers," *IEEE Trans Nucl Sci*, vol. 42, no. 4, pp. 601-605, 1995.

[White, 1994] T. A. White, *SPECT reconstruction directly from photomultiplier tube signals*, Ph.D. Dissertation, University of Arizona, Tucson, Arizona, 1994.

[Weber, 2002] M. J. Weber, "Inorganic scintillators: today and tomorrow," *J. Lums*, vol. 100, pp. 35-45, 2002.

[Wilson, 2000] D. W. Wilson, E. W. Clarkson, H. H. Barrett, "Reconstruction of two- and three-dimensional images from synthetic collimator data," *IEEE Trans Med Im*, vol. 19, no. 5, pp. 412-422, 2000.

[van Eijk, 2002] van C. W. E. Eijk, "Inorganic scintillators in medical imaging," *Phys Med Biol*, vol. 47, pp. R85-R106, April 21, 2002

Chapter 3

Detectors for Small-Animal SPECT II

Statistical Limitations and Estimation Methods

Harrison H. Barrett*
barrett@radiology.arizona.edu

1. Introduction

In Chapter 2 we gave a broad overview of detectors for small-animal SPECT. At several points in that discussion, we alluded to the need for understanding the noise and other statistical factors that limit detector performance, and we saw that it was necessary to perform position estimation and other data-processing tasks that required definite statistical models. In this chapter, we introduce the statistical tools needed for these purposes.

Although there is considerable commonality between scintillation and semiconductor detectors in terms of statistics and data processing, we concentrate here on scintillation devices. Our goal is to look in detail at the statistical limitations of scintillation detectors and understand how to incorporate statistical models optimally into the data processing. Then, at the end, we shall indicate briefly how to extend the methodology to semiconductor detectors.

A key reference for this chapter is Barrett and Myers [2004], to which the reader is referred for many details and derivations. In particular, we shall rely on material from Chapter 11 of Barrett and Myers on Poisson statistics and from Chapter 12 on noise in detectors.

After a relatively non-mathematical discussion in Section 2 on the role of statistics in scintillation cameras, we provide a summary of the key properties of Poisson random variables, vectors, and processes in Section 3. In Section 4, we give a similar summary of random amplification, such as the gain processes that take place in PMTs.

In Section 5, we introduce maximum-likelihood estimation methods, and finally, in Section 6, we apply this background to scintillation cameras. The extension to semiconductors is presented in Section 7, and some unsolved problems and future directions are delineated in Section 8.

*The University of Arizona, Department of Radiology, Tucson, Arizona

2. Role of statistics

Consider a gamma-ray camera consisting of multiple optical detectors viewing a scintillator. The optical detectors can be discrete photomultiplier tubes (PMTs), they can be the various anodes in a multi-anode PMT, or they can be avalanche photodiodes (see Chapter 2). They can even be individual pixels in a CCD camera onto which the scintillator is imaged with a lens. For definiteness, however, we shall refer to the optical detectors simply as PMTs.

The raw data delivered by the camera are the signals from the PMTs. What information do we wish to extract from these signals and how can we obtain that information optimally? To address these questions, we shall first enumerate the diverse statistical inference tasks we might pose, then we inquire into the data needed to perform each task, and finally we look at what statistical models are required and what random effects they need to include.

2.1 Inference tasks for scintillation cameras

The most familiar inference task with scintillation cameras is 2D position estimation; from the PMT signals for a particular scintillation event, we wish to infer the 2D coordinates $(x,\ y)$ of the gamma-ray interaction. In most cases, we also want to estimate the energy $\mathcal{E}$ of the event. Further, as noted in Chapter 2, when the camera is used with pinholes or coded apertures, it is desirable to estimate the depth of interaction z.

To make matters more interesting, there may be more than one site within the detector at which energy is deposited for a single gamma-ray event. If the initial interaction is photoelectric absorption of the gamma ray by a K electron, the resulting K-shell vacancy is filled rapidly by an electronic transition from a higher shell. The x ray produced by this transition can be reabsorbed or scattered within the crystal at another location. Similarly, if the initial interaction is a Compton scatter event, then the scattered photon can be reabsorbed or scattered again.

If we have two sites of energy deposition, the estimation problem can be stated as 8D: x, y, z, $\mathcal{E}$ for each of the two sites. Alternatively, we can regard the parameters for the second interaction as nuisance parameters and not attempt to estimate them, reducing the problem back to 4D. Even in that case, however, the presence of the second site influences the estimate of the coordinates for the first site; thus, it should be taken into account.

Another statistical-inference task in gamma-ray imaging is classifying the detected photon as scattered or unscattered. This common step is more subtle than it might appear, because the scattering in question might occur in either the body of the patient (or animal) or in the detector itself. A photon that has scattered in the patient carries little information about its point of origin, and most approaches to SPECT attempt to reject such photons. There is, however, no reason in principle to reject photons that undergo Compton scatter in the detector; if we can accurately estimate their interaction locations in the detector, then they are still quite useful in the final tomographic reconstruction. Hence, the goal of the inference should be joint classification and estimation: decide if the photon was scattered in the detector, and if so, where.

Another goal, mentioned briefly in Chapter 2, is fluence estimation. The term fluence describes the mean number of photons per unit area incident on the camera face, so that the fluence can be thought of as the noise-free 2D image. A more precise definition will be given in Section 3 of this chapter.

A related goal is spectral estimation. By analogy to fluence, a spectrum is the mean number of photons per unit energy. Often a spectrum is estimated as a prelude to classification of the individual photons. Fluence and spectral estimation can be combined into spatio-spectral fluence estimation, where the objective is to infer the mean distribution of the detected photons as a function of both spatial coordinates (2D or 3D) and energy.

Finally, tomographic reconstruction itself is often formulated as a statistical inference process.

2.2 Data needed for inference tasks

For estimation of the 2D or 3D position of a single gamma-ray interaction, and also for energy estimation, we need in principle all of the PMT signals produced by that interaction. In practice, some subset of this data set might be used, but there is a risk of poorer estimation performance in those cases.

Classifying a detected gamma-ray photon as scattered or unscattered is often done on the basis of some *ad hoc* energy estimate, such as the sum of the PMT signals, but it is preferable to use the ML energy estimate. It is also possible to do the classification from the original data set, namely all of the PMT signals for that interaction. Indeed, it is essential to use all of the signals if one wants to distinguish scattering in the detector from scattering in the patient or animal.

Fluence and spectral distributions are properties of single tomographic projections of a 3D object. The simplest way of estimating the fluence is simply to bin the 2D position estimates for one projection into a 2D image, forming what we will call a histogram estimate. A more sophisticated approach, however, is to use all of the PMT signals for all interactions in one camera head at one orientation. Maximum-likelihood (ML) fluence estimates can be obtained from these PMT data. Similarly, a spectrum can be estimated by binning energy estimates for individual events, or it can be estimated directly by using the PMT signals for all events in one projection.

For tomographic reconstruction itself, we normally use the histogram estimates of the individual projection fluences, but it is also possible to use the ML fluence estimates, and it is even possible to do a full 3D reconstruction directly from the PMT signals for all photons hitting all cameras, without the intermediary of either position estimation or fluence estimation.

No matter what inference task we consider, it can always be performed from some set of PMT signals; if it is not done with these raw data, we need to inquire as to how much information loss has occurred.

2.3 Statistical models needed

To carry out the inference tasks listed above, we need first to characterize the statistical properties of the PMT signals and how those properties depend on the quantities we wish to estimate. As we shall argue in Section 5, ML estimates and ML decisions have several desirable features; therefore, we concentrate in this chapter on likelihood-based inferences and on likelihood models.

For an estimation task, the likelihood is the probability of the data (or probability density function if the data can take a continuous range of values), conditioned on the parameters we wish to estimate. Thus, the general form of a likelihood for discrete data is Pr(data | parameters). Note that we use $\Pr(\,\cdot\,)$ for probabilities and $\mathrm{pr}(\,\cdot\,)$ for probability density functions (PDFs) in the continuous case.

To be more specific to the problem at hand, consider a scintillation camera with K PMTs. We denote the set of (continuous-valued) PMT signals as $\{V_k, k = 1, .., K\}$, or as the $K \times 1$ vector $\mathbf{V}$. For different inference tasks, we need different conditional PDFs of $\mathbf{V}$. When we need to distinguish PMT signals for different events, we shall add another subscript; hence, $\mathbf{V}_j$ is the $K \times 1$ vector of signals for the jth event, and V_{kj} is the signal from the kth PMT for that event.

For 2D position estimation on the jth event, we need a likelihood of the form $\mathrm{pr}(\mathbf{V}_j|x, y)$; for 3D estimation, we need $\mathrm{pr}(\mathbf{V}_j|x, y, z)$. To estimate position and energy of an event simultaneously, we need $\mathrm{pr}(\mathbf{V}_j|x, y, \mathcal{E})$ or $\mathrm{pr}(\mathbf{V}_j|x, y, z, \mathcal{E})$. For photon classification, we need one of the latter two likelihoods plus some knowledge of the spectrum of scattered photons.

For fluence estimation, we need the PDF for all events in one camera head at one projection angle. For the 2D case, we denote the requisite likelihood as $\mathrm{pr}(\{\mathbf{V}_j\}|x, y)$, where the brackets denote a set, but because the events are independent (see Section 3), we can also write this likelihood as a product of single-event likelihoods, $\prod_{j=1}^{J} \mathrm{pr}(\mathbf{V}_j|x, y)$, where J is the total number of events in the set

2.4 Random effects in scintillation cameras

To enumerate the random effects that can influence the likelihoods listed above, we need only trace the sequence of events leading from the initial gamma-ray interaction to the measured signals.

The initial interaction takes place at a random location in the scintillator; at that location, it randomly undergoes either a Compton or photoelectric interaction. As discussed in Chapter 2, this event produces both a high-energy electron and an additional high-energy photon (either the Compton-scattered photon or a K x ray). The photon can, with some probability, escape the scintillator, or it can be reabsorbed at some random location, and the process can continue with production of more high-energy electrons and photons. Because of the random possibility of photon escape, the total energy deposited in the scintillator by the gamma ray is a random variable.

At each location where a high-energy electron is produced, it dissipates its energy by production of low-energy optical photons (the scintillation light) and phonons (lattice vibrations or heat). The number of optical photons produced is a key random variable describing the scintillation process.

After the optical photons are produced, they propagate randomly to the photocathodes of the various PMTs that make up the scintillation camera, and at each photocathode they randomly produce photoelectrons. The gain mechanism in the PMTs is another important random effect.

Although these various random effects seem very diverse, Poisson statistics play a critical role in all of them. That is not to say that all of the resulting random variables are Poisson distributed; they can have much more complicated statistics, but in every case the theory of Poisson random variables and processes is key to their analysis.

It follows that optimal statistical inference with data from scintillation cameras, or gamma-ray detectors more broadly, requires knowledge of Poisson theory. The main points of that theory are summarized in Section 3.1.1.

3. Poisson statistics

A Poisson random variable is an integer-valued random variable that follows the Poisson probability law. A Poisson random vector is a collection of these random variables. A Poisson point process is a collection of N Dirac delta functions, where N is a Poisson random variable. The thing that connects these Poisson entities is that the events which produce them are statistically independent. Indeed, the author goes so far as to tell his students that Poisson is French for independent.

As we shall see, Poisson random variables, vectors and processes all arise in the analysis of scintillation cameras. The three subsections in this section summarize material from Barrett and Myers [2004] on the three Poisson constructs.

3.1 Poisson random variables

There are two broad principles from which Poisson statistics arise. As already mentioned above, Poisson statistics stem from assumptions of statistical independence, formalized as a set of three postulates that lead to the Poisson law. These postulates and their generalizations and consequences are discussed in Section 3.1.1.

The other general principle is an approximate one, akin to the central-limit theorem that makes Gaussian statistics so prevalent. That theorem says that the sum of a large number of independent continuous-valued random variables tends to a Gaussian or normal distribution as the number being summed increases, no matter what the PDFs of the quantities being summed. Similarly, if we have an integer number of items and delete most of them randomly and independently, the resulting number of remaining items tends towards the Poisson law. The math behind this statement will be explained in Section 3.1.2.

Other important topics to be treated here include binomial selection of a Poisson (Section 3.1.3) and doubly stochastic Poisson random variables (Sections 3.1.4 and 3.1.5).

3.1.1 Poisson and independence. The postulates that lead to the Poisson law are:

(a) The number of events in any time interval is statistically independent of the number in any other *nonoverlapping* interval.

(b) If we consider a very small time interval of duration ΔT, the probability of a single event in this interval approaches some constant a times ΔT, i.e.,

$$\Pr(1 \text{ in } \Delta T) = a\Delta T. \tag{3.1}$$

(Note that a has dimensions of reciprocal time; it will soon be interpreted as a rate.)

(c) The probability of more than one event in a small interval ΔT is zero:

$$\Pr(1 \text{ in } \Delta T) + \Pr(0 \text{ in } \Delta T) = 1. \tag{3.2}$$

If the postulates are satisfied with a = constant, then it can be shown (see, for example, Barrett and Myers, 2004) that

$$\Pr(N \text{ in } T) = \frac{(aT)^N}{N!} \exp(-aT). \tag{3.3}$$

This is the familiar form of the Poisson probability law, where the mean of N is given by $\overline{N} = aT$. Thus, the mean number of events is aT, justifying the interpretation a as the mean number per unit time or the mean rate. It is a well-known property of Poisson random variables that the variance equals the mean: $\mathrm{Var}(N) = \langle (N - \overline{N})^2 \rangle = aT - \overline{N}$

The independence of the events is maintained if the rate is a *nonrandom* function of time $a(t)$. In that case, it is found that the number of events in $(0, T)$ is still a Poisson random variable:

$$\Pr[N \text{ in } (t, t+T)] = \frac{\overline{N}^N}{N!} \exp(-\overline{N}), \tag{3.4}$$

where $\overline{N}$ is now a function of time given by

$$\overline{N} = \int_t^{t+T} a(t')\, dt'. \tag{3.5}$$

Despite the time-varying rate, the variance still equals the mean, and all other properties of the Poisson law still hold. The variation in rate does not spoil the independence of the events and hence their "Poissonicity," provided the rate is not random. The case of a random rate is discussed later in Section 3.1.4.

3.1.2 Poisson and rarity. Consider a set of M Bernoulli trials (e.g., coin flips), where the probability of success (e.g., heads) is p. The total number N of successes in M trials is given by the binomial law

$$\Pr(N|M,p) = \begin{pmatrix} N \\ n \end{pmatrix} p^n q^{N-n}, \tag{3.6}$$

where $q = 1 - p$ is the probability of failure (tails). The mean number of successes is given by $\overline{N} = Mp$ and the variance is Mpq.

Now let M become very large and p become very small in such a way that Mp (or $\overline{N}$) remains constant. Poisson himself showed that

$$\lim_{M\to\infty} \Pr(N|M,p) = \frac{(\overline{N})^N}{N!} \exp(-\overline{N}). \tag{3.7}$$

This result can be summarized by saying "Rarity begets Poissonicity".

3.1.3 Binomial selection of a Poisson. In many applications of the binomial law, the number of trials M is random. An important example for our purposes is radiation detection by an inefficient photon-counting detector. Suppose M photons are incident on the detector in time T and that each has a probability η (called the *quantum efficiency*) of producing a photoelectron. If the photoelectric interactions are statistically independent, then the *conditional* probability $\Pr(N|M)$ for obtaining N photoelectrons is a binomial. The marginal probability $\Pr(N)$, however, is given by

$$\Pr(N) = \sum_{M=N}^{\infty} \Pr(N|M)\Pr(M). \tag{3.8}$$

Now suppose that the photons satisfy the three postulates so that M is a Poisson random variable. With $\Pr(N|M)$ being binomial, we have

$$\Pr(N) = \sum_{M=N}^{\infty} \Pr(N|M)\Pr(M)$$

$$= \sum_{M=N}^{\infty} \binom{M}{N} \eta^N (1-\eta)^{M-N} \exp(-\overline{M}) \frac{\overline{M}^M}{M!}. \tag{3.9}$$

A change of variables, $K = M - N$, and a little algebra shows that

$$\Pr(N) = \exp(-\eta\overline{M}) \frac{(\eta\overline{M})^N}{N!}. \tag{3.10}$$

Thus, N obeys a Poisson law with mean $\overline{N} = \eta\overline{M}$.

This important result is often called the *binomial-selection theorem*. It states that the binomial selection of a Poisson yields a Poisson, and that the mean of the output of the selection process is the mean of the input times the binomial.

An interesting corollary is that the number of times that the photon is *not* detected is also a Poisson random variable. Moreover, the number of nondetections is statistically independent of the number of detections.

These conclusions may seem counterintuitive if one thinks in terms of coin flipping. If the number of flips is fixed, the number of tails is completely determined by the number of heads. If, however, the number of flips is random, then the number of heads is independent of the number of tails if and only if the number of flips is a Poisson random variable.

The binomial-selection theorem can be applied to a cascade of selection processes. As an example very relevant to this chapter, consider a point source that emits a Poisson number of photons randomly in all directions. Some of the photons fall on the photocathode of a photomultiplier tube and some of these produce photoelectrons. We assume that the photon emissions are independent with mean $\overline{M}$ and that the photon directions are independent and isotropic. Thus the fraction of photons that fall on the PMT is just $\Omega/4\pi$, where Ω is the solid angle subtended by the PMT at the source point. When the photons reach the PMT, they produce photoelectrons randomly and independently; the fraction of incident photons that produce photoelectrons is the quantum efficiency η.

Hence, we have a Poisson source and two binomial selections in this problem. Because binomial selection of a Poisson yields a Poisson, we know at once that N follows a Poisson law where the mean number of photoelectrons is given by

$$\overline{N} = \eta \, \frac{\Omega}{4\pi} \, \overline{M}. \tag{3.11}$$

We can continue this process indefinitely, including other binomial selections such as absorption and reflection. The key point is that a Poisson source followed by any number of binomial selections gives a Poisson. All we need to do is compute the final mean, and then we will have the full probability law for the final number of events.

3.1.4 Doubly stochastic Poisson variables. Often we need to consider Poisson random variables where the Poisson mean is random. As one example, we can argue that gamma rays produce a Poisson number of photoelectrons (denoted N) in the PMT of a scintillation detector *if* all gamma-ray photons have the same energy, but the distribution of energies causes variation in $\overline{N}$. The photopeak is governed by Poisson statistics, but the overall pulse-height spectrum is not.

A second example is the random depth of interaction of a gamma ray in a scintillation camera; the depth controls the mean amount of light reaching the PMT and hence the mean number of photoelectrons.

Even when N is a discrete random variable with only integer values, its mean $\overline{N}$ can take on any value in $(0, \infty)$. Thus, random $\overline{N}$ must be described by a probability density function $\mathrm{pr}(\overline{N})$. The mean number of photoelectrons is now given by

$$\Pr(N) = \int_0^\infty d\overline{N} \, \Pr(N|\overline{N}) \, \mathrm{pr}(\overline{N}). \tag{3.12}$$

The variable N is said to be *doubly stochastic* because two random effects are involved.

Specifically, if $\Pr(N|\overline{N})$ is Poisson, N is a *doubly stochastic Poisson random variable*, and its probability law is

$$\Pr(N) = \frac{1}{N!}\int_0^\infty d\overline{N}\, \overline{N}^N \exp(-\overline{N})\, \mathrm{pr}(\overline{N}). \tag{3.13}$$

This expression is called the *Poisson transform* of $\mathrm{pr}(\overline{N})$.

We can use (3.13) to compute the mean and variance of a doubly stochastic Poisson random variable. The mean is denoted $\overline{\overline{N}}$, where the double overbar indicates two separate averages, one with respect to $\Pr(N|\overline{N})$, another with respect to $\mathrm{pr}(\overline{N})$.

The variance of N is given by

$$\mathrm{Var}(N) = \left\langle (N - \overline{\overline{N}})^2 \right\rangle = \overline{\overline{N}} + \mathrm{Var}(\overline{N}). \tag{3.14}$$

The first term is the Poisson variance appropriate to the average value of the mean. The second term, often called the *excess variance*, is the result of randomness in the Poisson mean.

3.1.5 Binomial selection, non-Poisson source. Now we combine the results from the two previous subsections and discuss binomial selection (with probability η) of a doubly stochastic Poisson random variable (of mean $\overline{\overline{M}}$). An example would be a non-Poisson light source illuminating a photocathode of efficiency η.

The overall mean of the number of photoelectrons is $\overline{\overline{N}} = \eta\, \overline{\overline{M}}$, and it can be shown that the variance is given by

$$\mathrm{Var}(N) = \eta\, \overline{\overline{M}} + \eta^2\, \mathrm{Var}(\overline{M}). \tag{3.15}$$

Note that the Poisson part of the variance scales as η, while the excess variance scales as η^2. The key point is that a small efficiency reduces the excess variance relative to the Poisson part. Again, rarity begets Poissonicity.

3.2 Poisson random vectors

Consider an array of photon-counting detectors, with g_j counts in the jth detector. The data thus consist of the set $\{g_j, j = 1, 2, ..., J\}$. If individual counts g_j are Poisson (i.e., independent), then the multivariate probability law is

$$\Pr(\{g_j\}) = \prod_{j=1}^{J} \Pr(g_j) = \prod_{j=1}^{J} \exp(-\overline{g}_j)\frac{\overline{g}_j^{\,g_j}}{g_j!}. \tag{3.16}$$

3.2.1 Covariance matrix. Independent counts are necessarily uncorrelated, and the variance equals the mean; therefore, the covariance matrix of a Poisson random vector has elements

$$K_{jk} = \left\langle [g_j - \overline{g}_j][g_k - \overline{g}_k] \right\rangle = \overline{g}_j\, \delta_{jk}. \tag{3.17}$$

A useful alternative notation is to define a $J \times 1$ data vector g with components $\{g_1, g_2, ..., g_J\}$. The covariance matrix can then be written as

$$[\mathbf{K}_\mathbf{g}] = \left\langle [\mathbf{g} - \overline{\mathbf{g}}] \, [\mathbf{g} - \overline{\mathbf{g}}]^t \right\rangle = \text{diag}\,(\overline{\mathbf{g}}), \tag{3.18}$$

where superscript t denotes transpose, and diag $(\overline{\mathbf{g}})$ indicates a diagonal matrix with the components of the mean vector $\overline{\mathbf{g}}$ as diagonal elements.

3.2.2 Doubly stochastic random vectors. Now suppose that each g_j is a doubly stochastic Poisson random variable. Then the overall covariance matrix becomes

$$[\mathbf{K}_\mathbf{g}]_{ik} = \overline{\overline{g}}_i \, \delta_{ik} + [\mathbf{K}_{\overline{\mathbf{g}}}]_{ik} \, , \tag{3.19}$$

or, in vector notation

$$\mathbf{K}_\mathbf{g} = \text{diag}\,(\overline{\overline{\mathbf{g}}}) + \mathbf{K}_{\overline{\mathbf{g}}}. \tag{3.20}$$

The key point is that the overall covariance $\mathbf{K}_\mathbf{g}$ can now be nondiagonal. It becomes diagonal if the means are nonrandom, if the source is Poisson, or if the probability of detection is low.

3.3 Poisson random processes

As noted in the introduction to this section, Poisson random processes are sums of Dirac delta functions, where the number of terms in the sum is a Poisson random variable. The delta functions can be functions of time, space, energy, or direction, and all of these cases have application in discussing scintillation cameras. We begin with temporal delta functions.

3.3.1 Temporal point processes. A random temporal point process is defined by

$$z(t) = \sum_{n=1}^{N} \delta(t - t_n), \qquad (0 < t \leq T). \tag{3.21}$$

This function can describe the random occurrence of N events at random times $\{t_n\}$, where the number of events in time T, denoted N, can also be random. If the Poisson postulates hold and the rate a = constant, then we already know that N is a Poisson random variable with mean aT.

Under the Poisson assumptions, the mean of this process is simply $\langle z(t) \rangle = a$. (Note that the delta functions have dimensions of reciprocal time.) Not surprisingly, the variance of $z(t)$ is infinite, but the autocovariance function is given by

$$K_z(t, t') = \langle [z(t) - a][z(t') - a] \rangle = a\,\delta(t - t'). \tag{3.22}$$

In the limit as $T \rightarrow \infty$, the process becomes wide-sense stationary. By the Wiener-Khinchine theorem, the power spectral density is the Fourier transform of the autocovariance in that case; hence, $S_{\Delta z}(\nu) = a$. Indeed, *all* statistical properties of $z(t)$ are determined by the rate a.

If the Poisson postulates hold and the rate $a(t)$ is a nonrandom function, then we know from Section 3.1.1 that N is still Poisson, with a probability law given by (3.4) and (3.5) as

$$\Pr(N \text{ in } T) = \frac{\left[\int_0^T dt'\, a(t')\right]^N}{N!} \exp\left[-\int_0^T dt'\, a(t')\right]. \tag{3.23}$$

As noted earlier, the rate determines the mean and hence all properties of N, but it also determines all properties of the random process $z(t)$. For example, if the Poisson postulates hold, then the mean and autocovariance of $z(t)$ are given by

$$\langle z(t) \rangle = a(t)\,, \qquad K_z(t, t') = a(t)\, \delta(t - t'). \tag{3.24}$$

The variance is infinite, and the power spectral density is not defined in this nonstationary case.

In addition, the PDF on the times of occurrence is given by

$$\mathrm{pr}(t_n) = \frac{a(t_n)}{\int_0^T dt\, a(t)}. \tag{3.25}$$

Note the multiple interpretations of $a(t)$: It is the instantaneous rate, it is the mean of $z(t)$; it determines the autocovariance function; its integral over some time interval is the mean number of events in that interval, and it is the PDF on the times of occurrence. If the events are independent, all we ever need to know about $z(t)$ is the rate $a(t)$.

3.3.2 Spatial point processes. The spatial counterpart of the temporal point process $z(t)$ is denoted $g(\mathbf{r})$ and defined by

$$g(\mathbf{r}) = \sum_{n=1}^{N} \delta(\mathbf{r} - \mathbf{r}_n), \tag{3.26}$$

where $\mathbf{r}$ is a spatial position vector. For example, $g(\mathbf{r})$ could describe the pattern of photon interactions on a piece of film or the (unbinned) output of an Anger camera.

This function is a spatial Poisson process if the spatial counterparts of the Poisson postulates are satisfied. Specifically, the postulates are:

(a) The number of counts in any area A_1 is statistically independent of the number in any other nonoverlapping area A_2.

(b) If we consider a very small area ΔA contained in A and centered on point $\mathbf{r}$, the probability of a single count in this area during an observation time approaches a deterministic function $b(\mathbf{r})$ times ΔA

$$\Pr(1 \text{ in } \Delta A) = b(\mathbf{r}) \Delta A, \tag{3.27}$$

(c) The probability of more than one count in a small area ΔA is zero.

Note that we have allowed $\Pr(1 \text{ in } \Delta A)$ to be a function of position, but $b(\mathbf{r})$ is a fixed function and not yet a random process.

The properties of spatial Poisson processes can be stated by analogy to the temporal case. Under the Poisson assumptions, the probability of N counts in a finite area A is Poisson with mean

$$\overline{N} = \int_A d^2r\, b(\mathbf{r}), \tag{3.28}$$

so $b(\mathbf{r})$ is the mean number per unit area or fluence.

The fluence also determines the spatial distribution of the individual events; the PDF for the random locations $\mathbf{r}_n$ is

$$\mathrm{pr}(\mathbf{r}_n) = \frac{b(\mathbf{r}_n)}{\int_A d^2r\, b(\mathbf{r})}. \tag{3.29}$$

The mean and covariance of the random process are

$$\langle g(\mathbf{r}) \rangle = b(\mathbf{r}), \qquad K_{\mathbf{g}}(\mathbf{r}, \mathbf{r}') = b(\mathbf{r})\, \delta(\mathbf{r} - \mathbf{r}'). \tag{3.30}$$

As in the temporal case, all properties of the spatial Poisson process are determined by $b(\mathbf{r})$, the photon fluence.

3.3.3 Doubly stochastic spatial processes. In many practical circumstances, the fluence is a random function. An important example concerns imaging of random objects. The pattern of detected photons $g(\mathbf{r})$ is Poisson for repeated imaging of one object, but it is not Poisson when we average over many objects.

If the postulates are satisfied for a given fluence, but the fluence itself is random, then $g(\mathbf{r})$ is a doubly stochastic Poisson point process. The autocovariance is modified to

$$K_{\mathbf{g}}(\mathbf{r}, \mathbf{r}') = \overline{b}(\mathbf{r})\, \delta(\mathbf{r} - \mathbf{r}') + K_{\mathbf{b}}(\mathbf{r}, \mathbf{r}'). \tag{3.31}$$

The first term represents the average Poisson random process, and the second term is the autocovariance of the fluence $b(\mathbf{r})$.

4. Random amplification

To complete the discussion of random effects in scintillation cameras, we need to discuss the gain processes that occur in the PMTs and in the scintillation material itself. As in Barrett and Myers [2004], to which the reader is referred for details, we first discuss amplification in single-element devices such as PMT, then we move on to amplification of point processes in order to obtain the appropriate formalism for scintillators and fluorescent screens.

Finally, we briefly mention a situation that does not appear to involve amplification, namely the position estimation step in a scintillation camera; as we shall see, this process is just a special case of random amplification.

4.1 Amplification in single-element detectors

Consider a non-imaging detector such as a photomultiplier or avalanche photodiode in which the input is photons ("primaries") and the output is electrons ("secondaries").

If N primaries are absorbed in time T and the nth primary produces k_n secondaries, then the total number of secondaries is

$$K = \sum_{n=1}^{N} k_n. \tag{3.32}$$

Our goal is to determine the statistical properties of K from those of N and the set $\{k_n\}$.

We begin with some definitions. The conditional probability of K secondaries for exactly one primary is defined as

$$\Pr(K|N=1) = \gamma(K). \tag{3.33}$$

The function $\gamma(K)$ can be regarded as the output pulse-height spectrum for the detector.

In terms of $\gamma(K)$, the mean and variance of the number of secondaries for one primary are given by

$$\mathrm{E}\{K|N=1\} = \sum_{K=0}^{\infty} K\,\gamma(K) \equiv m_1\,, \qquad \mathrm{Var}\{K|N=1\} = m_2 - m_1^2, \tag{3.34}$$

where m_j is the jth moment of $\gamma(K)$.

The remaining step is to average over the number of primaries. When this is done, the mean total number of secondaries (for all primaries) is

$$\mathrm{E}\{K\} = \overline{N} m_1, \tag{3.35}$$

The overall variance is given by

$$\mathrm{Var}(K) = \overline{N}\,\mathrm{Var}(k_n) + \overline{k}_n^2\,\mathrm{Var}(N). \tag{3.36}$$

This result is often referred to as the *Burgess variance theorem.*

For a Poisson input, $\mathrm{Var}(N) = \overline{N}$, so the variance becomes

$$\mathrm{Var}(K) = \overline{N}\left[\mathrm{Var}(k_n) + \overline{k}_n^2\right] = \overline{N} m_2, \tag{3.37}$$

It is instructive to combine the expressions for means and variances into signal-to-noise ratios (SNRs), where an SNR is defined as the mean of a random variable divided by its standard deviation. For a single-element amplifiers with a Poisson-distributed number of primaries, the Burgess variance theorem yields

$$[\mathrm{SNR_{out}}]^2 = [\mathrm{SNR_{in}}]^2\,\frac{m_1^2}{m_2}. \tag{3.38}$$

The ratio m_1^2/m_2 is known as the *Swank factor*.

If $m_2 = m_1^2$, then the Swank factor is unity, the variance of k_n is zero, and the gain mechanism is noise-free; therefore, $\text{SNR}_{\text{out}} = \text{SNR}_{\text{in}}$ for a Poisson input N. This does not mean, however, that the output K is also Poisson. Instead, $\text{Var}(K) = m_1\overline{K} = \overline{k}_n^2\overline{N}$, so the variance is increased by the square of the gain, while the mean is increased only linearly. Rarity begets Poissonicity, but amplification (even noise-free amplification) inevitably destroys it. Because the secondaries come in bursts, they are not independent.

4.2 Amplified point processes

A theory of random amplification can also be developed for point processes. A point process consisting of N delta functions is amplified to produce another point process with K delta functions, with $K >> N$ if the gain is large.

The main radiographic application of this theory is integrating detectors such as film-screen systems, but it also describes the distribution of optical photons on a PMT face for one gamma ray interacting in a scintillation camera.

A sample function of the amplified point process is given by

$$y(\mathbf{r}) = \sum_{n=1}^{N}\sum_{k=1}^{k_n} \delta(\mathbf{r} - \mathbf{r}_{nk}) = \sum_{n=1}^{N}\sum_{k=1}^{k_n} \delta(\mathbf{r} - \mathbf{R}_n - \Delta\mathbf{r}_{nk}), \tag{3.39}$$

where $\mathbf{R}_n$ is the location at which the nth primary is absorbed, $\mathbf{r}_{nk}$ is the location for the kth secondary produced by that primary, and $\Delta\mathbf{r}_{nk}$ is the random displacement. Calculation of statistical properties such as the mean or autocovariance function for $y(\mathbf{r})$ requires averaging over all of these random variables.

After many pages of math, the autocovariance function has the form

$$K_{\mathbf{y}}(\mathbf{r}, \mathbf{r}') = \left[\mathcal{H}_1\overline{\mathbf{b}}\right](\mathbf{r})\,\delta(\mathbf{r} - \mathbf{r}') + \left[\mathcal{H}_2\overline{\mathbf{b}}\right](\mathbf{r}, \mathbf{r}') + \left[\mathcal{H}_1 K_{\mathbf{b}}\mathcal{H}_1^{\dagger}\right](\mathbf{r}, \mathbf{r}'). \tag{3.40}$$

(See Barrett and Myers for details and definitions of operators $\mathcal{H}_1$ and $\mathcal{H}_2$.) The delta-correlated term arises because the amplified point process is still a sum of delta functions. The second term arises from the amplification process, and the third is the contribution from the doubly stochastic nature of the source.

4.3 Mislocation without gain

A scintillation camera maps the interaction position $\mathbf{r}$ to an estimated position $\hat{\mathbf{r}}$. We can think of this process as fitting into the formalism for amplified point processes but with no amplification. One primary produces exactly one secondary.

If we set $\text{Var}(k_n) = 0$ and $\overline{k}_n(\mathbf{R}) = 1$ and neglect randomness in the fluence, then the autocovariance function becomes

$$K_{\mathbf{y}}(\mathbf{r}, \mathbf{r}'|\mathbf{b}) = \left[\int_\infty d^2R\, \text{pr}_{\Delta\mathbf{r}}(\mathbf{r} - \mathbf{R}|\mathbf{R})b(\mathbf{R})\right]\delta(\mathbf{r} - \mathbf{r}'). \tag{3.41}$$

This expression is just what we would have for a Poisson random process and an ideal detector, except that the fluence pattern is blurred. The point spread function for the blurring is just the PDF on the random displacements, $\mathrm{pr}_{\Delta\mathbf{r}}(\mathbf{r}|\mathbf{R})$. Note, however, that the individual delta functions that make up the point process are not blurred, and the output process remain delta-correlated.

Moreover, because the points remain independent (for repeated imaging of a single object), the (unbinned) output of a scintillation camera is a Poisson random process, for any estimation method and any degree of blur. With binning into a finite image array, the output is a Poisson random vector.

5. Approaches to estimation

Although many books on estimation theory are available, we summarize here the main points that we will need in discussing scintillation cameras.

Estimation is basically a mapping from what we have measured to what we want to know. Suppose we are given an $M \times 1$ data vector $\mathbf{g}$ and we know that the probability law on $\mathbf{g}$ is specified by a $K \times 1$ parameter vector $\boldsymbol{\theta}$. (For example, $\mathbf{g}$ is a set of measured PMT signals; $\boldsymbol{\theta}$ is the unknown interaction position.)

The measurement of $\mathbf{g}$ is a stochastic mapping; $\boldsymbol{\theta}$ determines the probability law from which the random $\mathbf{g}$ is drawn. Estimation of $\boldsymbol{\theta}$, on the other hand, is a deterministic mapping; from the measured $\mathbf{g}$ we want a rule or algorithm that returns an estimate of $\boldsymbol{\theta}$, denoted $\hat{\boldsymbol{\theta}}(\mathbf{g})$ or simply $\hat{\boldsymbol{\theta}}$ for short.

To find the optimal mapping, we need to:

- Define optimal;
- Develop a stochastic model for the data, $\mathrm{pr}(\mathbf{g}|\boldsymbol{\theta})$; and
- Specify the prior knowledge, $\mathrm{pr}(\boldsymbol{\theta})$ (if any).

Stochastic models for scintillation-camera data have already been introduced in Sections 3 and 4. Performance measures for the estimation mapping are summarized below in Section 5.1, and ML estimation and the sense in which it is optimal will be discussed in Section 5.2. As we shall see, ML methods do not use any prior knowledge about the parameter being estimated; Bayesian methods that do bring in a prior are discussed briefly in Section 5.3.

5.1 Performance measures

5.1.1 Cost and risk. A general approach to specifying an optimal estimator is to define a *cost function* $C(\boldsymbol{\theta}, \hat{\boldsymbol{\theta}})$ that depends on both the true value of the parameter and on the estimate. For example, a quadratic risk is the squared norm of the difference between $\boldsymbol{\theta}$ and $\hat{\boldsymbol{\theta}}$. Then one defines a *risk* or average cost by averaging $C(\boldsymbol{\theta}, \hat{\boldsymbol{\theta}})$ in some way, and the estimation rule is chosen to minimize the risk.

Different estimation methods, and indeed different schools of statistics, are defined by the choice of the cost function and the method of averaging. The frequentist school assumes that there is a single — though unknown — value for the parameter to be estimated; hence, the average to be used in computing the risk is over repeated realizations of the data for a fixed value of the parameter. By contrast, the Bayesian school asserts that there is no need to consider data sets other than the one actually observed; thus, the average is over values of $\boldsymbol{\theta}$, as specified by the prior $\mathrm{pr}(\boldsymbol{\theta})$, with g fixed.

Thus, to a frequentist, the risk is a function of $\boldsymbol{\theta}$, while to a pure Bayesian the risk is a function of g. A pragmatic alternative to either school is to average over both $\boldsymbol{\theta}$ and g, making the risk simply a scalar and not a function at all.

5.1.2 Bias and variance. The most common approach to specifying the performance of an estimator is to state its bias and variance. In common parlance, an estimation procedure is a measurement, the bias is the systematic error in the measurement, and the variance is the random error. In other words, the bias is the accuracy and the variance is the precision.

Stated more mathematically, the bias in an estimate of a scalar parameter (denoted by θ rather than the vector $\boldsymbol{\theta}$) is defined by

$$B(\theta) \equiv \left\langle \hat{\theta} - \theta \right\rangle_{\mathrm{g}|\theta} , \tag{3.42}$$

and the variance is defined as

$$\mathrm{Var}(\hat{\theta}) \equiv \left\langle \left[\hat{\theta} - \left\langle \hat{\theta} \right\rangle \right]^2 \right\rangle_{\mathrm{g}|\theta} , \tag{3.43}$$

where $\langle \cdot \rangle_{\mathrm{g}|\theta}$ indicates a frequentist average over repeated realizations of g for a fixed true value of θ.

Note that the variance is the mean-square variation of the estimate from its mean value, not from the true value of the parameter. If we (as frequentists) want to specify the deviation from the true value, we can define a total mean-square error (MSE) by

$$\mathrm{MSE}(\hat{\theta}) \equiv \left\langle \left[\hat{\theta} - \theta \right]^2 \right\rangle_{\mathrm{g}|\theta} . \tag{3.44}$$

Thus, this form of MSE is the risk associated with a quadratic cost function and frequentist averaging.

Vector generalizations of these scalar definitions are straightforward.

5.1.3 Bounds on variance. There is a minimum value, called the *Cramér-Rao lower bound*, for the variance of any estimate. An unbiased estimator that achieves the bound is called *efficient*.

Sometimes it cannot be determined what the optimal estimator is, or we cannot compute the MSE even if we do know the estimator. In those circumstances, a reasonable alternative is to use the Cramér-Rao bound as a figure of merit. All that is required to compute the bound is knowledge of the likelihood $\mathrm{pr}(\mathbf{g}|\boldsymbol{\theta})$. Thus, scintillation cameras (or other imaging systems) can be designed and compared on the basis of the bound rather than on the actual MSE achieved by some particular estimator.

5.2 ML estimation

One possible estimation rule is to choose the value of $\boldsymbol{\theta}$ that maximizes the likelihood. Formally,

$$\hat{\boldsymbol{\theta}}_{ML} = \underset{\boldsymbol{\theta}}{\mathrm{argmax}} \left\{ \mathrm{pr}(\mathbf{g}|\boldsymbol{\theta}) \right\}, \tag{3.45}$$

where the argmax operator returns the value of the $\boldsymbol{\theta}$ argument that maximizes the quantity in brackets for the observed value of $\mathbf{g}$.

An equivalent rule is to maximize the logarithm of the likelihood:

$$\hat{\boldsymbol{\theta}}_{ML} = \underset{\boldsymbol{\theta}}{\mathrm{argmax}} \left\{ \ln \left[\mathrm{pr}(\mathbf{g}|\boldsymbol{\theta}) \right] \right\}. \tag{3.46}$$

For Gaussian data, the log-likelihood is a quadratic functional of the data; therefore, ML estimation reduces to some form of least-squares fitting.

5.2.1 Rationale for ML estimation.

Maximum-likelihood estimates have many nice properties. They are:

- Efficient if an efficient estimator exists;
- Asymptotically efficient;
- Asymptotically unbiased;
- Generally simple and intuitive;
- Unresponsive to prior information.

In much of the statistics literature, the word "asymptotically" implies that a large number of independent realizations of the same data set have been obtained. Because Poisson random processes involve independent events, we can regard each event as its own data set; hence, "asymptotically" can mean that the number of events is large. For example, in a scintillation camera the asymptotic limit is approached as the number of photoelectrons increases. Thus, in the context of this chapter, we can often expect that ML estimates are in fact efficient and unbiased.

5.3 Bayesian estimation

To a Bayesian, $\mathbf{g}$ is fixed once it is measured, and the only remaining random quantity is the unknown parameter $\boldsymbol{\theta}$ itself. If we know a prior density on the parameter, $\mathrm{pr}(\boldsymbol{\theta})$, we can use Bayes' rule to write the posterior probability of $\boldsymbol{\theta}$ as

$$\mathrm{pr}(\boldsymbol{\theta}|\mathbf{g}) = \frac{\mathrm{pr}(\mathbf{g}|\boldsymbol{\theta})\ \mathrm{pr}(\boldsymbol{\theta})}{\mathrm{pr}(\mathbf{g})} = \frac{\mathrm{pr}(\mathbf{g}|\boldsymbol{\theta})\ \mathrm{pr}(\boldsymbol{\theta})}{\int d^M g\ \mathrm{pr}(\mathbf{g}|\boldsymbol{\theta})\ \mathrm{pr}(\boldsymbol{\theta})}. \tag{3.47}$$

All Bayesian estimates are based on this posterior; different Bayesian estimates, however, use different cost functions.

The most common choice of cost function in Bayesian estimation is the uniform cost, where all errors for which the norm $||\hat{\boldsymbol{\theta}} - \boldsymbol{\theta}||$ exceeds some threshold ϵ are assigned the same cost, and then ϵ is allowed to approach zero. The optimal estimator under this cost function is called the *Maximum a posteriori*, or MAP estimator, and is given by

$$\hat{\boldsymbol{\theta}}_{MAP} = \underset{\boldsymbol{\theta}}{\mathrm{argmax}} \left\{\mathrm{pr}(\boldsymbol{\theta}|\mathbf{g})\right\} = \underset{\boldsymbol{\theta}}{\mathrm{argmax}} \left\{\mathrm{pr}(\mathbf{g}|\boldsymbol{\theta})\ \mathrm{pr}(\boldsymbol{\theta})\right\}, \tag{3.48}$$

where the last step follows because $\mathrm{pr}(\mathbf{g})$ is independent of $\boldsymbol{\theta}$.

The MAP estimator in (3.48) has the same form as the ML estimator in (3.45) except that the likelihood is weighted by the prior. If all values of $\boldsymbol{\theta}$ are equally probable *a priori*, then $\mathrm{pr}(\boldsymbol{\theta})$ is a constant and MAP estimation reduces to ML.

6. Application to scintillation cameras

We can now bring together everything we have learned about basic statistics and estimation methods and develop a rigorous approach to position and energy estimation in scintillation cameras.

Section 6.1 summarizes the relevant statistical models for PMT signals and discusses various simplifying assumptions. Section 6.2 uses these models to formulate various ML estimation principles, and Section 6.3 discusses ways of using these principles to find the ML estimates. Some practicalities related to data compression are treated in Section 6.4, and methods of scatter rejection are discussed in Section 6.5.

6.1 Statistical models

As we know from Section 2.4, a complete statistical model for a scintillation camera must include models for the initial interaction and any subsequent interactions, the statistics of the scintillation light and the resulting photoelectrons, and the PMT gain process. We will now see how all of these effects can be incorporated into overall models of the PMT outputs.

6.1.1 The initial interaction. For simplicity, we consider monoenergetic gamma rays passing through a parallel-hole collimator onto the face of the camera. Because the gamma rays are independent and because they travel in the z direction (normal to the detector face), they are fully described by a 2D Poisson random process with fluence $b(\mathbf{r})$, where $\mathbf{r} = (x, y)$.

We know from (3.29) that the PDF on the 2D interaction position $\mathbf{r}_{int}$ is just a normalized version of the fluence. From Beer's law, the PDF on the depth of interaction z_{int} is a simple exponential and for homogeneous detector material, z_{int} is statistically independent of $\mathbf{r}_{int}$. Thus, we have at once that

$$\mathrm{pr}(\mathbf{r}_{int}, z_{int}) = \frac{b(\mathbf{r}_{int})}{\int_A d^2r\, b(\mathbf{r})}\, \alpha_{tot}\, \exp[-\alpha_{tot} z_{int}], \tag{3.49}$$

where α_{tot} is the total attenuation coefficient.

To obtain a more compact notation, we let the 3D vector $\mathfrak{r}_{int}$ denote the 3D position of interaction in the scintillation crystal, so $\mathfrak{r}_{int} = (x_{int}, y_{int}, z_{int})$. Then the PDF in (3.49) can also be written as $\mathrm{pr}(\mathfrak{r}_{int})$.

To analyze the statistics of the scintillation light, we need to know not only the PDF for the location of the initial interaction but also the one for the energy deposited there. The energy deposited is random because the event is randomly either photoelectric or Compton, and in the latter case the scattering angle and hence the energy imparted to the electron is random.

As we saw in Chapter 2, the range of the photoelectron is of order 20 μm, and that of a Compton electron is even less. These ranges are almost always small compared to the detector dimensions and the achievable spatial resolution; hence, it is a good approximation to assume that the electron energy is deposited exactly at the interaction location.

If we further assume that the detector is a homogeneous material, then the energy deposited by the electron is statistically independent of the interaction location, and we can write

$$\mathrm{pr}(\mathfrak{r}_{int}, \mathcal{E}_{int}) = \mathrm{pr}(\mathfrak{r}_{int})\, [\mathrm{pr}(\mathcal{E}_{int}|\mathrm{C})\, \mathrm{Pr}(\mathrm{C}) + \mathrm{pr}(\mathcal{E}_{int}|\mathrm{pe})\, \mathrm{Pr}(\mathrm{pe})]\,, \tag{3.50}$$

where C and pe denote Compton and photoelectric interactions, respectively. The individual factors in (3.50) can be evaluated from the basic physics (averaging over scattering angles for the Compton case and, if desired, averaging over electron shells for the photoelectric case).

6.1.2 Multiple interaction sites. To account for reabsorption of a K x ray or Compton-scattered photon, we need to define a secondary site of energy deposition, yielding a total of 8 random variables (x, y, z, and $\mathcal{E}$ for each of the two sites).

Consider the case where the first interaction is Compton and the scattered photon is reabsorbed. The joint PDF for the 8 random variables in this case can be written usefully as

$$\mathrm{pr}(\mathfrak{r}_{int}, \mathcal{E}_{int}, \mathfrak{r}_{sec}, \mathcal{E}_{sec}|\mathrm{C}) = \mathrm{pr}(\mathfrak{r}_{sec}, \mathcal{E}_{sec}|\mathfrak{r}_{int}, \mathcal{E}_{int}, \mathrm{C})\, \mathrm{pr}(\mathfrak{r}_{int}, \mathcal{E}_{int}|\mathrm{C}), \tag{3.51}$$

where *int* now refers to the initial interaction, and *sec* refers to the secondary one. The point of writing it this way is that $pr(\mathfrak{r}_{sec}, \mathcal{E}_{sec}|\mathfrak{r}_{int}, \mathcal{E}_{int}, \mathrm{C})$ can be determined from the physics of Compton scattering. If we know the location of the scattering event and the energy it deposits, we know the scattering angle, and therefore we know (just as in a Compton camera) that the scattered photon must travel along a cone with vertex at $\mathfrak{r}_{int}$. Thus, $pr(\mathfrak{r}_{sec}, \mathcal{E}_{sec}|\mathfrak{r}_{int}, \mathcal{E}_{int}, \mathrm{C})$ must be zero unless $\mathfrak{r}_{sec}$

lies on this cone and within the detector crystal. The exact form of the PDF then follows from the Klein-Nishina formula for the differential scattering cross section.

To get the full PDF on $(\mathbf{r}_{int}, \mathcal{E}_{int}, \mathbf{r}_{sec}, \mathcal{E}_{sec})$ it is necessary to write another PDF similar to (3.51) but conditioned on the initial event being photoelectric and to perform a weighted sum of the two as in (3.50). A second weighted sum is also needed since the secondary interaction itself can be either Compton or photoelectric. The final expression is messy but tractable.

6.1.3 Statistics of scintillation light. As discussed in Chapter 2, scintillation is a two-step process: the high-energy electron from the initial interaction produces electron-hole pairs which in turn produce optical photons. Both steps are inefficient, with only about 10% of the kinetic energy of the high-energy electron going into optical photons in NaI(Tl). Competing processes are mainly phonon generation.

In the first step, the minimum energy required to generate an electron-hole pair is the bandgap energy $\mathcal{E}_g$; therefore, a photoelectron of kinetic energy $\mathcal{E}_{kin}$ could in principle produce $\mathcal{E}_{kin}/\mathcal{E}_g$ pairs, but because of phonon generation, a smaller number will be produced on average. We define the mean energy expended per electron-hole pair, $\mathcal{E}_{eh}$, such that the mean number of pairs is

$$\overline{N}_{eh} = \frac{\mathcal{E}_{kin}}{\mathcal{E}_{eh}}. \tag{3.52}$$

Next we examine the distribution of N_{eh} about its mean. If there were no phonon generation, conservation of energy would require that $N_{eh} = \mathcal{E}_{kin}/\mathcal{E}_g$, which is not a random number at all. At the opposite extreme, if only a small fraction of the electron energy goes into creation of electron-hole pairs, the pairs would be generated independently, and N_{eh} would be a Poisson.

Thus, $0 < \text{Var}\{N_{eh}\} \leq \overline{N}_{eh}$. To describe this range, we define the *Fano factor* F_{eh} as

$$F_{eh} = \frac{\text{Var}(N_{eh})}{\overline{N}_{eh}}. \tag{3.53}$$

A value of $F_{eh} < 1$ implies sub-Poisson behavior.

In Si and Ge, $F_{eh} \approx 0.07$ to 0.15. Values of F_{eh} for scintillators are not known because the hole-electron pairs are not observed directly, but they are expected to be larger because of the larger bandgaps.

We still need to consider the second step, conversion of electron-hole pairs to light. This step is inefficient also; hence, the number of optical photons N_{opt} is more nearly Poisson and the Fano factor is nearer to one. It should be a good approximation to assume that the Fano factor for the number of optical photons, F_{opt}, is close to one. Even this factor, however, is not directly measurable in scintillators because what we observe is photoelectrons in some photodetector, not the optical photons themselves.

6.1.4 Statistics of the photoelectrons. Two more inefficient steps are necessary to obtain from the number of optical photons generated in the initial gamma-ray interaction to the number of photoelectrons generated in a PMT.

If we assume that there is only one site of energy deposition, $\mathbf{r}_{int}$, then the light must propagate from that point to the PMT. In a scintillation camera, the probability of a photon reaching the kth PMT is necessarily a strong function of the scintillation position, and we denote it as $\beta_k(\mathbf{r}_{int})$. This number can vary from perhaps 25% for a PMT close to the scintillation event to a small fraction of a percent for distant PMT.

Second, an optical photon that reaches the PMT has a probability η_k (the quantum efficiency) of producing a photoelectron. With current vacuum PMTs, this efficiency is around 25-30%, although it can be much larger with silicon-based photodiodes.

Because both of these steps are binomial selections, the mean number of photoelectrons produced in the kth PMT is the mean number of optical photons times the two binomial probabilities,

$$\overline{n}_k(\mathbf{r}_{int}, \mathcal{E}_{int}) = \eta_k \, \beta_k(\mathbf{r}_{int}) \, \overline{N}_{opt}(\mathcal{E}_{int}) \,. \tag{3.54}$$

Note that the energy deposition affects the mean number of optical photons but not the probability that they will arrive at the PMT and produce photoelectrons, so $\beta_k(\mathbf{r}_{int})$ is independent of $\mathcal{E}_{int}$. We can also assume that $\overline{N}_{opt}(\mathcal{E}_{int})$ is independent of $\mathbf{r}_{int}$ for a homogeneous crystal.

We argued above that the number of optical photons is likely to be approximately Poisson, and if so it follows from the binomial-selection theorem that n_k is also Poisson. Even if the number of optical photons is not Poisson, however, n_k would still approach a Poisson if $\eta_k \, \beta_k(\mathbf{r}_{int}) \ll 1$, which it almost always is. Thus, it is an excellent approximation to assume that

$$\Pr(n_k|\mathbf{r}_{int}, \mathcal{E}_{int}) \approx \frac{(\overline{n}_k)^{n_k}}{n_k!} \exp\left(-\overline{n}_k\right) . \tag{3.55}$$

Moreover, even with the inefficient steps, we often have $\overline{n}_k >> 1$, so another possibility is to approximate the Poisson with a Gaussian:

$$\Pr(n_k|\mathbf{r}_{int}, \mathcal{E}_{int}) \approx \frac{1}{\sqrt{2\pi\overline{n}_k}} \exp\left[-\frac{(n_k - \overline{n}_k)^2}{2\overline{n}_k}\right] . \tag{3.56}$$

This Gaussian approximation may break down for PMTs far from the scintillation event, where $\beta_k << 1$, but the Poisson form is certainly valid in that case.

It is important to note that these probabilities depend on the interaction position and on the energy deposited in the interaction. To obtain either the Poisson form or its Gaussian approximation, we must assume that the energy $\mathcal{E}_{int}$ is deposited at one 3D location $\mathbf{r}_{int}$, which means either a photoelectric interaction with negligible range for both the photoelectron and K x ray, or a Compton interaction with photon escape. More generally, we need to average over energy-deposition points.

6.1.5 PMT gain process. To complete the statistical description of scintillation cameras, we must consider the randomness in the PMT gain process. We denote the signal from the kth PMT as V_k and the whole set of signals from the K

PMTs as the $K \times 1$ vector $\mathbf{V}$. We need the multivariate PDF on this vector as a function of the interaction position and energy.

The gain fluctuations in one PMT have no effect on those in another PMT, and we have already argued that the photoelectrons are Poisson and hence independent. Thus, the PMT signals must be statistically independent, and we can write

$$\mathrm{pr}(\mathbf{V}|\mathbf{r}_{int}, \mathcal{E}_{int}) = \prod_{k=1}^{K} \mathrm{pr}(V_k|\mathbf{r}_{int}, \mathcal{E}_{int}). \tag{3.57}$$

We emphasize that this result is valid only conditionally; randomness in the interaction location or energy deposition will introduce statistical dependencies.

It is rather difficult to give a specific form for the PDF of a PMT signal if only a single photoelectron is produced at the photocathode, but we can take advantage of the fact that each scintillation event makes multiple, independent photoelectrons. By the central-limit theorem, therefore, we can expect the overall PDF of $\mathbf{V}$ to be multivariate normal; therefore, all we need in order to specify $\mathrm{pr}(\mathbf{V}|\mathbf{r}_{int}, \mathcal{E}_{int})$ is the relevant mean vector and covariance matrix.

The conditional mean for the kth signal is given by

$$\overline{V}_k(\mathbf{r}_{int}, \mathcal{E}_{int}) = G_k\, \overline{n}_k(\mathbf{r}_{int}, \mathcal{E}_{int}) = G_k\, \eta_k\, \beta_k(\mathbf{r}_{int})\, \overline{N}_{opt}(\mathcal{E}_{int}), \tag{3.58}$$

where G_k is the average gain of the PMT and any associated electronics. It follows from (3.57) that the covariance is conditionally diagonal,

$$\mathbf{K}_{\mathbf{V}|\mathbf{r}_{int}, \mathcal{E}_{int}} = \mathrm{diag}\, \{\mathrm{Var}(V_k|\mathbf{r}_{int}, \mathcal{E}_{int})\}. \tag{3.59}$$

Now we need an expression for the conditional variance of each signal.

We can obtain the variance from the Burgess variance theorem (see Section 4.1) if we assume that the number of photoelectrons is Poisson (for a given $\mathbf{r}_{int}$ and $\mathcal{E}_{int}$). From (3.38) we find that

$$\mathrm{Var}(V_k|\mathbf{r}_{int}, \mathcal{E}_{int}) = G_k\, \overline{V}_k\, \frac{m_2}{m_1^2}, \tag{3.60}$$

where m_1 and m_2 are the first and second moments of the gain distribution, respectively. The factor m_2/m_1^2 is the reciprocal of the Swank factor associated with the PMT gain.

6.1.6 Scaled Poisson model. In high-quality PMTs, it is often useful to assume that the Swank factor is near unity and hence that most of the variance in the PMT signal is from the variance in the number of photoelectrons n_k. If the Swank factor were exactly unity, we could determine n_k simply by dividing the measured V_k by the gain G_k. Even if the Swank factor is not exactly unity, this normalization is still useful to obtain the signals into units of photoelectrons. An integer-valued random variable U_k can always be defined for each PMT by

$$U_k = \mathrm{NINT}\left\{\frac{V_k}{G_k}\right\}, \tag{3.61}$$

where the NINT$\{\cdot\}$ operator returns the nearest integer to its argument. If the PMT gain fluctuates symmetrically about its mean, the mean of U_k is $\overline{n}_k$.

A reasonable model for the multivariate probability law for the set of all $\{U_k\}$ (or the vector $\mathbf{U}$) is

$$\Pr(\mathbf{U}|\mathbf{r}_{int}, \mathcal{E}_{int}) = \prod_{k=1}^{K} \frac{(\overline{n}_k)^{U_k}}{U_k!} \exp\left(-\overline{n}_k\right), \tag{3.62}$$

where $\overline{n}$ is to be interpreted as $\overline{n}_k(\mathbf{r}_{int}, \mathcal{E}_{int})$

We shall refer to (3.62) as the *scaled Poisson model* for the PMT signals. A variant on the theme is to approximate the Poisson by a Gaussian as in (3.56), and in that case we can omit the NINT step.

6.1.7 Random interaction parameters. As we have emphasized, all of our nice models with Poisson probabilities and statistically independent signals assume that there is a single, nonrandom interaction site and a single, nonrandom amount of energy deposited there. In practice, of course, both $\mathbf{r}_{int}$ and $\mathcal{E}_{int}$ are beyond our control. We usually have a spectrum of photon energies incident on the detector, and even if we use a monoenergetic source, we cannot control the depth of interaction of a photon in the crystal. This observation does not invalidate the models constructed up to now, but it does mean that they need to be regarded as conditional models.

Consider, for example, the random depth of interaction z_{int}. When the detector is used with a parallel-hole collimator, z_{int} is a nuisance parameter, but in pinhole SPECT or in PET, z_{int} is something we would like to know in order to avoid blurring when photons strike the detector obliquely.

If we want to estimate the depth of interaction, then of course a PDF conditioned on z_{int} is exactly what we want in a likelihood function (see Section 5.2).

If, on the other hand, z_{int} is an uninteresting nuisance parameter, then we have several options [Barrett and Myers, 2004, Chapter 13]. The one favored in much of the estimation literature is to estimate the nuisance parameter anyway and then throw away the result. A better option is to average or marginalize the density over the nuisance parameter and then estimate only the parameters of interest. Barrett and Myers showed that this option minimizes the Bayes risk for a uniform cost function, provided we have a verifiable prior PDF on the nuisance parameter; in the case of depth of interaction, the needed prior is just Beer's law, as in (3.49). Other options are to attempt to make the system insensitive to the nuisance parameter, for example by design of the coupling optics in a scintillation camera, or to assign it some typical value, such as $z_{int} = 1/\alpha_{tot}$.

Suppose that we choose to marginalize over the random depth of interaction, so that the inference task is to estimate the two lateral coordinates and the energy of the scintillation event. Recalling that $\boldsymbol{\mathfrak{r}}_{int} = (\mathbf{r}_{int}, z_{int})$, we can write

$$\begin{aligned}\mathrm{pr}(\mathbf{V}|\mathbf{r}_{int}, \mathcal{E}_{int}) &= \int_0^L dz_{int}\, \mathrm{pr}(\mathbf{V}|\mathbf{r}_{int}, z_{int}, \mathcal{E}_{int})\ \mathrm{pr}(z_{int}) \\ &= \int_0^L dz_{int} \left[\prod_{k=1}^{K} \mathrm{pr}(V_k|\mathbf{r}_{int}, z_{int}, \mathcal{E}_{int})\right] \mathrm{pr}(z_{int}). \quad (3.63)\end{aligned}$$

With this form, the PMT outputs are no longer independent (unless the density $\mathrm{pr}(V_k|\mathbf{r}_{int}, z_{int}, \mathcal{E}_{int})$ is independent of z_{int}). If we wish to use a multivariate normal approximation, we must have off-diagonal elements in the covariance. Even if we use the scaled Poisson model, the random depth of interaction makes it doubly stochastic; hence, the components are not independent.

Similar considerations apply to random energy. In small-animal imaging, we may be willing to neglect scatter and accept all photons regardless of their energy, so that the energy becomes a nuisance parameter. Marginalizing over it is a matter of adding one more integral to (3.63), and, again, the effect is to introduce statistical dependence.

Finally, as we have seen, multiple interaction sites introduce additional parameters (see Section 6.1.2). Usually we have no interest in the parameters of the secondary interaction, so we can regard them as nuisance parameters. On the other hand, if we do estimate the parameters of both sites, it is possible in principle to construct a Compton camera in a single detector [Lehner, 2003].

6.2 ML estimation principles

In Section 2.1, we listed some of the statistical inference tasks relevant to scintillation cameras, and in Section 6.1, we developed a variety of statistical models for describing the data available from the cameras. Now we begin to bring these pieces together and state some important ML estimation principles. In addition to developing some useful formulas, we shall also take stock of what information is needed to implement them.

6.2.1 3D estimation, normal models. Suppose we want to estimate all three coordinates of the scintillation event as well as its energy. Assume further that there is only one interaction site. For notational convenience, we drop the *int* subscripts and assume that energy $\mathcal{E}$ is deposited at a point designated by the 3D vector $\boldsymbol{\mathfrak{r}}$.

With these assumptions and the discussion above, we know that the photomultiplier signals are statistically independent (see Section 6.1.5). If we model the likelihood as a multivariate normal, the covariance matrix is diagonal.

The general form of the multivariate normal likelihood for this problem is

$$\begin{aligned}\mathrm{pr}(\mathbf{V}|\boldsymbol{\mathfrak{r}}, \mathcal{E}) &= (2\pi)^{-\frac{1}{2}K} [\det \mathbf{K}_V(\boldsymbol{\mathfrak{r}}, \mathcal{E})]^{-\frac{1}{2}} \\ &\times \exp\left\{-\tfrac{1}{2}[\mathbf{V} - \overline{\mathbf{V}}(\boldsymbol{\mathfrak{r}}, \mathcal{E})]^t\, \mathbf{K}_V^{-1}(\boldsymbol{\mathfrak{r}}, \mathcal{E})[\mathbf{V} \quad \overline{\mathbf{V}}(\boldsymbol{\mathfrak{r}}, \mathcal{E})]\right\}. \quad (3.64)\end{aligned}$$

This expression can be simplified by use of (3.59) and (3.60), and it is also useful to take its logarithm. Because the determinant is the product of the diagonal elements for a diagonal matrix, we can write the log-likelihood as

$$\log[\mathrm{pr}(\mathbf{V}|\mathfrak{r},\mathcal{E})] = -\tfrac{1}{2}\sum_{k=0}^{K}\left\{\log\left[A_k\overline{V}_k(\mathfrak{r},\mathcal{E})\right] + \frac{\left[V_k - \overline{V}_k(\mathfrak{r},\mathcal{E})\right]^2}{A_k\overline{V}_k(\mathfrak{r},\mathcal{E})}\right\}, \quad (3.65)$$

where $A_k \equiv G_k m_1^2/m_2$ is the mean gain divided by the Swank factor, and an irrelevant constant has been dropped.

ML estimation requires

$$\log[\mathrm{pr}(\mathbf{V}|\mathfrak{r},\mathcal{E})] = \max \text{ at } \mathfrak{r} = \hat{\mathfrak{r}}_{ML} \text{ and } \mathcal{E} = \hat{\mathcal{E}}_{ML}. \quad (3.66)$$

Often we can assume that $\sum_k \log\left[A_k\overline{V}_k(\mathfrak{r},\mathcal{E})\right]$ is a slowly varying function of its arguments and treat it as approximately a constant. In that case, maximizing the log-likelihood is equivalent to minimizing the quadratic form in (3.65):

$$\sum_{k=0}^{K}\frac{\left[V_k - \overline{V}_k(\mathfrak{r},\mathcal{E})\right]^2}{A_k\overline{V}_k(\mathfrak{r},\mathcal{E})} = \min \text{ at } \mathfrak{r} = \hat{\mathfrak{r}}_{ML} \text{ and } \mathcal{E} = \hat{\mathcal{E}}_{ML}. \quad (3.67)$$

Since the mean signals are nonlinear functions of their arguments, (3.67) states a nonlinear weighted least-squares problem.

To use this approach, we must know the mean of each signal as a function of 3D position and energy, and we must also know A_k for each PMT.

The mean signals cannot be measured directly since we cannot control the depth of interaction, but they are amenable to analysis or simulation. From (3.58) we know that $\overline{V}_k(\mathfrak{r},\mathcal{E}) \propto \beta_k(\mathfrak{r})\,\overline{N}_{opt}(\mathcal{E})$, and the propagation factor $\beta_k(\mathfrak{r})$ can be calculated by optical ray-tracing or Monte Carlo simulation. Most scintillators are at least approximately linear, so $\overline{N}_{opt}(\mathcal{E}) = \mathcal{E}/W$, where W is the mean energy expended per optical photon, a characteristic of the particular scintillator material. With this knowledge, the gain and Swank factors can be estimated by curve-fitting a pulse-height spectrum obtained with a collimated beam of known energy; only a single such spectrum is needed because the factors being estimated are independent of position and energy.

6.2.2 2D estimation, normal model. As we have emphasized, the statistical independence of the signals is destroyed by random depth of interaction. If we want to estimate the 2D coordinates of the scintillation event (denoted $\mathbf{r}$ rather than $\mathfrak{r}$) plus the energy, the relevant likelihood is $\mathrm{pr}(\mathbf{V}|\mathbf{r},\mathcal{E})$, and if we use a normal model, we require the mean and covariance as a function of 2D position and energy.

Again neglecting the slowly varying log-determinant, we can write the ML principle as [*cf.* (3.67)]

$$\sum_{k=0}^{K}\sum_{k'=0}^{K}\left[V_k - \overline{V}_k(\mathbf{r},\mathcal{E})\right]\left[\mathbf{K}_V^{-1}(\mathbf{r},\mathcal{E})\right]_{kk'}\left[V_{k'} - \overline{V}_{k'}(\mathbf{r},\mathcal{E})\right]$$
$$= \min \text{ at } \mathbf{r} = \hat{\mathbf{r}}_{ML} \text{ and } \mathcal{E} = \hat{\mathcal{E}}_{ML}. \quad (3.68)$$

This expression is more computationally intensive than (3.67) because it requires inversion of a $K \times K$ matrix. It is practical for modular cameras where K may be 4 or 9, but less so for large clinical cameras.

Unlike the 3D case, the mean and covariance as 2D functions can be directly measured. Monoenergetic photons from a collimated source are directed at the scintillation crystal at 2D position $\mathbf{r}$, and a set of samples of the PMT signals is acquired in list mode. Then the sample mean and covariance matrix are computed for each $\mathbf{r}$, and the dependence on $\mathcal{E}$ is obtained by assuming that the scintillator is linear. For details on the measurement procedure, see the chapter by Chen and Barrett in this volume, and for more on list-mode acquisition, see the chapter by Furenlid.

A further simplification results if the camera response is insensitive to the depth of interaction z, or if we just choose to ignore this dependence and the resulting off-diagonal elements of the covariance. Then the ML estimate is given by (3.67), but the important difference is that the required mean $\overline{V}_k(\mathbf{r}, \mathcal{E})$ is directly measurable.

6.2.3 2D estimation, scaled Poisson. With the scaled Poisson model introduced in Section 6.1.6, we normalize the PMT signals by the gain to get them in units of photoelectrons, and then we convert them to integers so that the likelihood is a probability rather than a PDF. The new signals are denoted $\{U_k\}$, and ML estimation requires knowledge of the mean $\overline{U}_k(\mathbf{r}, \mathcal{E})$.

If we again assume that the camera response is insensitive to z and that the scintillator is linear in energy, we can write

$$\overline{U}_k(\mathbf{r}, \mathcal{E}) = \mathcal{E} f_k(\mathbf{r}), \tag{3.69}$$

and the function $f_k(\mathbf{r})$ is directly measurable as described above.

The ML principle is derived from the assumption that U_k is Poisson. After a bit of algebra, we find

$$\sum_{k=1}^{K} \{U_k \ln [\mathcal{E} f_k(\mathbf{r})] - \mathcal{E} f_k(\mathbf{r})\} = \min \text{ at } \mathbf{r} = \hat{\mathbf{r}}_{ML} \text{ and } \mathcal{E} = \hat{\mathcal{E}}_{ML}. \tag{3.70}$$

This equation describes the procedure we use most often with the modular scintillation cameras at the Center for Gamma-ray Imaging (CGRI).

6.3 Scatter rejection

In addition to position estimation, another important inference task is classifying the photon as scattered or unscattered. In this section, we survey three different approaches to this problem, and then we discuss some ways of comparing the methods. For more details, see Chen [1995, 1997].

6.3.1 Energy window. The conventional way of discriminating against scattered radiation in nuclear medicine is to estimate the energy of the photon absorbed in the detector and to compare the estimate to an energy window, rejecting the event if the estimate falls outside the window.

In a scintillation camera, the usual energy estimate is merely the sum of the PMT signals; this estimate is valid (consistent and unbiased) only if the total amount of light collected by the PMT array is independent of position, which is not true for the modular cameras under development at CGRI and only approximately true for commercial cameras.

We can improve on the energy windowing procedure if we have accurate likelihood models for our detectors. As discussed above, we can perform a joint ML estimate of scintillation position and energy, and both estimates are nearly unbiased if our model is correct. Thus, when we compare our energy estimates to a window, we can be confident that we are using unbiased estimates.

6.3.2 Likelihood window. An alternative to energy windowing is likelihood windowing. In this method, we do not perform a joint estimation of position and energy. Instead, we estimate the position *assuming* $\mathcal{E} = \mathcal{E}_0$, where $\mathcal{E}_0$ is the energy of an unscattered photon. Explicitly, in the 2D case we maximize $\mathrm{pr}(\mathbf{V}|\mathbf{r}, \mathcal{E}_0)$, and then we accept the event if the resulting maximized likelihood exceeds a threshold: $\mathrm{pr}(\mathbf{V}|\mathbf{r}, \mathcal{E}_0) > L_0$.

An immediate practical advantage to the likelihood window is that it requires only a 2D (x, y) search instead of a 3D $(x, y, \mathcal{E})$ search for the ML estimate.

A potential disadvantage of the likelihood window is that the mean number of unscattered photons that pass the test might be a function of position, leading to flood-field nonuniformity. If that is the case, the likelihood threshold can be made to depend on position in such as way as to accept a constant fraction of unscattered photons.

6.3.3 Bayesian window. Both the energy window and the likelihood window test the null hypothesis (H_0) that the photon is unscattered; neither specifies the alternative hypothesis (H_1).

Bayesian optimal decisions minimize a risk that depends on both hypotheses. No matter how the risk is defined, it always turns out [Barrett and Myers, 2004, Chapter 13] that the decision should be based on a likelihood ratio,

$$\Lambda \equiv \frac{\mathrm{Pr}(\mathrm{data}|H_1)}{\mathrm{Pr}(\mathrm{data}|H_0)}. \tag{3.71}$$

The optimal strategy is always to compute Λ and compare it to a threshold that depends on prior knowledge and assigned costs for correct and incorrect decisions.

In the present problem, the data are the PMT signals $\mathbf{V}$ and the null hypothesis is that photon is unscattered. We must figure out how to evaluate the numerator and denominator in Λ.

Suppose we have prior knowledge of the probability P_{sc} that a photon is scattered and of the normalized scatter spectrum $S_{sc}(\mathcal{E})$, defined as the PDF for $\mathcal{E}$ given that the photon is scattered. Then the PDF of *actual* photon energies (not estimates) is

$$\mathrm{pr}(\mathcal{E}) = P_{sc}\, S_{sc}(\mathcal{E}) + (1 - P_{sc})\, \delta(\mathcal{E} - \mathcal{E}_0). \tag{3.72}$$

We assume for simplicity that the entire energy $\mathcal{E}$ is deposited at the interaction site.

Under these assumptions, the numerator in Λ can be written as

$$\Pr(\mathbf{V}|H_1) = \int_0^{\mathcal{E}_0^-} d\mathcal{E}\ \mathrm{pr}(\mathbf{V}|\mathbf{r},\mathcal{E})\, S_{sc}(\mathcal{E}), \tag{3.73}$$

and the likelihood-ratio test is to classify the photon as scattered if

$$\frac{\int_0^{\mathcal{E}_0^-} d\mathcal{E}\ \mathrm{pr}(\mathbf{V}|\mathbf{r},\mathcal{E})\, S_{sc}(\mathcal{E})}{\Pr(\mathbf{V}|\mathbf{r},\mathcal{E}_0)} > \frac{P_{sc}}{1-P_{sc}}. \tag{3.74}$$

Because we do not know the interaction position $\mathbf{r}$, we can replace it with the ML estimate $\hat{\mathbf{r}}$ calculated under H_0, or we can maximize the numerator and denominator separately with respect to $\mathbf{r}$ before taking the ratio.

Bayesian windowing is computationally more demanding than energy windowing or likelihood windowing, but it has the advantage of incorporating prior knowledge of the scattered spectrum.

6.3.4 Photon ROC curves. In signal-detection problems, an ROC (receiver operating characteristic) curve is a plot of the true-positive fraction (probability of detection) vs. the false-positive fraction (false-alarm rate). In scatter-rejection problems, the ROC curve is a plot of the probability of accepting an unscattered photon vs. the probability of accepting a scattered photon, with points on the curve generated by varying the acceptance threshold.

In both cases, the area under the ROC curve (AUC) can be used as a figure of merit [Chen, 1995, 1997]. Perfect detection or perfect scatter rejection corresponds to AUC =1.

In the scatter application, AUC depends on the method of scatter discrimination and on the properties of the detector. For example, with ML energy windowing, the AUC depends on the energy resolution of the detector, which in turn depends on the light output of the scintillator and the quantum efficiency of the PMTs. With energy estimates based on the sum of PMT values, the AUC is likely to be reduced by the variation in total collected light with interaction position.

For more details on photon ROC curves and examples of their application to modular scintillation cameras, see Chen [1995, 1997].

6.4 Finding the estimates

We have stated several versions of the ML principle for 2D or 3D position estimation. Now we look at some computational details for actually applying these principles.

6.4.1 Exhaustive search. The brute-force approach to ML estimation is to evaluate the log-likelihood at all points on a 2D or 3D grid and possibly for a set of energies. This approach is most feasible for 2D position estimation and a likelihood window. For example, to estimate position on a 64×64 grid, we need 4,096 evaluations for each event. Exhaustive search is much less feasible if estimation of energy and/or depth of interaction is needed.

6.4.2 Subset search. The computational expense of an exhaustive search can be reduced by narrowing down the range of possible values of $\mathbf{r}$ (and $\mathcal{E}$ if desired) before evaluating the likelihood.

To narrow the range of possible interaction positions, we could choose some coarse initial estimate $\hat{\mathbf{r}}_0$ and search within a preset radius R of this point. For example, $\hat{\mathbf{r}}_0$ could be chosen as the location of the center of the PMT that gives the largest signal, or it could be determined by standard Anger arithmetic.

Similarly, we can compute an Anger-like estimate of energy [*cf.*, (3.69)],

$$\hat{\mathcal{E}}_0 = \frac{\sum_{k=1}^{K} U_k}{\sum_{k=1}^{K} f_k(\mathbf{r})}, \tag{3.75}$$

and search only energies near this value. This approach works well if $\sum_{k=1}^{K} f_k(\mathbf{r})$ is nearly independent of $\mathbf{r}$; otherwise, we can use $\mathbf{r} = \hat{\mathbf{r}}_0$ or update $\mathbf{r}$ in the energy search as the position search goes on.

6.4.3 Nested search. If we plan to use the likelihood window for scatter rejection (see Section 6.3.2), we do not need to search over $\mathcal{E}$, and we can reduce the search region in $\mathbf{r}$ by eliminating points that will not pass the likelihood test.

With the scaled Poisson model, the relevant likelihood for 2D position estimation and the likelihood window is $\Pr(\mathbf{U}|\mathbf{r}, \mathcal{E}_0)$. Because of the independence of the normalized signals, this likelihood factors as [*cf.* (3.62)]

$$\Pr(\mathbf{U}|\mathbf{r}, \mathcal{E}_0) = \prod_{k=1}^{K} \Pr(U_k|\mathbf{r}, \mathcal{E}_0) \tag{3.76}$$

Even if the point $\mathbf{r}$ turns out to maximize $\Pr(\mathbf{U}|\mathbf{r}, \mathcal{E}_0)$, it will nevertheless be rejected by the likelihood window unless

$$\Pr(\mathbf{U}|\mathbf{r}, \mathcal{E}_0) > L_0, \tag{3.77}$$

where L_0 is the likelihood threshold.

Because the factors in (3.76) are probabilities (not PDFs) and hence less than or equal to unity, the product of likelihoods cannot exceed the threshold L_0 if any factor is less than L_0. Moreover, each factor has a maximum possible value $P_{max} < 1$, and in practice L_0 will be set to a value much less than P_{max}^K.

If we look at a single PMT and assume that all other signals take on that maximum value, we see that a point $\mathbf{r}$ can be accepted by the likelihood window only if

$$\Pr(U_k|\mathbf{r}, \mathcal{E}_0)\, P_{max}^{K-1} > L_0. \tag{3.78}$$

This condition defines a set of points that might be accepted ML position estimates, based just on the kth PMT.

To use this knowledge to reduce the computational expense of searching for the estimate that maximizes the overall likelihood $\Pr(\mathbf{U}|\mathbf{r}, \mathcal{E}_0)$ and satisfies (3.77), we can start with the PMT that gives the highest signal and search for values of $\mathbf{r}$

consistent with (3.78) for that PMT. Then we consider the PMT with the second-highest signal and search *among values that survived the first test* for $\mathbf{r}$ consistent with (3.78) for the second PMT. We repeat this procedure for all PMTs (with an ever-shrinking set size), and finally search the smallest set for the true ML point that maximizes (3.76); only then do we apply (3.77) and accept or reject the event.

6.4.4 Directed search. So far we have discussed only search methods that evaluate likelihoods for all points in some set. Most of the optimization literature, however, deals with methods that require far fewer function evaluations. Methods such as steepest descent and conjugate gradient attempt to minimize an objective function (such as the negative of the log-likelihood) by traversing a systematic path in the parameter space with ever-decreasing values of the function.

Conjugate gradient, in particular, can converge in remarkably few iterations; if the function is quadratic and the parameter space is N-dimensional, this algorithm is guaranteed to find the true minimum in N steps or less.

A disadvantage of a gradient search is that it might get stuck in a local minimum if the function being minimized is not a convex function of the parameters. Choosing a good starting point $(\hat{\mathbf{r}}_0, \hat{\mathcal{E}}_0)$ as described in Section 6.4.2 can ameliorate this problem.

6.4.5 Precomputation. All of the methods for ML position and energy estimation require many evaluations of likelihood or log-likelihood functions; for gradient-search methods, derivatives of these functions with respect to the parameters being estimated are also needed. It would be prohibitive to start these calculations anew for each gamma-ray event, but fortunately there are several factors that are independent of the specific data that can be computed in advance.

For example, with 2D position estimation and the scaled Poisson model, the quantity to be maximized is given by (3.70) as

$$\lambda(\mathbf{r}, \mathcal{E}) = \sum_{k=1}^{K} \{U_k \ln [\mathcal{E} f_k(\mathbf{r})] - \mathcal{E} f_k(\mathbf{r})\}. \tag{3.79}$$

For a likelihood window, we can set $\mathcal{E} = \mathcal{E}_0$ and write

$$\lambda(\mathbf{r}, \mathcal{E}_0) = \sum_{k=1}^{K} U_k\, A_k(\mathbf{r}) - B(\mathbf{r}), \tag{3.80}$$

where

$$A_k(\mathbf{r}) \equiv \ln [\mathcal{E}_0\, f_k(\mathbf{r})]\,, \qquad B(\mathbf{r}) \equiv \mathcal{E}_0 \sum_{k=1}^{K} f_k(\mathbf{r}). \tag{3.81}$$

The quantities $A_k(\mathbf{r})$ and $B(\mathbf{r})$ can be precomputed and stored for all $\mathbf{r}$ on a regular grid. For example, if $\mathbf{r}$ is estimated on a 128×128 grid, each function requires just 32 kB of storage (16 kB each for x and y), and for a modular scintillation camera with 9 PMTs, 10 such functions are needed. Derivatives of $A_k(\mathbf{r})$ and $B(\mathbf{r})$

are also required for gradient-search methods, but even then the required storage is less than 1 MB.

6.5 Lookup tables and data compression

Even with all of the tricks discussed above, position and energy estimation is still computationally demanding, and it must be done for each of the events in a full SPECT acquisition.

A much more rapid approach is to compute ML estimates for all possible combinations of PMT signals in advance and to look up the answer when an event comes along. At CGRI, we use this approach for modular scintillation cameras with 4 PMTs, but it is not so obvious that it can be extended to larger cameras.

In this section, we examine the practicalities of using lookup tables for the final ML estimates, and then we touch on methods of data compression that could make it feasible in a general case.

6.5.1 Size of the table. Consider a camera with K PMTs, each digitized to B bits. The number of possible combinations of PMT signals is

$$N = 2^{KB} \tag{3.82}$$

For example, with 4 PMTs each digitized to 6 bits, $N = 2^{24}$ or about 16 million locations. For 2D estimation on a 128×128 grid, we require 14 bits of storage for the estimates $\hat{x}$ and $\hat{y}$, and one additional bit can be used to determine whether the event passes a likelihood or energy window. Thus, we need 2 bytes per location or 32 MB of memory per camera, which is readily feasible with today's computers.

If we use 4 PMTs but increase the digital precision to 8 bits, we get $N = 2^{32}$ or about 4 billion locations. This example requires 8 GB of memory per camera, which is difficult with current technology but could become feasible soon.

The modular cameras currently in use at CGRI, however, have 9 PMTs, and each output is digitized to 12 bits, so $N = 2^{108}$, a number so large that we dare not invoke Moore's law.

There are several measures we can take to reduce the size of the lookup tables. An obvious one is not to store zeros. Most combinations of PMT signals do not have any measurable likelihood of being produced by scintillation events of any position or energy, so there is no point in computing the ML estimates in the first place, much less storing the results. Even in a 4-PMT camera, far less than 1% of the possible addresses would contain valid events. A more complicated addressing scheme is needed if ML estimates for invalid events are not stored, but the benefit can be large.

The second useful measure is to reduce the number of bits B used for each PMT. If this is done cleverly, as discussed in Section 6.5.2, the loss in camera performance can be minimal.

Finally, we can reduce the number of signals used to compute the ML estimates from the number of PMTs K to some smaller number J. An *ad hoc* way to do this is simply to use the J PMTs with the largest signals, but this is almost certain to entail unacceptable loss in performance if J is significantly less than K. A better approach, sketched in Section 6.5.3, is to look for approximate *sufficient statistics*.

6.5.2 Square-root compression. How do we choose B, the number of bits used in digitizing each PMT signal? If we consider only the cost and availability of analog-to-digital converters, we may well opt to make B large in order to mitigate any information loss in the digitization; that is how we arrived at $B = 12$ in the current 9-PMT modular cameras at CGRI. If, on the other hand, we want to use lookup tables for the final ML estimation, we should make B as small as possible; intuitively we should be safe if we make the least significant bit (LSB) smaller than the standard deviation of the noise in the PMT signals.

The problem is that this noise level depends on the mean signals because PMT noise is dominated by Poisson statistics. If we choose B such that the LSB is, say, half a standard deviation at the lowest mean signal we are likely to encounter, then it is far less than a standard deviation at the highest mean, and we are wasting bits there. In the CGRI cameras, the mean signal for an event directly under one PMT is about 50 times greater than for the most distant event, and this ratio is likely to increase as the number of PMTs increases.

The solution used with the 4-PMT cameras at CGRI is to compute the square root of the PMT signal before coarse digitization. If $y \equiv \sqrt{n}$ and n is a Poisson random variable, then it is a curious fact that $\mathrm{Var}(y) \approx \frac{1}{4}$ independent of the mean of n. As a consequence, we can use fewer bits if we digitize y rather than a signal proportional to n. In practice, we use surprisingly few bits, just $B = 5$ or 32 levels of quantization.

Square-root compression is useful for the 4-PMT cameras but it falls far short of making lookup tables feasible with 9 or more PMTs.

6.5.3 Sufficient statistics. A *statistic* is any function of the data. A *sufficient statistic* is one that is just as good as the data for performing some estimation task. A sufficient statistic is useful if it reduces the amount of storage needed or, in our case, if it reduces the size of a lookup table. Thus, we can think of sufficient statistics as lossless data compression.

As an example, suppose we form linear combinations of the PMT signals:

$$T_j = \sum_{k=1}^{K} w_{jk} V_k\,, \qquad j = 1, ..., J. \tag{3.83}$$

We can then do ML position and energy estimation with the new $J \times 1$ data vector $\mathbf{T}$. If $K = 9$ but $J = 3$ or 4, a lookup table becomes feasible for the 9-PMT camera. The crucial question is how to choose the weights so that there is minimal or no loss in camera performance as defined, say, by spatial and energy resolution. Should this turn out not to be possible, the next question is whether we can use nonlinear functions of the V_k as sufficient statistics.

The estimation literature provides some guidance in answering these questions (see, for example, Lehmann, 1991). By definition, $\mathbf{T}(\mathbf{g})$ is a sufficient statistic for estimation of $\boldsymbol{\theta}$ if and only if $\text{pr}(\mathbf{g}|\mathbf{T},\boldsymbol{\theta})$ is independent of $\boldsymbol{\theta}$. In scintillation cameras, $\mathbf{g}$ is a vector of PMT signals $\mathbf{V}$, and $\boldsymbol{\theta}$ corresponds to interaction position and possibly energy, so this definition says that the probability of occurrence of some combination of PMT signals is fully determined by the sufficient statistic without requiring additional knowledge of the interaction position and energy.

A useful result from estimation theory is the *factorization theorem*: $\mathbf{T}(\mathbf{g})$ is a sufficient statistic for estimation of $\boldsymbol{\theta}$ if and only if there exist non-negative functions k and h such that

$$\text{pr}(\mathbf{g}|\boldsymbol{\theta}) = k\left[\mathbf{T}(\mathbf{g}),\boldsymbol{\theta}\right]h(\mathbf{g}). \tag{3.84}$$

It follows from this theorem that ML estimation can be done by maximizing $k\left[\mathbf{T}(\mathbf{g}),\boldsymbol{\theta}\right]$ rather than the likelihood $\text{pr}(\mathbf{g}|\boldsymbol{\theta})$, provided the factorization can be achieved.

In most cases, however, we cannot write the likelihood in the form (3.85), and hence no exact sufficient statistic exists. In these cases, we need to be content with searching for *approximate sufficient statistics*.

In broad terms, the procedure is to generate some trial functions of the PMT signals and test them for sufficiency. Tests for approximate sufficiency can be derived from the definition or from the factorization theorem, but the most direct approach is to test how effective the trial statistics are in terms of bias and variance of the resulting estimates.

To this end, we need the likelihood for the sufficient statistic, $\text{pr}(\mathbf{T}|\boldsymbol{\theta})$, which can often be obtained from transformation laws for PDFs. It is straightforward to do this transformation for linear statistics of the form (3.83), especially if we use a Gaussian model for the original data; a linear combination of Gaussians is a Gaussian.

From the likelihood for a trial sufficient statistic, we can compute the Fisher information matrix and the Cramér-Rao bound on the variances of position and energy estimates. Alternatively, we can simulate samples of the PMT signals and compare ML estimates performed either on the basis of these sample or from the trial statistics; the degree of sufficiency is related to how closely the estimation performance from the statistic approximates that from the original PMT samples.

7. Semiconductor detectors

Although this chapter has concentrated on scintillation cameras, the statistical and data-processing issues are remarkably similar with semiconductor arrays. In Section 7.1, we delineate some of these similarities by discussing the data sets and what information we want to extract from them. In Section 7.2, we indicate some new random effects that need to be incorporated into the statistical models for semiconductors, and in Section 7.3 we present a multivariate Gaussian likelihood that includes these effects.

7.1 Data sets and estimation tasks

As we saw in Chapter 2, semiconductor imaging detectors can be either arrays of individual elements or monolithic semiconductor crystals with arrays of electrodes.

Individual elements are almost always operated in a triggered or event-driven mode, producing an output pulse for each gamma-ray interaction. The data associated with the interaction is the pulse waveform, and the main data-processing task is to estimate the energy deposited in the interaction. It often happens that the waveform is sensitive to the random depth of interaction of the gamma ray, z_{int}, but this parameter is usually treated as a nuisance parameter, something to be estimated in order to improve the energy estimate but not of intrinsic interest itself. No attempt is made to estimate the lateral coordinates x_{int} and y_{int}, and the lateral resolution is limited by the element size.

If an electrode array is used with a monolithic crystal, the electronics can be either event-driven or integrating. An event-driven array is triggered by a gamma-ray interaction and produces some set of output signals in response to it. In principle, the measured data could be full waveforms for one or more elements in the array, but it is easier to incorporate a pulse-shaping circuit at each pixel; in that case, the data for each event would consist of a single number (the pulse height) for the element that triggered the readout and possibly for neighboring elements as well. If only a single element is read out, there is little difference between a monolithic crystal with an electrode array operated in an event-driven mode and an array of independent detector elements.

By contrast, an integrating array such as the Arizona hybrid accumulates charge for a fixed time T and reads out frames whether or not an event has occurred. Thus, an $N \times N$ pixel array that views a source for a total time of JT produces a huge data set consisting of J $N \times N$ arrays of numbers.

The first step in the data processing for integrating monolithic arrays is to parse each frame for events. This is a detection problem where the events to be detected are random both in the amount of charge they deposit and in their spatial location. To make matters more complicated, the number of events per frame is unknown, and at high gamma-ray fluxes two or more events can produce charge in the same detector pixel.

At low fluxes, we might be able to neglect overlap [Furenlid, 2000] and assume that each detector pixel receives charge from at most one event. In that case, one possible way of parsing the frame is to look for subarrays of pixels, say 3×3 or 5×5, that have accumulated a total charge greater than a preset threshold. Because several overlapping subarrays can pass this test for a single event, we can search for one where the largest pixel signal is at the center of the subarray. The data recorded for the event thus consist of the address of this central pixel and the charges accumulated in that pixel and its neighbors.

After this initial event-detection step, the remaining data-processing task for each event is to estimate the coordinates of the interaction site in two or three dimensions and to estimate the deposited energy. A simple approach would be to forget about depth of interaction, estimate the 2D coordinates of the interaction by the location of the center pixel, and estimate the energy either by the charge accumulated in the center pixel or the total charge in the neighborhood around that pixel. Needless to say, these *ad hoc* methods are not optimal.

7.2 Random effects in semiconductors

The data set from an integrating array is remarkably similar to that from a scintillation camera. In both cases, each event produces signals on an $N \times N$ array of sensors (electrodes in a semiconductor camera, PMTs in a scintillation camera). Additionally in both cases, these signals are random because of the random interaction position and energy, the random production of low-energy secondary particles (electrons and holes in semiconductors, optical photons in scintillators), and random propagation of these secondaries to the sensors.

There are, however, some noteworthy differences in the basic physics. Optical photons can be refracted or reflected at interfaces, but they are not appreciably absorbed in high-quality optical materials or scintillation crystals. Electrons and holes are not refracted or reflected, but they can be trapped or recombined in the bulk of the semiconductor. On the other hand, optical photons produce an output signal only if they reach a PMT and produce photoelectrons. but electrons and holes can induce charge on an electrode even if they do not reach it. The effect of the trapped charge is described by an electrostatic Green's function, often called a weighting potential in the detector literature.

There are also two important quantitative differences between scintillators and semiconductors. First, the Fano factors are quite different. In scintillators, we saw that the statistics of production of electron-hole pairs were quite unimportant; because of the inefficiencies of conversion of electron-hole pairs to optical photons, propagation of the photons to PMTs and conversion to photoelectrons, we argued that the particles being sensed – the photoelectrons – should follow Poisson statistics to an excellent approximation.

In semiconductors, the particles being sensed are the holes and electrons themselves, so the Fano effects are more important. In addition, the Fano factors for the number of electron-hole pairs are smaller in semiconductors because the bandgaps are smaller; Fano factors around 0.05 are routinely reported for silicon, and a value of 0.15 has been reported for cadmium zinc telluride.

The second quantitative difference is the role of readout noise. Photomultipliers have a large gain, so noise in the electronics that follows is usually irrelevant. Moreover, as we saw in Sections 6.1.5 and 6.1.6, noise in the gain process itself leads to a multiplicative factor near unity in the signal variance [see (3.60)], and it is a good approximation to think of the PMT as a noise-free amplifier.

Semiconductor detectors do not have internal gain, so the amplifier noise is much more important. Johnson (thermal) noise and flicker (1/f) noise in the circuitry are significant, as is a kind of noise called kTC noise, associated with the gated integrator.

7.3 A Gaussian model

The only practical way of accounting for all of these random effects appears to be through a multivariate Gaussian model. As with most invocations of Gaussian statistics, the justification proceeds from the central-limit theorem. Electronic noise is Gaussian to an excellent approximation because it results from the motion of a large number of electrons in the circuit components. Similarly, a large number of electrons and holes are produced by each gamma-ray interaction; thus, their net effect should be well described by Gaussian statistics.

Suppose we wish to estimate the interaction position and energy for a single event from the signals on an $N \times N$ electrode array. The specific Gaussian model we need for that purpose is an N^2-dimensional PDF conditioned on the position and energy. Because multivariate Gaussian PDFs are fully specified by their mean and covariance, we need an $N^2 \times 1$ mean vector and an $N^2 \times N^2$ covariance matrix that accurately account for all the random effects discussed in Section 7.2.

Details of the analysis can be found in Barrett and Myers [2004], Chapter 12, but to give the flavor of the results, we present the expression for the covariance matrix for estimation of 3D position with data from an integrating array:

$$\begin{aligned}
&[\mathbf{K}_V(\mathbf{r}_{int}, \mathcal{E}_{int})]_{mm'} = \\
&\quad \left(\frac{e}{C}\right)^2 \overline{N}_{eh} \int_\infty d^3\mathbf{r}\ [\mathrm{pr}_e(\mathbf{r}|\mathbf{r}_{int}) + \mathrm{pr}_h(\mathbf{r}|\mathbf{r}_{int})]\ \Phi_m(\mathbf{r})\ \Phi_{m'}(\mathbf{r}) \\
&\quad + \left(\frac{e}{C}\right)^2 (F-1)\, \overline{N}_{eh} \int_\infty d^3\mathbf{r}\ \mathrm{pr}_e(\mathbf{r}|\mathbf{r}_{int})\ \Phi_m(\mathbf{r}) \times \\
&\quad \int_\infty d^3\mathbf{r}'\ \mathrm{pr}_e(\mathbf{r}'|\mathbf{r}_{int})\ \Phi_{m'}(\mathbf{r}') \\
&\quad + \left(\frac{e}{C}\right)^2 (F-1)\, \overline{N}_{eh} \int_\infty d^3\mathbf{r}\ \mathrm{pr}_h(\mathbf{r}|\mathbf{r}_{int})\ \Phi_m(\mathbf{r}) \times \\
&\quad \int_\infty d^3\mathbf{r}'\ \mathrm{pr}_h(\mathbf{r}'|\mathbf{r}_{int})\ \Phi_{m'}(\mathbf{r}'). \qquad (3.85)
\end{aligned}$$

In this expression, indices m and m' run from 1 to N^2 and indicate the electrode, C is the capacitance used in the integrating circuit at each electrode, e is the charge on the electron, $\overline{N}_{eh}$ is the mean number of hole-electron pairs (proportional to the deposited energy $\mathcal{E}_{int}$), and F is the Fano factor. The PDFs $\mathrm{pr}_e(\mathbf{r}|\mathbf{r}_{int})$ and $\mathrm{pr}_h(\mathbf{r}|\mathbf{r}_{int})$ describe the spatial distribution of charge at the end of the integration period, and $\Phi_m(\mathbf{r})$ is the weighting potential for the mth electrode.

As written, (3.85) does not account for electronic noise, but simple addition of a multiple of the unit matrix will solve that problem if we can assume that the noise in different electronic amplifiers is independent and has the same variance.

The covariance expression in (3.85) can be evaluated if we assume a homogeneous semiconductor material. The weighting potentials can be expressed in terms of image charges [Barrett and Myers, 2004], and the PDFs $\mathrm{pr}_e(\mathbf{r}|\mathbf{r}_{int})$ and $\mathrm{pr}_h(\mathbf{r}|\mathbf{r}_{int})$ are just exponential terms to account for trapping plus delta functions to account for the charge that propagates to the electrodes. The integrals can then be evaluated numerically for all points $\mathbf{r}_{int}$ on a 3D grid and used in a likelihood analogous to (3.64) for ML estimation.

8. Summary and conclusions

For scintillation cameras, we have seen that accurate statistical models can be derived from basic knowledge of Poisson processes and random gain. These models can then be used for rigorous ML estimation of 2D or 3D interaction position and energy of individual gamma-ray events. They also can be used for estimating the fluence on the camera, though that topic was not discussed here.

Another topic not treated in any detail was the use of segmented scintillator crystals, where the task is classification rather than estimation, but the same basic statistical models apply in that case also. Further research is needed on this topic.

For semiconductor detectors, we cannot rely on Poisson statistics to simplify our likelihood models, but we expect multivariate Gaussians to work well. In principle we know how to compute the relevant mean vectors and covariance matrices, though in practice it is necessary to assume a homogeneous slab of semiconductor material. Real materials, especially cadmium zinc telluride, are notoriously inhomogeneous, and a pressing need in the field is calibration methods to account for the inhomogeneities.

Another need with integrating detectors is more investigation of methods of parsing a frame for events. Similarly, we need statistical models that apply at higher gamma-ray fluxes and do not neglect overlapping events.

For both scintillators and semiconductors, the methods described here are computationally demanding but feasible. They all require recording signals from multiple sensors for each event, but the list-mode acquisition methods described by Furenlid in this volume make that step feasible. As the number of sensors increases, however, there will be an increasing need for data reduction without information loss; thus, the theory and practice of sufficient statistics will be key.

References

[Barrett, 2004] H. H. Barrett, K. J. Myers, *Foundations of Image Science*, New York, John Wiley and Sons, 2004.

[Chen, 1995] J. C. Chen, "Modular gamma cameras: Improvements in scatter rejection and characterization and initial clinical application," Ph.D. Dissertation, University of Arizona, 1995.

[Chen, 1997] J. C. Chen, "Scatter Rejection in Gamma Cameras for Use in Nuclear Medicine," *Biomed Eng Appl Basis Comm*, vol. 9, pp. 20-26, 1997.

[Furenlid, 2000] L. R. Furenlid, E. Clarkson, D. G. Marks, H. H. Barrett, "Spatial pileup considerations for pixellated gamma-ray detectors," *IEEE Trans. Nucl. Sci.*, vol. 47, pp. 1399-1402, 2000.

[Lehner, 2003] C. E. Lehner, Z. He, F. Zhang, "4π Compton Imaging Using a 3-D Position-Sensitive CdZnTe Detector via Weighted List-Mode Maximum

Likelihood," *Proc IEEE Med Imag Conf*, 2003.

[Lehmann, 1991] E. L. Lehmann, *Theory of Point Estimation*, Pacific Grove, California, Wadsworth & Brooks, 1991.

Chapter 4

The Animal in Animal Imaging

Gail Stevenson*

1. Introduction

With the development of new imaging modalities, techniques, and radiotracers, it is easy to get caught up in the excitement of the equipment and the pictures. Yet the value in imaging lies primarily in the benefit it brings to human lives. That potential value is determined first by studies in animals. This paper will focus on the care and handling of rodents as they make up over 90% of the animal research done. However, many of the concepts we will be discussing could be applied to any species. Whatever species you work with, take time to learn about them and their specific needs; it will pay compounding dividends.

Although you may be more aware of a multi-thousand dollar transgenic, I also want to impart the importance of monitoring even the two-dollar "garden-variety" mouse. The cost of buying the animal is only a small part of your overall expense. You can calculate other numbers such as lost technician time, wasted radiotracers, lost machine time, and your time (which is becoming an increasingly precious commodity). More importantly, how do you calculate the effect of poor data gathered from an animal that may have outwardly appeared fine, but whose physiological parameters were far from "normal"? I recall a graduate student who was seriously impacted by the discovery that a particular physiological function they had studied for two years was due to a one-degree temperature change that occurred while the animal was under anesthesia. Heart rate, respiratory rate, and body temperature are all affected by anesthetics and sedatives; these, in turn, affect cardiac output, acid-base balance, and perfusion of all the tissues. Poor perfusion or an acid-base imbalance affects uptake and washout of the radiotracer and drugs given. "Physiological stability also impacts on interstudy variability as well as intrastudy variability" [Qiu, 1997]. The more we know about what is happening, the more we can strive for a more physiologically normal parameter, and the more applicable our findings are. Before leaving this topic, I will mention the most important reason for careful monitoring of each animal because I feel it serves as a compliment to the fine researchers I have had the opportunity to work with over the past 20 years: we

*The University of Arizona, Department of Radiology, Tucson, Arizona

are given stewardship over the species that we work with; they are to be valued for the contribution they make to our lives and are to be cared for responsibly and with compassion. As I often tell the students who I am working with, "If you don't feel anything for the animal you are working with, it's time to change professions."

2. Health surveillance programs

Monitoring of the animal in research begins even before it arrives at your institution. Vendors and institutions have a variety of health surveillance programs to identify infectious organisms. At the University of Arizona, vendors are placed on an approved list when they meet or exceed the guidelines used here. Animals coming from these vendors can enter into use within a few days after arrival. (There is an adjustment period of at least two days, and preferably five days, after arrival to allow the animal to recover from the stress of shipment and adjust to a new location. If animals are placed into an experiment before their stress responses have returned to normal, physiological responses will be altered.) However, it is not unusual that animals coming to our facility for imaging have spent time at another facility with a differing set of guidelines. More and more mice are originating from noncommercial sources with the development of unique genetically altered models. In some of these situations, the health status is unknown. "Although most rodent infections may not cause clinical signs, such infectious agents can still alter physiological parameters and influence experimental results, thus increasing the number of animals needed to compensate for statistical variability and avoid misinterpretation of the data" [Martin-Caballero, 2002]. Subclinical infections, such as the mouse parvovirus, may not be an issue to one investigator's study, but could significantly impact other research such as involving the immune system. Your imaging system may serve as an ongoing source of infection once infected animals are placed within it. Rat pinworms have plagued many facilities and these relatively sticky eggs are frequently spread on fomites. Once introduced to your facility, you can expect weeks of treatment and disinfection causing serious delays to your research and the addition of new variables.

3. Species specifics

As already mentioned, the more you know about the animals you work with, the more effective you can be with designing your experiment, controlling variables, monitoring changes, and producing meaningful results. Laboratory Animal Medicine by Fox, et al. [2002] may be a valuable resource. Tables from this text provide a reference on normative data for the mouse and rat. This information is general, but can guide you. Whenever possible, gather more specific information for the strain and sex you are working with. Here are some interesting facts to keep in mind:

1 Mice thrive in a narrow ambient temperature range of 21-25°C (70-77°F). Due to their high ratio of body surface to body mass, they would go into shock from dehydration if they depended on evaporation for cooling. Consequently,

they have no sweat glands and they cannot pant. In the wild, they depend on burrowing to help regulate body temperature, but this is essentially unavailable to the laboratory rodent. They do not tolerate nocturnal cooling well, and they will begin to die at ambient temperatures of 37°C (98.°F). They can partially adapt to moderate increases in temperature by increasing their body temperature, decreasing their metabolic rate, and increasing the blood flow to their ears [Fox, 2002]. These changes are likely to affect experimental results.

2 In rats, prolonged exposure to temperatures as low as 26.6°C (80°F) can result in male infertility, which can be irreversible [Fox, 2002].

3 A rodent's metabolic rate is high, and it accommodates for this with several factors, including a rapid respiratory rate (163/min for a mouse) and short air passages. Consider these factors when ventilating rodents under anesthesia. Because a long tracheal tube creates a significant increase in dead space, keep the tubes as short as practical.

4 "Mice excrete only a drop or two of urine at a time, and it is highly concentrated" [Fox, 2002]. The filtering system per gram of tissue is twice that of the rat. They can concentrate urine to 4300 mOsm/liter compared to 1160 mOsm/liter for people. Large amounts of protein in the urine are normal, including creatinine, which is different from other mammals [Fox, 2002].

5 "Heart rates from 310-840/min have been recorded for mice, and there are wide variations in rates and blood pressure among strains." [Fox, 2002].

6 Light-dark cycles (rodents are nocturnal), pheromones, social grouping, and room changes noticeably affect animals. Some of the behavior studies that I have participated in required that animal cages remain in the same location on racks, and that only same sex animals be in a room. I have personally recorded weight loss in rats that were placed on the top shelves of racks where the lighting was more intense.

7 Olfaction is a critical sense in rodents. It only takes a quick look at the rat brain to realize that an inordinate percentage is devoted to the olfactory lobes. Compared to many species, man is olfactory impaired. These animals live in a world where fragrant clouds surround them, mingle, and pass by. They extract huge amounts of information from these odors, including danger, food availability, kinship, social status, and sexual status.

8 Rats can vocalize in the ultrasonic range. "Stress-induced vocalization can make handling more difficult for other rats within hearing range." [Fox, 2002].

9 "Rat eyes are exophthalmic, which increases the risk of injury from trauma and drying during anesthesia." [Fox, 2002]. Liberally apply ophthalmic ointment when under anesthesia.

10 The Harderian gland of a rat secretes a red substance, porphyrin, when the animal is stressed. This reddish discharge around the eyes or nose is a signal to check for problems.

11 "Incisors grow continuously. If the incisors are not worn evenly or are misaligned due to gingivitis or congenital defects, the resulting malocclusion may lead to nonfunctional, spiral elongation of the incisors, injury to the palate, and reduced food intake." [Fox, 2002]. Consider this if your rodents are placed on a soft diet, have decreased food intake, or have an injury or fall. This is not an uncommon problem in older animals as well. These overgrown or irregular incisors should be trimmed back.

12 Rats cannot vomit. This is due to a fold in the stomach that lies where the esophagus enters [Fox, 2002]. You do not need to withhold food or water prior to surgery; this is an advantage due to their increased metabolic rate and susceptibility to dehydration.

13 The rat does not have a gall bladder. The bile ducts from each lobe of the liver form the common bile duct, which dumps into the small intestine. (The mouse does have a gall bladder.)

14 Most rats are fed *ad libitum* (free choice). However, there are numerous reports demonstrating that this significantly increases the incidence of neoplasia and reduces longevity when compared to rats fed $\sim$ 80% of the free choice amount. Food restriction does require daily weight records.

15 Rodents are designed to physiologically function in a horizontal position. Although vertical positioning can be used for short-term procedures, they are compromised. In longer studies, we have seen an increase in mortality.

These are just a few of the interesting facts with rodents. Hopefully, it will perk your interest to look into the details of the system you are working with, and possibly even some of the specifics of the strains you work with.

4. On arrival

Once animals arrive at your institution, animal care technicians will look them over briefly as they are placed in cages; it is ideal if a staff member can give them a physical examination as well. The extent of the examination varies with the general condition of the animals, their age, and health risks. Daily weight sheets help detect early loss of appetite. Weight loss will often precede other clinical signs such as decreased mobility or hunched appearance. Supplementation may prevent a stress-induced weight loss from spiraling into mortality. Applesauce, butter, and mash (moistened rodent food) can be offered in small restaurant metal dishes. A high-calorie vitamin supplement such as STAT (PRN Pharmacal, Pepsicola, FL) can be added for an additional boost; it is also highly palatable. A couple of hints:

1 Moistened pet food must be kept refrigerated and should be replaced every couple of days. These foods readily grow bacteria and spoil.

2 Rodents are neophobic. Even if the food you give them is tasty, they will often only eat a small bite the first day it is offered. In practical terms, let them taste and learn to like your supplement before you need it in a crisis.

3 When making mash, presoak the pellets overnight in the refrigerator, as they are hard and absorb water slowly.

4 Rodents have continually growing teeth and must have something hard to gnaw on to prevent tooth overgrowth and resultant mouth injuries. Keep some dry food available, and trim the teeth if needed.

5. Anesthetics

Experimental protocols are as variable as the mind can imagine. Yet they consistently measure a change. If that change is in an animal, realize that it will likely affect the anesthetics and imaging of that animal. Any change of function is reflected in the animal's ability to metabolize and/or excrete medications or other chemicals. The following discussion of anesthetic programs offers guidelines for rodents. These guidelines can act as a starting point from which you can tailor your experimental needs. Pilot studies can then verify the application.

Preanesthetics are rarely used in rodents. Anticholinergics such as atropine and glycopyrrolate can be administered to reduce salivary and bronchial secretions and protect the heart from vagal inhibition [Flecknell, 1996]. However, these medications also increase the viscosity of these secretions, which can result in obstruction in these narrow airways. When they are used, the airways should be periodically suctioned [White, 1987]. It is also feasible to give sedatives prior to the anesthetic. This may reduce the stress of transporting the animal to the surgical or imaging center. Many of these products have advantages of providing analgesia and reducing the dose of the general anesthetic. However, because they do require more handling of the animal, they are often incorporated into a single combination injection with the anesthetic. The anesthetic agents themselves can be delivered either parenterally (by injection) or by inhalation. Parenteral administration is usually IP (intraperitoneal) for several reasons: it is relatively easy to do, a small volume of potentially irritating drug is placed in a well-perfused space with a large surface area, and many programs have been developed for IP use. IM (intramuscular) drug delivery is usually done in one of the larger muscle masses, typically the thigh muscle. IV (intravenous) injections are usually done in the lateral tail vein. This technique requires some practice. The animal is placed in a restraining device, and the tail is warmed (by a warm pad, heat lamp, or warm water). For a mouse, we prefer a 30-gauge needle, though a 27-gauge needle can be used. There is a margin of error in this procedure even with experienced personnel, and post-injection images frequently show some deposit of tracer around the injection site, possibly from leakage at the penetration point. The use of indwelling catheters can help, but also require practice.

Inhalation anesthesia is becoming increasingly popular as investigators discover they have greater control over the depth and duration of anesthesia, greater survivability, and minimal metabolic effect, thus reducing the variables in their experiments [Kohn, 1997]. Scavenging systems to remove waste anesthetic gases must be provided for these systems. Where exhausting to the outside is not feasible, activated carbon filter systems can be employed. Remember that nitrous oxide, if used as a part of the program, is not filtered by activated carbon systems [Fox, 2002].

Each of the texts listed in the references and V. Lukasik's review article provide tables with a variety of anesthetic programs and dosages for both mice and rats. The number of animals used, the duration of the procedure, the depth of anesthesia required, and the equipment available will influence each investigator's choice. Our protocols for imaging allow for a variety of programs so that we can complement the programs being used by our collaborators. A few notes for your consideration follow [Fox, 2002]:

1 Barbiturates produce general anesthesia with muscle relaxation, but they also produce a dose-related respiratory and cardiovascular depression that worsens over time. Cardiac output can be decreased up to 50%, and hypotension can be profound.

   (a) Sodium pentobarbital (Nembutal) is often used as an IP injection to induce anesthesia in rats. For imaging studies, the level of anesthesia may be adequate, but the dose needed for a surgical plane of anesthesia is close to a lethal dose. Given IP, it causes appreciable abdominal inflammation [Spikes, 1996]. It is even less predictable in mice.

   (b) Propofol (Diprivan, Rapinovet) is a "novel" hypnotic with a rapid onset and short duration (unless given by continuous infusion.) It must be given IV, and the cardiac and respiratory effects are significant if it is used alone [Kohn, 1997].

2 Ketamine is a dissociative agent which produces some analgesia and immobility, but without muscle relaxation. Although respiratory depression is minimal, a release of catecholamines results in tachycardia and increased blood pressure [Lukasik, 2003]. It is typically combined with tranquilizers and sedatives.

3 The alpha2-adrenergic agonists include xylazine (Rompun) and medetomidine (Domitor). These drugs have both sedative and analgesic effects. Xylazine is combined frequently with ketamine to enhance the analgesia and provide muscle relaxation. However "they also may cause hyperglycemia, bradycardia, peripheral vasoconstriction, hypothermia, and diuresis." An interesting side effect of these drugs is a biphasic effect on blood pressure. Initially, there is an increase in arterial pressure for 20-45 minutes, but this is soon followed by profound hypotension [Shalev, 1997b, Lukasik, 2001a]. Consequently, processes affected by blood pressure such as perfusion of tissues could fluctuate. These drugs can be reversed using yohimbine or atipamezole (Antisedan).

4 Etomidate, an imidazole 5-carbonic acid derivative, provides minimal analgesia, but does allow good cardiovascular stability. It causes adrenal cortical depression for 6 hours, and it is expensive [Lukasik, 2001a]. It is usually combined with an opioid.

5 Anesthetic adjuvants available include:

   (a) the phenothiazine tranquilizers, especially acepromazine. Phenothiazines produce increased sedation, but without analgesia. Notably, the phenothiazines drop blood pressure and are contraindicated in cases of hypotension or hypovolemia. They should also be avoided in anemic animals because they can decrease the circulating red blood cells by up to 50% within 30 minutes. They cause respiratory depression, excessive vagal tone and bradycardia, and may trigger seizures [Shalev, 1997a, Lukasik, 2001a].

   (b) The benzodiazepines, diazepam (Valium) and midazolam (Versed), also produce some increased sedation without analgesia. They have virtually no cardiac effects, but can cause mild respiratory depression [Lukasik, 2001a]. An advantage of the benzos is that they can be reversed using flumazenil (Romazicon).

   (c) Opioids (such as buprenorphine, butorphanol, fentanyl, oxymorphone, etorphine, and morphine), on the other hand, are moderate sedatives, do provide analgesia, and have only mild cardiovascular effects [Lukasik, 2001a]. However, there is some respiratory depression. These agents can also be reversed by using naloxone [Kohn, 1997].

6 Dr. Janyce Cornick-Seahorn recommends that when using combinations, use only one agent from each general class [Cornick-Seahorn, 2000].

7 "Inhalation anesthesia circumvents many of the difficulties associated with injectable agents. Because the agents are used to effect, issues of dose calculation and variations in response do not arise. These agents are not controlled substances and also escape the burden of detailed record keeping required for barbiturates, opioids, benzodiazepines, and ketamine. Available agents include enflurane, halothane, isoflurane, sevoflurane, and desflurane. In general, the... agents are characterized by rapid induction and recovery. To varying degrees, all inhalation anesthetics cause dose-related cardiovascular and respiratory depression, but these effects are frequently less severe than equipotent doses of injectable agents. ... Currently, isoflurane probably possesses the best combination of properties in term of expense and safety of personnel and patient."

8 One exception on isoflurane: "In humans, isoflurane has been reported to cause transient postoperative immunosuppression, which also occurs in mice. This study suggests that isoflurane should not be used for surgeries directly preceding immunologic research studies in mice." [Kohn, 1997].

In many situations, these drugs are combined to offset adverse effects and maximize the desired anesthesia and analgesia. In our facility, inhalation anesthesia appears to be the safest program for the animal, allows the fastest recovery, and has the least influence on the experiment. As with most research, it is not always possible to judge the duration of anesthesia that will be needed for a particular imaging session. With inhalation anesthesia, we can extend or shorten the program as needed. We are currently using isoflurane in a nonrebreathing system with a modified Bain mask on the rodent. (A system similar to ours is described in the reference by [Horne, 1998].) Depth of anesthesia can be adjusted from a deeper plane to allow for placement of a jugular catheter to a lighter plane, which maintains position during imaging. With isoflurane anesthesia, an animal can be induced quickly, maintained for short or long periods, and recovered quickly. This provides the flexibility we need and the safety to even repeat anesthetics in the same day. For those who would like more information on commercial inhalation systems available, refer to [Diven, 2003].

6. Animal monitoring

One of the areas of animal care that we are striving to improve in our facility is the ability to monitor the animal while it is being imaged. Visual monitoring is limited to respiratory rate once the animal is in the imager; and reflex responses (such as the toe pinch and muscle tone) are no longer accessible. We are left with some of the following options [Flecknell, 1996]:

1 Respiratory system

   (a) Visual observation of the rate, depth, and pattern of respirations. This can be done directly or via a camera placed within the imaging compartment.

   (b) Tidal volume is difficult to monitor in rodents, but it is sometimes controlled by using a ventilator. "People using ventilators should know that carbon dioxide is the main stimulus for respiration, and that if the arterial carbon dioxide level is reduced below 35-40mm Hg, the animal will not attempt to breathe. They should appreciate how altering the ventilator settings changes arterial carbon dioxide levels. A common mistake is to underventilate so that the animal fights the ventilator. This is misinterpreted as the animal being too light, and more anaesthetic is given. The end result is a hypercapnic animal that is too deeply anaesthetised. Inappropriate ventilator settings also lead investigators to use neuromuscular blocking agents when they are not necessary." [Young, 1999].

   (c) Electronic monitors are now sensitive enough to detect movement of the mouse chest wall.

   (d) Chestwall movement still does not indicate whether there is lung gas exchange. Obstructions in the airways or tubing could have blocked actual air movement. (The character of the respiration does change with total occlusion. With normal respiration, both the abdomen and chest expand simultaneously. Try taking a couple breaths with your hand occluding your mouth and nose; you will notice that your chest expands while your abdomen moves in [Young, 1999].)

i Pulse oximeters: used to measure the percentage saturation of arterial blood. In rodents, a clip can usually be placed on an ear or hind foot. "In general, a saturation of $> 95\%$ is good. If it falls to $< 90\%$, then the anaesthetist should take note but corrective action may not be necessary, especially if the cause is known and self-limiting. When the saturation falls below 80%, action should be taken to improve oxygenation." [Young, 1999]. "An oxygen saturation of 90% is equivalent to a PaO2 of 60 mmHg." [Kohn, 1997].

ii End-tidal carbon dioxide: used to measure the concentration of carbon dioxide in the exhaled gas. "The level of carbon dioxide at the end of expiration is normally within a few mmHg of the arterial carbon dioxide level." [Young, 1999]. Typical values would be $4 - 8\%$. High levels are an alert to possible respiratory failure. If the trace does not return to 0, the animal is rebreathing exhaled gases (increase the flow rate or cut down on the dead space). If values are too low, hyperventilation or hypotension with decreased cardiac output may be involved. Sudden decreases indicate an airway obstruction or cardiac arrest.

iii Blood gas analysis: "is the gold standard for assessing respiratory function." [Young, 1999]. This analyzer will measure the partial pressure of oxygen and carbon dioxide and the pH of the blood. It does require an arterial sample, and the instrument corrects for body temperature so that must be supplied. These instruments are generally expensive. Arterial samples from an animal breathing room air should be: 28-40 mmHg for P CO2; 82-94 mm Hg for P O2; and a pH of 7.35-7.45.

2 Cardiovascular system

(a) Again, the visual evaluation of the mucous membrane and touch for evaluating peripheral temperature are not available. Before the animal enters the imaging unit, capillary refill time should be < 2 seconds. Membranes should be pink, though admittedly cyanosis does not occur until the oxygen level has dropped dangerously low. Pale gums may indicate hypovolemia, anemia, or circulatory failure.

(b) ECG (electrocardiogram): monitors the electrical activity in the heart. Electrodes are generally placed on both forelimbs and the right hind limb. Pediatric pads can be taped to the foot in rodents. The electrical activity is essential for the diagnosis and treatment of arrhythmias

[Young, 1999], but do not make the mistake of assuming this is also the actual pumping of the heart. In veterinary school, we observed ECG patterns for up to 15 minutes after an animal's heart had stopped.

(c) Blood pressure:

i Direct: placing a catheter in an artery and connecting it to a transducer.

ii Indirect: inflating a cuff around the limb or tail. These systems do exist for rodents but are challenging to work with [Young, 1999].

iii The mean arterial pressure (MAP) primarily tells how well tissues are perfused. Typical values are 60-70 mm Hg. "Prolonged moderate hypotension (mean arterial presssre <60mmHg) produces renal shutdown." If systolic and diastolic arterial pressure values are available, they give information about "the degree of vasoconstriction and the adequacy of ventricular ejection." [Young, 1999].

3 Body Temperature

(a) Temperature is usually measured by a rectal or esophageal probe. "Rectal temperatures may be 1-2 degrees lower than core temperature due to loss of muscle tone." [Lukasik, 2001b]

(b) Normal value for a mouse is 37.4°C and 37°C for a rat.

(c) All anesthetics interfere with thermoregulation.

(d) Hypothermia is common in rodents and has numerous physiological effects:

i "Immune system depression–impaired leukocyte mobility and phago cytosis, decreased T-cell antibody production, depressed nonspecific host defenses.

ii Post-operative infection rate–increased to three times normal rate in patients experiencing intra-operative mild hypothermia.

iii Coagulopathy–independent of clotting factor levels, more severe in factor-deficient patients.

iv Blood viscosity–increased, sludging can occur.

v Systemic vascular resistance–increased (also increased afterload).

vi CO2 production–is decreased and may lead to alkalemia if IPPY is not adjusted.

vii Respiratory drive–diminished response to hypoxemia and hypercarbia.

viii CND–delayed recovery from anesthesia, confusion, stupor, coma.

ix Hyperglycemia–due to catecholamine release.

x Hypovolemia–due to cold diuresis, may be seen as profound hypotension after rewarming has occurred.

xi MAC–decreased approximately 5% per degree centigrade, anesthetic overdose can easily occur.

xii Drug metabolism–can be significantly delayed.

xiii Liver metabolism–can be greatly decreased, can lead to drug toxicity." [Lukasik, 2001b].

(e) Our current system of keeping rodents warm throughout the procedure employs a warm-water circulating blanket. These are safe for the animal, and the pads are thin enough to allow imaging.

(f) We are currently exploring the possibility of having an ambient temperature controlled warm air system or possibly a core temperature controlled warm air system.

Dr. Lukasik recently tested an MRI compatible monitoring system that we hope to introduce to the Center for Gamma-Ray Imaging as well. This system allows for simultaneous monitoring of ECG, temperature, respiratory rate, internal blood pressure, and end tidal carbon dioxide. Results are displayed on the computer in a Windows manner, which allows for monitoring several parameters simultaneously. Again, the more we know, the more we can adjust for deviations, and the more meaningful the experimental results.

Great care is given to selecting an appropriate anesthetic and monitoring the animal. Once an appropriate radiotracer is selected, the route of administration is determined. Intradermal injections have been used for lymphatic studies. However, the vast majority of our radiotracer injections are given IV. With any of the other methods of injection, uptake of the tracer is ongoing over a prolonged time period; IV administration allows us to pinpoint the time that tracer entered the circulation and image that immediate effect. Dynamic images are accomplished by placing a tiny catheter (PE 90 on a 27- or 30-gauge blunted needle) in the external jugular vein. The catheter is made long enough to extend out of the imaging system once the animal is positioned. Injections are now done using an automated syringe pump to standardize the timing and consistency of the injection. Limitations exist for the volume of radiotracer that can be given. This is typically more of a concern in mice; a 25-30g mouse can receive approximately 0.2cc over a 1-2 minute injection. (Remember that the use of any other IV-delivered medications, including anesthetics, will reduce the volume of radiotracer that can be administered.)

Every effort is made to maintain an animal within normal parameters throughout an imaging session. Heat loss is minimized using a Delta-phase pad (Braintree Scientific, Braintree, MA) or warm-water circulating pad. (If you are fortunate enough to have good thermostatic control of the lab's ambient temperature, that is important too.) Bubble wrap is helpful but must be loose, and it does obstruct view of respiratory movement. Be cautious with lamps; anesthetized animals cannot move away from excessive heat, and a burn will not be immediately obvious due to their hair. We do not restrict food or water prior to anesthesia. (Remember that rodents do not vomit.) Typically, the procedure is not of a duration that requires supplemental fluid or energy. If you have older animals or the procedure is prolonged, warm fluids can be administered either subcutaneously or intraperitoneally (1-2 ml/30g mouse and 5 ml/200g rat). Isotonic saline (0.9%), dextrose-saline (4% dextrose-0.18% saline), and Lactated Ringers are options [Flecknell, 1996]. As previously mentioned, ocular lubricants are important to prevent corneal damage, particularly in rats [Rand, 2001]. Do not replace the animal on conventional bedding until they are alert and moving. Shavings can be inhaled and may stick to the nose or mouth. Remember that the anesthetic will inhibit their ability to thermoregulate, and rodents are sensitive to temperature changes. Regulate their ambient temperature; incubators can be excellent for this. Return to animal quarters is done only after the animal is ambulatory, and even then give consideration to maintaining body temperature, easy access to food and water, and periodic checkups.

If euthanasia is an endpoint, guidelines are provided in the Report of the American Veterinary Medical Association's Panel on Euthanasia [AVMA, 2000].

7. Regulations

I have saved the discussion of the regulations involved with animal imaging for last, but those of you involved with this process know that nothing happens until guidelines are met and protocols are approved. Our role as an imaging center has brought me into a working relationship with three different regulatory groups on campus: the animal care group, which also includes IACUC (Institutional Animal Care and Use Committee), the radiation control group, and the biosafety group. Their guidelines must be coordinated with the investigator's experiment before we can proceed. Because good research is always on the "cutting edge", there are times when specific issues have not yet been addressed. An animal checklist can help coordinate some of the information that expedites an imaging experiment.

For those of you writing your first animal imaging protocols, contact your institution's animal care division or IACUC for their guidelines. Federally funded projects are governed by the Animal Welfare Act (rodents are not currently regulated by this act, but this may change) and the Public Health Service Policy. The Public Health Service Policy is the law that supports the use of the Guide for the Care and Use of Laboratory Animals [NRC, 1996]. This guide is used by research institutions to set their standards. In addition, some funding is guided by The Good Laboratory Practices Act, specifically projects funded by the Environment Protection Agency and products developed for approval by the Food and Drug Administration. Some private funding agencies have their own specific requirements [IACUC, 1998].

This process takes time and can be frustrating. However, the goal of each of the regulatory groups is to assure that the well-being of all people and animals is given careful consideration. Although I may argue that some of the particulars are cumbersome and duplicative, I cannot argue their principle.

As you learn more about the physiology of the animals you work with and the pharmacology of the anesthetics and imaging agents, the quality of your research can only improve. This is reflected in more effective and efficient use of all your resources. Thank you for taking this first step; it is the courage to keep taking one step forward that makes science meaningful and valuable. Thank you, too, from these furry and not-so-furry critters.

References

[AVMA, 2000] "2000 Report of the AVMA Panel on Euthanasia," *Journal of the American Veterinary Medical Association*, vol. 218, pp. 669-696, 2001.

[Cornick-Seahorn, 2000] J. Cornick-Seahorn, "How to Mix the Preemptive Analgesic Cocktail," *Veterinary Forum*, March, pp. 33-36, 2000.

[Diven, 2003] K. Diven, "Inhalation Anesthetics in Rodents," *Lab Animal*, vol. 32, pp. 44-47, 2003.

[Flecknell, 1996] P. Flecknell, *Laboratory Animal Anesthesia*, Second Edition, Academic Press, San Diego, California, 1996.

[Fox, 2002] J. Fox, L. C. Anderson, F. M. Loew, F. W. Quimby, *Laboratory Animal Medicine*, Second Edition, Academic Press, San Diego, California, 2002.

[NRC, 1996] *Guide for the Care and Use of Laboratory Animals*, National Research Council, National Academy Press, 1996.

[Hartsfield, 1996] S. Hartsfield, J. Cornick-Seahorn, S. Cuvelliez, J. Gaynor, C. McGrath. "Commentary and recommendations on control of wast anesthetic gases in the workplace," *The Journal of the American Veterinary Medical Association*, vol. 209, pp. 75-77, 1996.

[Horne, 1998] D. Horne, B. Ogden, J. Houts, A. Hall. "A Nonrebreathing Anesthetic Delivery System for Mice," *Lab Animal*, vol. 27, pp. 32-34, 1998.

[IACUC, 1998] *The University of Arizona Institutional Animal Care and Use Committee Handbook*, IACUC, University of Arizona, 1998-1999.

[Kohn, 1997] D. F. Kohn, S. K. Wixson, W. J. White, G. J. Benson. *Anesthesia and Analgesia in Laboratory Animals*, Academic Press, New York, New York, 1997.

[Lukasik, 2001a] V. M. Lukasik, "Cadiovascular and respiratory effects of anesthetic drugs," *High-Resolution Imaging in Small Animals*, Rockville, Maryland, 2001.

[Lukasik, 2001b] V. M. Lukasik, "Inadvertent hypothermia," *High-Resolution Imaging in Small Animals*, Rockville, Maryland, 2001.

[Lukasik, 2003] V. M. Lukasik, "Animal anaesthesia for *in vivo* magnetic resonance," *NMR in Biomedicine*, vol. 16, pp. 459-467, 2003.

[Martin-Caballero, 2002] J. Martin-Caballero, A. Naranjo, E. de la Cueva. "Genetically Modified Mouse Health Reporting: A Need for Global Standardization," *Lab Animal*, vol. 32, pp. 38-45, 2002.

[Qiu, 1997] H. H. Qiu, G. P. Cofer, L. W Hedlund, G. A. Johnson. "Automated Feedback Control of Body Temperature afor Small Animal Studies with MR Microscopy," *IEEE Transactions on Biomedical Engineering*, vol. 44, pp. 1107-1113, 1997.

[Rand, 2001] M. S. Rand, "Handling, Restraint, and Techniques of Laboratory Rodents" Department of Animal Care, University of Arizona, May 2001.

[Shalev, 1997a] M. Shalev, "Resource, drugs for animal use, Acepromazine," *Lab Animal*, vol. 26, pp. 35-39, 1997.

[Shalev, 1997b] M. Shalev, "Resource, drugs for animal use, Xylazine," *Lab Animal*, vol. 26, pp. 35-39, 1997.

[Spikes, 1996] S. E. Spikes, S. L. Hoogstraten-Miller, G. F. Miller. "Comparison of Five Anesthetic Agents Administered Intraperitoneally in the Laboratory Rat," *Contemporary Topics by the American Association for Laboratory Animal Science*, vol. 35, pp. 53-56, 1996.

[White, 1987] W. J. White, K. J. Field. "Anesthesia and Surgery of Laboratory Animals," *Veterinary Clinics of North American: Small Animal Practice*, vol. 17, pp. 989-1015, 1987.

[Young, 1999] S. S. Young, "Anesthesia Monitoring Systems," 1999 ACLAM Forum.

Chapter 5

Objective Assessment of Image Quality

Matthew A. Kupinski and Eric Clarkson*

1. Introduction

Small-animal imaging has shown great promise in the areas of oncology, cardiology, molecular biology, drug discovery and development, and genetics [Green, 2001]. The demand for small-animal imaging has increased greatly with the recent advances in biomolecular research. Examples include functional genomics, functional protenomics, and molecular targeting of tumor cells or cells with other abnormalities. SPECT and PET imaging are of particular interest because these systems intrinsically image function instead of anatomy. Traditional thought has precluded SPECT and PET imaging of small animals because of the lack of resolution of these systems. In recent years at CGRI and other research facilities, numerous fast, high-resolution and high sensitivity SPECT imaging systems designed specifically for imaging small animals have been developed. These systems produce three-dimensional images of the distribution of radiotracers within the animal and, because these systems have no moving parts, dynamic studies can be readily performed. However, there are many components of such imaging systems that need to be optimized in order to best perform small-animal imaging studies.

Much of the recent research in medical imaging has dealt with the design of imaging systems or of image-processing techniques to produce "better" images [Chang, 2002, Kao, 2002, Penney, 2002, Oudkerk, 2002, Ludwid, 2002, Imbriaco, 2001, Kato, 2000, Yavuz and Fessler, 1999]. Thus, regardless of the imaging modality involved or the image-processing techniques used, a definition of what constitutes a "better" image is required. One common approach to the assessment of image quality is visual comparison by human observers. That is, an observer views a few images and then states whether she or he thinks the images produced by one system are better or worse than those produced by another system. This method is both subjective and irreproducible. Researchers also may focus on quantitative measures such as mean-squared error (MSE), resolution, sensitivity, or signal-to-noise ratio. However, there are many different definitions for each of these figures of merit, which impedes comparisons between different imaging systems, modalities,

*The University of Arizona, Optical Sciences Center, Department of Radiology, Tucson, Arizona

and researchers. Another problem associated with these figures of merit is that they are not always related to the performance of observers using the imaging systems on the tasks for which they are intended.

A more objective approach to assessing image quality is one based on task performance [Barrett, 1990, Barrett, 1995, Barrett, 1998, Metz, 1978]. To implement this approach, three elements must be specified: (a) the task for which the images are being produced, (b) the observer who will perform this task, and (c) the patient population being imaged. The primary tasks in small-animal imaging are classification and estimation. When there are only two classes, classification is usually referred to as detection. Detection tasks deal with determining whether an abnormality, usually a tumor, is present or not. Estimation tasks are those that require the observer to quantify a clinically relevant parameter of interest such as the cardiac ejection fraction or tumor location. The observer is usually a human observer for tumor-detection tasks and a computer observer or human-assisted computer observer for estimation tasks. However, we have previously shown that mathematically and statistically ideal observers are useful for performing imaging hardware optimizations [Barrett, 1998, Kupinski, 2003a]. We also have found that models of human observers can be used effectively to optimize imaging software and displays to maximize human-observer performance.

Modern imaging systems rely frequently on complicated hardware and sophisticated algorithms to produce useful digital images. It is essential that the imaging hardware used be optimized, enabling radiologists to best make decisions and quantify a patient's health status. This optimization of the hardware must take into account image-acquisition parameters such as the number of projection angles in SPECT. Hardware optimization also includes the physical design of the system, such as the design of the collimators in SPECT. Often, such system parameters are chosen via a trial-and-error approach or by using the results of simulation studies that do not incorporate a task-based figure of merit. A better approach would be to evaluate the system based on the performance of ideal observers performing a specific task with the raw data. This has the effect of optimizing the task-based information present in the data which the system produces. An alternative is to use human or human-model observer performance as a figure of merit for the optimization of hardware. However, a drawback to this approach is that the raw data from the imaging system must be processed through a reconstruction algorithm in order for these observers to make use of it.

In addition to hardware optimization, image reconstruction and processing algorithms are usually optimized based on subjective criteria or suspect figures of merit such as the MSE, a measure of image quality that does not take into account the continuous nature of the object functions being imaged. Because reconstructed images are intended for human observers and are produced for these observers to perform certain tasks, these algorithms should be optimized based on human or model-human observer performance on these tasks.

2. Image quality

The components necessary to carry out task-based assessment of image quality will be outlined in this section. We will describe the imaging chain from the continuous object to the final reconstructed image. We will also describe the types of tasks and observers that are relevant in small-animal imaging, and we will provide examples of figures of merit that measure observer performance on these tasks.

2.1 The imaging chain

We model imaging system using the equation

$$\boldsymbol{g} = \mathcal{H}\boldsymbol{f} + \boldsymbol{n}, \tag{5.1}$$

where $\boldsymbol{f}$ is the object being imaged (represented here as a function, or an infinite-dimensional vector[1]), $\mathcal{H}$ is an operator that describes how the imaging system maps the continuous object to discrete data, $\boldsymbol{n}$ is the noise in the system which is Poisson for SPECT system and, therefore, depends on $\boldsymbol{f}$), and $\boldsymbol{g}$ is the noisy image data returned by the imaging system. If we compare two different imaging systems ($\mathcal{H}_1$ and $\mathcal{H}_2$, for example), then we must accurately model all components of the imaging systems in order to properly measure the quality of the images produced on these systems.

The image data $\boldsymbol{g}$ may be an image ready for viewing or it may need processing before being viewed, such as with tomographic imaging systems. In the latter case, there is a further link in the imaging chain: the reconstruction algorithm $\mathcal{O}$, which produces an estimate $\hat{\boldsymbol{f}}$ of the original object $\boldsymbol{f}$ via

$$\hat{\boldsymbol{f}} = \mathcal{O}\boldsymbol{g}. \tag{5.2}$$

This estimate $\hat{\boldsymbol{f}}$ is an image intended for human viewing. This image may be an ordinary two-dimensional image, a three-dimensional reconstruction which may be viewed from different angles or slices, or it may be a four-dimensional reconstruction where the fourth dimension is time. There are other possibilities for added dimensions of the reconstructed images $\hat{\boldsymbol{f}}$, such as energy or wavelength.

2.1.1 Imaging operators. When the imaging operator $\mathcal{H}$ is applied to an object function $\boldsymbol{f}$, it produces the mean data vector averaged over noise realizations. Therefore, the operator $\mathcal{H}$ is determined by the physical characteristics of the imaging hardware. We will assume that $\mathcal{H}$ is a linear operator, although this is not necessary, and there are imaging modalities with nonlinear system operators. Nuclear-medicine imaging systems such as SPECT and PET are well described by linear operators.

For a linear imaging operator, the output at the mth detector element is given by the equation

$$g_m = \int_S h_m(\boldsymbol{r}) f(\boldsymbol{r})\, d\boldsymbol{r} + n_m, \tag{5.3}$$

where g_m and n_m are the mth elements of the vectors $\boldsymbol{g}$ and $\boldsymbol{n}$, respectively, $f(\boldsymbol{r})$ is the continuous object (now represented as a spatial function), $h_m(\boldsymbol{r})$ is the mth sensitivity function, and S is the field of view of the imaging system. There are M sensitivity functions $h_m(\boldsymbol{r})$ that together comprise the imaging operator $\mathcal{H}$.

The sensitivity functions $h_m()$ are often modeled by analytic expressions that are developed from a consideration of the geometry of the aperture-detector configurations, the physical processes involved in the detection of photons, and other physical effects, such as septal penetration. This is the usual procedure at CGRI when we are performing simulations in order to evaluate systems that have not been built yet. It is also the usual procedure in other laboratories before and after systems have been built. At CGRI, however, we usually measure the sensitivity functions for existing systems by measuring the detector outputs when a point source is moved around in the field of view. The advantages of this procedure are that it does not assume uniform detector response and perfect machining and alignment of apertures. These are all factors that are not accounted for in typical simulations but do not result in nonlinearities in the system operator.

2.1.2 Object ensembles. Observer performance is often limited by the normal background anatomy and not the noise in the imaging system. Thus, it is important to employ object models that can both interfere with the task of detection or estimation and are realistic. We have had recent experience with two object models: the lumpy object model [Rolland and Barrett, 1992, Kupinski, 2003, Kupinski, 2003a] and the clustered lumpy object model [Bochud, 1999, Chen and Barrett, 2003]. Both of these object models are composed of simple object components called "lumps." In general, these object models are characterized by a set of parameters that we denote with the vector $\boldsymbol{\Theta}$. These parameters include descriptors of the lump shape and values that characterize the distribution of the lumps within the object

Lumpy objects. The lumpy object model is generally composed of a random number of lumps placed randomly within the field of view (in either two or three dimensions). The lump function is often a Gaussian function but researchers have considered other lump functions as well [Gallas, 2001]. Two examples of lumpy objects are shown in Fig. 5.1. The two images shown were sampled from lumpy object models with different model parameters $\boldsymbol{\Theta}$. Lumpy backgrounds are desirable because statistical moments of the object ensemble can be computed analytically, and yet they are often a good representation of objects imaged in nuclear medicine. Another desirable property of lumpy backgrounds is that relatively complicated objects can be represented with a small number of parameters: the number and centers of the lumps for example. Finally, lumpy objects are easily mapped through the imaging equation (Eq. 5.3). Examples of planar nuclear-medicine images taken on a human patient are shown in Fig. 5.2. Regions within these images appear to follow a lumpy-object-like form.

Fitting object models. The object models we currently use have a set of parameters $\boldsymbol{\Theta}$ that characterize the statistics of the objects $\boldsymbol{f}$. These parameters

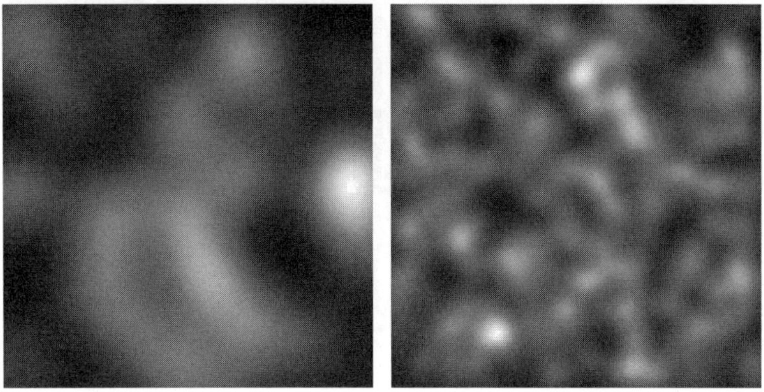

(a) (b)

Figure 5.1. Example of two-dimensional lumpy objects taken from two different object models (i.e., different Θ's).

include the mean number of lumps in the lumpy object model, as well as parameters describing the shape of the lumps. Because the objects sampled from these object models can be very different depending on the choice of Θ, it is important to choose the parameters of the object model such that the statistics of the simulated images match those of real images. That is to say, if our task is to detect tumors in nuclear medicine, then we must ensure that our object model statistically matches real background anatomy.

We have recently developed methods to determine the randomness in the objects being imaged using real images from a well-characterized imaging system [Kupinski, 2003]. These techniques determine the set of parameters Θ which produces images that best match (statistically) the images acquired by the real imaging system. All that is required is an accurate characterization of the imaging system ($\mathcal{H}$), which is usually obtained through simulation or measurement, and an understanding of the distribution of the noise in the imaging system. The techniques we have developed rely on knowledge of the characteristic functional of the object ensemble and a linear imaging system operator. With this information, we can analytically determine the characteristic function for the data produced by the imaging system and match it to the empirical characteristic function derived from data produced by the actual system.

The ability of an observer to perform a task such as detection or estimation is often limited by the background. Furthermore, to perform hardware optimizations, it is necessary to understand the statistical nature of the background object which produces the background image data. Hence, the methods we have developed will aid in providing accurate models of the backgrounds so that the imaging systems we are optimizing are as realistic as possible.

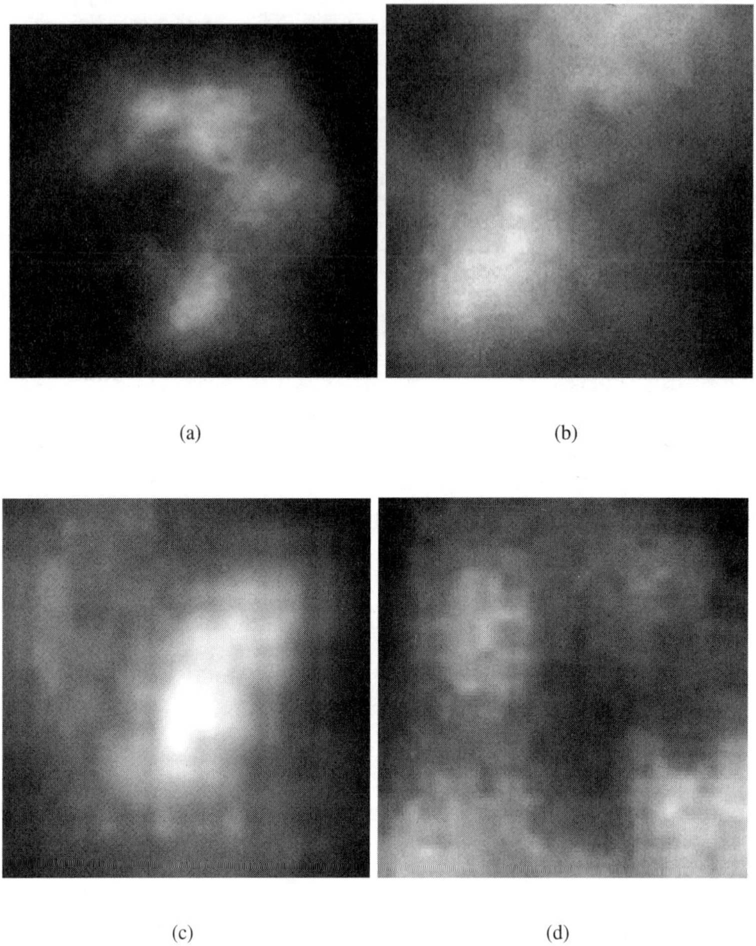

Figure 5.2. Real nuclear-medicine images that appear similar to lumpy objects.

2.2 Tasks

Any task in medical imaging can be framed as a classification task, an estimation task, or a combination of the two. For a classification task, there exists a finite number of classes from which the image is drawn at random. The goal in a classification task is to determine to which class the image belongs. The simplest classification task occurs when there are only two classes. This is often referred to as a detection task. Detection tasks are usually performed by humans or computer-assisted humans. The latter is often referred to as computer-aided diagnosis (CAD).

An estimation task is one in which the goal is to quantify some parameter of interest relating to the patient's health. The estimate is generally non-discrete and usually computed by a computer or a human-assisted computer. An example of an estimation task is determination of a patient's cardiac ejection fraction, the fraction of blood pumped out of the left ventricle at the end of each heart cycle. Another example is the determination of the width of a vessel when assessing the extent of stenosis.

A combination estimation/detection task requires the detection of an abnormality together with an estimate of some parameter of the abnormality. The detection of a tumor and the estimation of its location is one example of a combination estimation/detection task. Because these tasks involve detection, they are usually performed by humans or computer-assisted humans.

2.3 Observers

Defining the task is only one component necessary to perform a task-based assessment of image quality. Another necessary component is the specification of the observer performing the task. As we have alluded to earlier, observers can be human, model human, mathematically ideal, or computer observers. The observer is responsible for using the image to produce a decision in a classification task or a set of numbers in an estimation task.

The human observers in medical imaging are usually trained professionals such as radiologists or cardiologists. Trained professionals are often too expensive or too busy to aid in the assessment of image quality. Thus, naive observers are often employed to perform these studies. The time required to perform a study even with naive observers is often prohibitively long.

A model-human observer is a computer program designed to mimic the average performance of human observers. These model-human observers employ knowledge gained from neurological and psychophysical studies of the visual system. Model-human observers are usually task specific. It is difficult to model the performance of professional observers on a wide range of complicated tasks because they employ a large knowledge base in order to make their decisions. Thus, model-human observers are designed to mimic the performance of naive observers on relatively simple tasks. The most common example is the detection of a known signal at a known location. These observers can quickly analyze a large number of images, unlike human observers.

It is sometimes advantageous to use a mathematically ideal observer when quantifying the quality of an imaging system. Such an observers uses the raw data, which may not be an image, to make a decision or estimate a parameter. For hardware optimization, it is especially useful to use the performance of an ideal observer since it does not depend on the reconstruction algorithm or other image processing steps. There are generally two types of ideal observers for detection tasks: Bayesian ideal observers and ideal linear observers. For estimation tasks, one can employ the unbiased estimator with the smallest possible variance as the ideal estimator. For combined tasks, it is not clear at this point how to define an ideal observer unless the costs of various decisions are known.

Computer observers are programs that analyze images and produce decisions for classification tasks or parameter estimates for estimation tasks. Some of these observers are fully automatic in that they require no human intervention, while

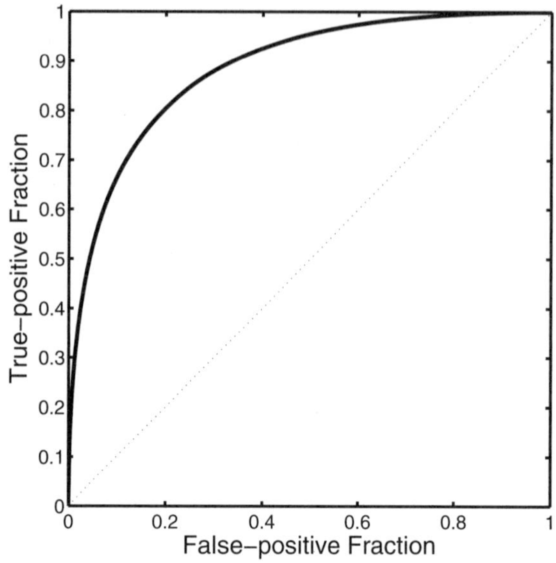

Figure 5.3. An example ROC curve. The closer the curve is to the upper-left corner, the better the performance of the observer. The dotted line shows the performance of a guessing observer.

others require some limited human assistance. An example of the latter situation is when a radiologist outlines a region of interest in an image, and the computer estimates the amount of activity in that region. The decisions of fully automatic computer observers, unlike those of human observers and human-assisted computer observers, are completely reproducible.

2.4 Figures of merit

For detection tasks, we wish to evaluate the performance of an observer attempting to detect abnormalities (such as tumors) in images. To compute this performance, we use the area under the receiver operating characteristic (ROC) curve [Egan, 1961, Egan, 1975, Metz, 1978, Metz, 1986, Metz, 1989, Metz, 1990] denoted by AUC (area under curve). The ROC curve is a plot of the true-positive fraction (TPF) versus the false-positive fraction (FPF) because the confidence threshold of the observer is varied from its lowest value to its highest value (see Fig. 5.3 for an example). The TPF is the probability that the observer will decide that a tumor is present when a tumor is actually present. The FPF is the probability that the observer will decide that a tumor is present when it is not present. The AUC is widely accepted as a measure of performance on tumor detection tasks [Hanley, 1989]. A perfect observer (never makes a mistake) has an AUC of 1, while a guessing observer has an AUC of 0.5. The AUC can be computed for human observers, mathematical observers, and, in many situations, the ideal observer [Clarkson and Barrett, 2000, Kupinski, 2003a].

We estimate the AUC for an observer in one of two ways. The first is to perform a two-alternative forced choice (2AFC) experiment in which the observer is presented two images and is forced to decide which image contains the signal. They know *a priori* that one of the images does not contain the signal and the other does. After presentation of a large number of pairs of images, the fraction of pairs where the observer correctly identified the abnormal image is an estimate of the AUC. The statistics of this estimate are well known as a function of number of images, number of observers, and true AUC value. The other method we employ to estimate the AUC is to perform a rating-scale experiment where the observer's output is not simply a decision but a number indicating their confidence that the signal is present in a single image. After many images have been rated, this type of data can be used to produce an estimate of the ROC curve which, in turn, is used to produce an estimate of the AUC.

A second figure of merit for detection tasks can be computed using confidence ratings. The SNR, or d' value, is defined as the ratio of the difference between the means of the two ratings under each class to the standard deviation of the ratings. For Gaussian decision-variable data, this figure of merit is known to have a one-to-one correspondence with AUC.

When measuring the performance of an observer performing an estimation task, we generally focus on two statistics of the estimator: the bias and the variance. The bias describes how close the observer is, on average, to estimating the true value of the parameter of interest (e.g., cardiac EF). The variance describes the reproducibility of the observer's estimates. One figure of merit that combines these two statistics is the mean-squared error (MSE) which measures, on average, the square of the difference between the estimate and the true value of the parameter. Mathematically, the MSE is a sum of the variance with the square of the bias. This is not to be confused with the MSE between the voxels in a reconstructed image and a voxelized object.

The Fisher information matrix is a valuable tool for determining a figure of merit for estimation tasks. One can use the Fisher information matrix to determine the minimum possible variance that an unbiased estimator could possibly have. (An unbiased estimator is one for which the bias is zero.) There are often estimators that come close to achieving this variance. Furthermore, maximum-likelihood estimators are known to always asymptotically approach this lower bound. One can also extend the Fisher information matrix formalism to account for biased estimators.

Another figure of merit for estimation tasks is the Bayes risk. To utilize this figure of merit, one must develop a formula that assigns a cost to every possible combination of true parameter value and estimate of that value. By averaging this formula over both the true parameter value and the estimates, one obtains the Bayes risk for that estimator. Often the cost formula used in Bayes risk is a function of the bias and the variance, although this is not necessary. For this figure of merit, one also needs to have a prior distribution on the true parameter that is being estimated.

3. The Hotelling observer

A complete treatment on the types of observers for both detection and estimation tasks is beyond the scope of this single chapter. Thus, we will focus on one class of observers used for signal-detection tasks that have been found to be both useful and practical: the Hotelling observers. These observers include: the Hotelling observer, the channelized Hotelling observer using anthropomorphic channels, and the channelized Hotelling observer using efficient channels. These three different observers can be used to mimic either the performance of a human observer or an ideal observer. The Hotelling observer will be discussed in this section, leaving the channelized variants of this observer for the next section.

The Hotelling observer is defined as the linear observer that maximizes the signal-to-noise ratio (SNR) of the observer's confidence ratings. This observer is defined as linear, implying that some template $\boldsymbol{w}$ is applied to each image $\boldsymbol{g}$ to produce the decision variable or confidence rating[2]. That is,

$$t = \boldsymbol{w}_{\text{Hot}}^{\dagger}\boldsymbol{g}, \tag{5.4}$$

where the vectors $\boldsymbol{w}_{\text{Hot}}$ and $\boldsymbol{g}$ have the same dimension, say $M \times 1$. To maximize the SNR of the confidence ratings, the Hotelling observer employs knowledge of the first- and second-order statistics of the image data. That is,

$$\boldsymbol{w}_{\text{Hot}} = K_g^{-1}\Delta\overline{\boldsymbol{g}}, \tag{5.5}$$

where K is the $M \times M$ covariance matrix, and $\Delta\overline{\boldsymbol{g}}$ is the difference in the means of $\boldsymbol{g}$ under both signal-present and signal-absent hypotheses. Using this information, the SNR can be computed as

$$d' = \sqrt{\Delta\overline{\boldsymbol{g}}^{\dagger} K_g^{-1} \Delta\overline{\boldsymbol{g}}}. \tag{5.6}$$

Equation 5.6 is often difficult to evaluate in practice because it involves knowledge of the first- and second-order statics on the image data. While the difference in the means might be relatively easy to estimate, the covariance matrix K may be difficult to estimate because it has M^2 elements. For example, if a planar imaging system produces image data that have 256×256 elements, then $M = 256^2$ and K is a $256^2 \times 256^2$ matrix. Not only must we estimate the covariance matrix K, we must also *invert* this large matrix. The issues involved in estimating and inverting this large covariance matrix are summarized in [Barrett, 2001].

4. The channelized Hotelling observer

Many of the computation difficulties associated with the Hotelling observer can be avoided by using the channelized Hotelling observer. The channelized Hotelling observer introduces a set of channels that reduce the dimensionality of the image data from an M-vector to a N-vector where N is the number of channels and $N \ll M$. Because a channel operator is a linear operator, it can be represented as a matrix multiplication, i.e.,

$$\boldsymbol{v} = T\boldsymbol{g}, \tag{5.7}$$

where $\boldsymbol{v}$ is the $N \times 1$ channel output for image $\boldsymbol{g}$, and T is the $N \times M$ channel operator. The Hotelling observer performance is now computed using channel outputs $\boldsymbol{v}$s instead of image-data $\boldsymbol{g}$s. That is,

$$d' = \sqrt{\Delta \overline{\boldsymbol{v}}^{\dagger} K_{v}^{-1} \Delta \overline{\boldsymbol{v}}}, \tag{5.8}$$

where K_v is the $N \times N$ channel covariance matrix, and $\Delta \overline{\boldsymbol{v}}$ is the different in the means of the channels under the two hypotheses. Because we have applied a dimensionality-reduction step, the estimation and inversion of the covariance matrix K_v is trivial (N is often between 3 and 15).

4.1 Efficient channels

So far, we have said nothing about the channel operator T other than it reduces dimensionality, which eases computation. There are two common types of channel operators: efficient and anthropomorphic. Efficient channels are designed to mimic the performance of the Hotelling observer. Thus, these channels are designed to extract all of the necessary information from the images (into the vectors $\boldsymbol{v}$) so that the SNR from the channelized Hotelling observer is approximately that of the Hotelling observer. In practice, this approximation is asymptotic as the number of channels increases. For signal-known-exactly (SKE) detection tasks, where the signal to be detected is radially symmetric, Gallas showed that Laguerre-Gaussian channels are efficient [Gallas, 2001]. In fact, he shows that only 10 Laguerre-Gaussian channels were needed to accurately approximate the performance of the Hotelling observer.

4.2 Anthropomorphic channels

The channel operator can also be chosen to mimic the performance of human observers. This is done using channels that are designed to mimic the way in which the human-visual system processes images. It is well known that the human-visual system contain frequency-selective channels. For radially symmetric signals and SKE detection tasks, these channels are radial, band-pass filters. The so-called difference-of-Gaussian channels have been shown to accurately mimic the performance of human observers for a wide variety of background statistics and image-noise statistics [Abbey and Barrett, 2001].

5. Summary

To improve medical imaging systems and algorithms, there must be a clear and quantitative definition of image quality. We take the approach that image quality should be based upon the performance of an observer performing a medically relevant task. In this chapter, we have presented the basic philosophy of task-based assessment of image quality. We have discussed the uses of task-based image quality measures for optimizing imaging hardware and reconstruction algorithms, the importance of background statistics and proper system modeling, and, finally, a practical and useful observer model called the Hotelling observer was presented.

The computational time required to objectively assess image quality is still far greater than the time required by subjective approaches or approaches that use measures not related to a task and an observer. Thus, the acceptance of these approaches in many areas of medical imaging has been slow. However, as these techniques become more advanced and more efficient, their use in medical imaging will increase. Clearly, task-based approaches to assessing image quality will play a vital role in future system developments and in properly understanding the strengths and limitations of various systems and algorithms.

Notes

1. Bold symbols denote vectors.

2. These observers may act on the raw image data $\boldsymbol{g}$ or on reconstructed images $\hat{\boldsymbol{f}}$. We use image data for simplicity.

References

[Abbey and Barrett, 2001] C. K. Abbey, H. H. Barrett. "Human- and model-observer performance in ramp-spectrum noise: Effects of regularization and object variability." *Journal of the Optical Society of America A*, vol. 18, pp. 473–488, 2001.

[Barrett, 1990] H. H. Barrett. "Objective assessment of image quality: Effects of quantum noise and object variability." *Journal of the Optical Society of America A*, vol. 7(7), pp. 1266–1278, 1990.

[Barrett, 1998] H. H. Barrett, C. K. Abbey, E. Clarkson. "Objective assessment of image quality. III. ROC metrics, ideal observers, and likelihood-generating functions." *Journal of the Optical Society of America A*, vol. 15, pp. 1520–1535, 1998.

[Barrett, 1995] H. H. Barrett, J. L. Denny, R. F. Wagner, K. J. Myers. "Objective assessment of image quality. II: Fisher information, Fourier crosstalk, and figures of merit for task performance." *Journal of the Optical Society of America A*, vol. 12, pp. 834–852, 1995.

[Barrett, 2001] H. H. Barrett, K. J. Myers, B. D. Gallas, E. Clarkson, H. Zhang. "Megalopinakophobia: its symptoms and cures." In Larry E. Antonuk and Martin J. Yaffe, editors, *Medical Imaging 2001: Physics of Medical Imaging*, pp. 299–307. SPIE, 2001.

[Bochud, 1999] F. Bochud, C. K. Abbey, M. Eckstein. "Statistical texture synthesis of mammographic images with clustered lumpy backgrounds." *Optics Express*, vol. 4(1), pp. 33–43, 1999.

[Chang, 2002] S. C. Chang, P. H. Lai, W. L. Chen, H. H. Weng, J. T. Ho, J. S. Wang, C. Y. Chang, H. B. Pan, C. F. Yang. "Diffusion-weighted MRI features of brain abscess and cystic or necrotic brain tumors - Comparison with conventional MRI." *Clin. Imaging*, vol. 26, pp. 227–236, 2002.

[Chen and Barrett, 2003] L. Chen, H. H. Barrett. "Optimizing lens-coupled digital radiographic imaging systems based on model observers performance." In

Dev. P. Chakraborty and Elizabeth A. Krupinski, editors, *Medical Imaging 2003: Image Perception, Observer Performance, and Technology Assessment*, pp. 63–70. SPIE, 2003.

[Clarkson and Barrett, 2000] E. Clarkson, H. H. Barrett. "Approximations to ideal-observer performance on signal-detection tasks." *Applied Optics*, vol. 39(11), pp. 1783–1794, 2000.

[Egan, 1961] J. P. Egan, G. Z. Greenberg, A. I. Schulman. "Operating characteristics, signal detectability, and the method of free response." *Journal of the Acoustical Society of America*, vol. 33, pp. 993–1007, 1961.

[Egan, 1975] J. P. Egan. *Signal Detection Theory and ROC Analysis.* Academic Press, New York, 1975.

[Gallas, 2001] B. D. Gallas. *Signal Detection in Lumpy Backgrounds.* Ph.D. dissertation, The University of Arizona, 2001.

[Green, 2001] M. V. Green, J. Seidel, J. J. Vaquero, E. Jagoda, I. Lee, W. C. Eckelman. "High resolution PET, SPECT, and projection imaging in small animals." *Computerized Medical Imaging and Graphics*, vol. 25(2), pp. 79–86, 2001.

[Hanley, 1989] J. A. Hanley. "Receiver operating characteristic (ROC) methodology: The state of the art." *Critical Review in Diagnostic Imaging*, vol. 29, pp. 307–335, 1989.

[Imbriaco, 2001] M. Imbriaco, S. Del Vecchio, A. Riccardi, L. Pace, F. Di Salle, F. Di Gennaro, M. Salvatore, A. Sodano. "Scintimammography with Tc-99m-MIBI versus dynamic MRI for noninvasive characterization of breast masses." *Eur. J. Nucl. Med.*, vol. 28, pp. 56–63, 2001.

[Kao, 2002] C. Kao, J. Feng, X. Pan, B. Penney. "Sinogram restoration filters for SPECT and PET reconstructions." *J. Nucl. Med.*, vol. 43, pp. 874, 2002.

[Kato, 2000] M. Kato, S. Saji, M. Kanematsu, D. Fukada, K. Miya, T. Umemoto, K. Kunieda, Y. Sugiyama, H. Takao, Y. Kawaguchi, Y. Takagi, H. Kondo, H. Hoshi. "Detection of lymph-node metastases in patients with gastric carcinoma: Comparison of three MR imaging pulse sequences." *Abdom. Imaging*, vol. 25, pp. 25–29, 2000.

[Kupinski, 2003] M. A. Kupinski, E. Clarkson, J. W. Hoppin, L. Chen, H. H. Barrett. "Experimental determination of object statistics from noisy images." *JOSA A*, vol. 20, pp. 421–429, 2003.

[Kupinski, 2003a] M. A. Kupinski, J. W. Hoppin, E. Clarkson, H. H. Barrett. "Ideal-observer computation in medical imaging using Markov-chain Monte Carlo." *JOSA A*, vol. 20, pp. 430–438, 2003.

[Ludwid, 2002] K. Ludwig, H. Lenzen, K. F. Kamm, T. M. Link, S. Diederich, D. Wormanns, W. Heindel. "Performance of a flat-panel detector in detecting artificial bone lesions: Comparison with conventional screen-film and storage-phosphor radiography." *Radiology*, vol. 222, pp. 453–459, 2002.

[Metz, 1978] Charles E. Metz. "Basic principles of ROC analysis." *Seminars in Nuclear Medicine*, vol. VIII, pp. 283–298, 1978.

[Metz, 1986] C. E. Metz. "ROC methodology in radiologic imaging." *Investigative Radiology*, vol. 21, pp. 720–733, 1986.

[Metz, 1989] C. E. Metz. "Some practical issues of experimental design and data analysis in radiological ROC studies." *Investigative Radiology*, vol. 24, pp. 234–245, 1989.

[Metz, 1990] C. E. Metz, J.-H. Shen, B. A. Herman. "New methods for estimating a binormal ROC curve from continuously-distributed test results." In *Joint Meeting of the American Statistical Society and the Biometric Society*, 1990.

[Oudkerk, 2002] M. Oudkerk, C. G. Torres, B. Song, M. Konig, J. Grimm, J. Fernandez-Cuadrado, B. O. de Beeck, M. Marquardt, P. van Dijk, J. C. de Groot. "Characterization of liver lesions with mangafodipir trisodiumenhanced MR imaging: Multicenter study comparing MR and dualphase spiral CT." *Radiology*, vol. 223, pp. 517–524, 2002.

[Penney, 2002] B. C. Penney, J. Feng, X. Pan. "Comparison of convolution and triple-energy-window spill-down and scatter correction in Tc-99m/In-111 SPECT." *J. Nucl. Med.*, vol. 43, pp. 907, 2002.

[Rolland and Barrett, 1992] J. P. Rolland, Harrison H. Barrett. "Effect of random background inhomogeneity on observer detection performance." *Journal of the Optical Society of America A*, vol. 9, pp. 649–658, 1992.

[Yavuz and Fessler, 1999] M. Yavuz, J. A. Fessler. "Penalized-likelihood estimators and noise analysis for randomsprecorrected PET transmission scans." *IEEE Trans. Med. Imaging*, vol. 18, pp. 665–674, 1999.

Chapter 6

SPECT Imager Design and Data-Acquisition Systems

Lars R. Furenlid, Yi-Chun Chen, and Hyunki Kim*

1. Introduction

In this chapter, we discuss the process of turning raw gamma-ray detector technology into a gamma-ray camera, how to combine one or more cameras with a mechanical gantry to form a complete small-animal imaging system, and how to obtain electrical signals digitized and into a form useable by position-estimation and three-dimensional reconstruction algorithms. We start with a survey of the optical image-forming principles available and discuss how they perform with short-wavelength (< 1 Å) radiation. We next consider materials and fabrication techniques that can be used to construct optical elements such as pinholes and collimators, and then discuss the critical tradeoffs between field-of-view, sensitivity, and magnification that characterize a small-animal SPECT imager's configuration. We discuss the merits of detailed calibration and describe the techniques adopted in our own laboratory for direct measurement of camera and system response.

In the second section of this chapter, we discuss the nature of the electric signals produced by currently available detector technologies and discuss strategies for readout. Included in this discussion are options for analog versus digital filtering and event detection. We compare and contrast list-mode and bitmap data accumulation and make some observations about how the rapid pace of advancements in computing and networking technology affect decisions about acquisition architecture. We conclude the chapter with short discussions of multi-modality imaging, dynamic imaging, and techniques for capturing and registering data from physiological monitors.

2. Gamma-ray optics

Virtually any of the physical processes that bend, block, or constrain the travel of light can be used to form an optical image. The effects available for exploitation are refraction, reflection, diffraction, and absorption (we ignore gravitational lensing because it is not suitable for the laboratory). While conventional optics used with the visible wavelengths, such as glass lenses, do not function with gamma rays,

*The University of Arizona, Department of Radiology, Tucson, Arizona

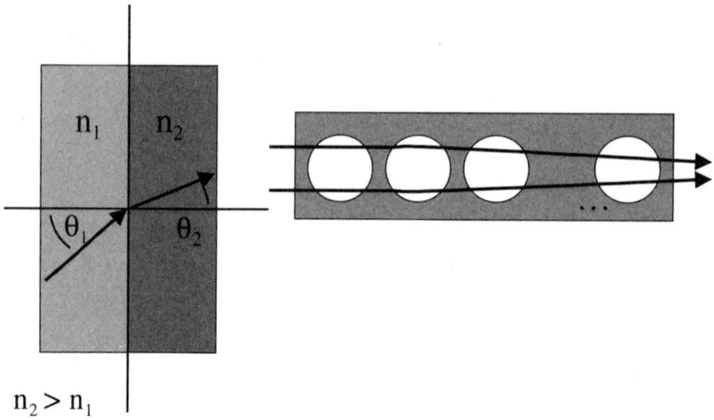

Figure 6.1. The geometry of refraction and the compound x-ray lens.

there are ways of affecting the paths of very short wavelength (< 1 Å) light if the right combinations of geometry and materials are used. Because the objective of this chapter is to discuss SPECT imager design, it is useful to consider what optical elements could be used as the link between the object and detector and why they are or are not feasible choices.

2.1 Refraction

Refraction is the bending of light moving through an interface between materials with different refractive indices. The complex refractive index describes the propagation velocity of light in the medium in the real part and the absorbance of light by the medium in the imaginary part. Both of these properties depend on the wavelength of the radiation, and it is convenient to write an energy-dependent index of refraction as

$$n(\lambda) = 1 - \delta(\lambda) - i\beta(\lambda). \tag{6.1}$$

Snell's law describes the angular change which a ray undergoes in traversing an interface in the geometry shown in Fig. 6.1. In the conventional scalar formulation, it is written as

$$n_1 \sin\theta_1 = n_2 \sin\theta_2. \tag{6.2}$$

Light is bent toward the interface normal when moving from an optically less dense to a more dense medium. The challenges with short-wavelength radiation are two-fold: 1) $\delta(\lambda)$ is typically $< 10^{-4}$ so that the angular deflections are very small, and 2) air is often a denser medium, optically, so concave lenses are required.

Nonetheless, a refractive lens for x rays and low-energy gamma rays has been invented [Snigirev, 1996] that may find future application in specialized small-animal SPECT systems. There are, however, a number of limitations. Because the angular deviation from traversing a single interface is small, compound (multi-element) lenses are required, each with a small radius of curvature. This results

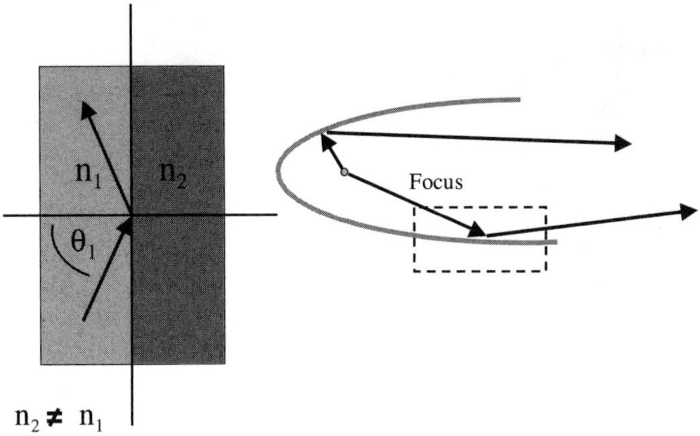

Figure 6.2. Left: The geometry of reflection. Right: Image formation via glancing angle reflection from an elliptical optic.

in an optic with an extremely large f-number ($\sim$ 1000), long focal length (1 m), and a consequently small field of view. Compound refractive lenses for x rays are currently used with synchrotron sources, but they may find use in emission tomography with further development.

2.2 Reflection

Reflection is the redirection of light rays about the normal at interfaces between media of different indices of refraction. When Snell's law can no longer be solved for a refracted ray, i.e.,

$$\sin \theta_1 = n_2/n_1, \tag{6.3}$$

total external or internal reflection occurs. (Internal versus external reflection are defined by whether $n_1 > n_2$ or vice versa.) Once again, the fundamental problem with short-wavelength radiation is that the refractive indices are so close to unity that the critical angles are very glancing. The reflectivity of the mirror also is a factor; for a given wavelength, it is a strong function of the materials chosen, the finish achieved, and the working angle of incidence.

The reflecting solid surface that brings light from a source point to a focal point is the ellipse of rotation. The geometry for image formation via glancing-angle reflection is shown in Fig. 6.2. The shape of the reflecting mirror is determined by the selected angle of incidence and the focal length. There are a number of challenges in fabricating glancing-angle mirrors, including the production of the aspheric reflecting surface, the polishing to atom-scale RMS smoothness, and the fact that significant angular acceptance requires substantial mirror length (tens of centimeters). As with the compound refractive x-ray lens, a single glancing-angle mirror is an optic with an extremely high f-number and consequently small field of view for practical arrangements.

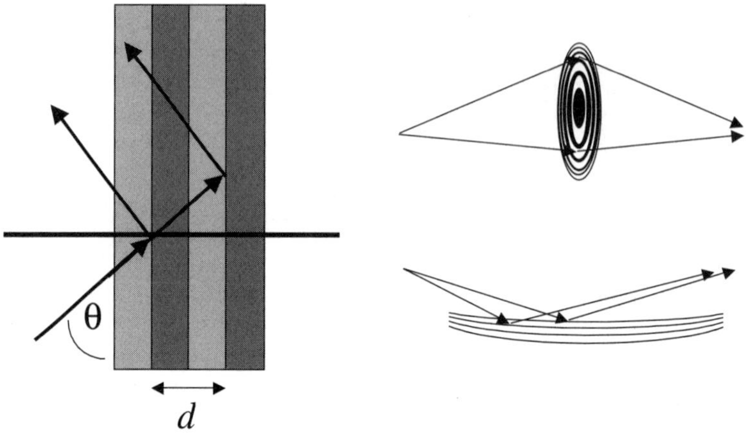

Figure 6.3. Left: The geometry of diffraction. Right: Image formation via Fresnel zone plate (above) and multilayer mirror (below).

It is possible to design a more efficient reflecting optic by creating an arrangement of thin shell mirrors, each capturing an annular segment of the emission [Serlemitsos, 1988, Serlemitsos, 1996]. Focal lengths remain long (> 1 meter), and a great deal of precision is required in fabrication to achieve a small focal spot. Nonetheless, small-animal imagers based on these kinds of mirror assemblies are under development.

An attractive alternative approach is the use of tapered microcapillaries. These work on a principle of total reflectance in much the same manner as optical fibers are used with visible wavelengths. They rapidly become less effective as wavelength decreases for the same reasons that single mirrors do: critical angles become very shallow, and surface roughness becomes increasingly significant.

2.3 Diffraction

Diffraction is the redirection of light by the constructive interference of reflections from a periodic structure. The criterion for constructive interference is given by Bragg's Law:

$$n\lambda = 2d \sin\theta \tag{6.4}$$

where $n(1, 2, 3 \ldots)$ is the "order", λ is the gamma-ray wavelength, d is the spacing between layers, and the geometry is as shown in Fig. 6.3.

Because λ is small for gamma rays and d is limited to approximately one atomic diameter and larger, $\sin\theta$ is small, and glancing angles are once again required. However, the benefits of constructive interference greatly increase the reflectivity over what could be achieved with a mirror at the same angle.

Conventional diffractive elements are perfect crystals, employed in either the Bragg (in which the incident and refracted rays are on the same side of the crystal) or Laue (in which the light passes through the crystal) geometries. However, unless the crystals are bent, they have no focusing or image-forming properties. There are, however, two fabricated diffractive optical elements that do find application for focusing short-wavelength light: Fresnel zone plates and multilayer mirrors [Hildebrandt, 2002].

The Fresnel zone plate has a set of concentric rings, typically produced with photolithographic etching techniques, with spacing that varies by radial distance such that the Bragg equation is satisfied for every ray originating at the object point. They are employed very successfully in x-ray microscopes, especially at 1 keV and lower photon energies, where the ring spacings are commensurate with standard photolithographic length scales. A Fresnel zone plate is always designed around an optimal wavelength, and its performance degrades rapidly as a function of the energy difference from the optimum.

The multilayer mirror is an elliptical optic fabricated via coating deposition techniques in such a way that the d-spacing matches the reflection angle for the design wavelength. When compared to a simple reflecting surface, the multilayer structure has much higher reflectivity at an extended range of angles. It can hence have shorter focal lengths (smaller radius of curvature) and wider angular acceptance. Creating an elliptical multilayer mirror is not an easy task; extraordinary control is required over layer thicknesses in combination with mirror figures. Vapor deposition coaters with built-in optical metrology are one technical approach.

All of the optical principles discussed so far have been demonstrated to work with photon energies in the sub-30 keV range, albeit with small fields of view and low efficiencies. They may thus be relevant for small-animal SPECT imaging using ^{125}I tracers, but further developments are necessary for work with the $>$100 keV gamma-ray emissions from clinical radioisotopes such as ^{99m}Tc or ^{111}In.

2.4 Absorption

Absorption is the least glamorous, but currently most effective, optical principle for image formation with singly emitted gamma rays. A pixel or area of detector is made sensitive to a particular volume of object space by simply blocking all other lines of sight. In practice, even absorption presents challenges as an image-forming principle at short wavelengths, because choice of materials and aperture designs play important roles in the optical performance.

The absorption of light by matter follows an exponential power law that depends on an energy-dependent absorption coefficient that at gamma-ray energies can be derived from the constituent atomic absorption coefficients weighted by relative amount, and the material density:

$$\frac{I(E)}{I_0(E)} = \exp\left[-\mu(Z, E)d\right], \tag{6.5}$$

where (Z, E) is the linear absorption coefficient, and d is the thickness of the material. Sample calculations based on tabulated cross-sections [McMaster, 1969] quickly reveal that the key to achieving absorption is high atomic number; attempting to block x rays or gamma rays with thick, but low Z, materials is never a good approach. Table 6.1 presents the absorption coefficients at 140 keV of some

Table 6.1. Properties of common elements used for shielding and aperture construction when used with 140 keV photons.

Element	Z	Absorption (cm^{-1})	Absorption Length (mm)	Transittance (1/8" material)
Pb	82	26.823	0.373	1/5,000
W	74	36.333	0.275	1/100,000
Au	79	42.629	0.235	1/1,000,000
Pt	78	43.831	0.228	1/1,000,000

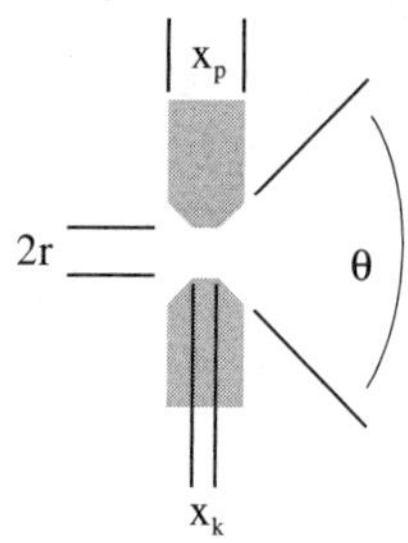

Figure 6.4. The geometric variables of a physical pinhole. r is aperture radius, x_p is overall pinhole thickness, x_k is keel-edge width, and θ is opening angle.

common elemental metals and rule-of-thumb numbers for what fraction of incident photons pass through an eighth-of-an-inch stock. These numbers can be used to demonstrate an important design principle: in order to have an effective absorbing aperture, the area of the opening must be large relative to the product of the area where light should be blocked and the transmittance. Otherwise, the image will be compromised by leakage photons.

2.5 Pinhole collimators

The three usual optical elements based on absorption are pinholes, collimators, and coded apertures. The pinhole is the simplest physical structure; the idealized version is an opening through an infinitely thin sheet of infinitely absorbing material. In practice, pinholes are a compromise of material choice, thickness, and shape arrived at by considering the desired clear opening, the angular acceptance, the extent of vignetting, and the tolerable amount of leakage. The geometric variables of a pinhole are shown in Fig. 6.4. In our laboratory, we currently manufacture pinholes as gold inserts for mounting in milled recesses in lead sheets or cylinders or in cast Cerrobend. We also work with machinable tungsten (W) alloys. For further discussion of pinhole design, see Chapter 5 in this book.

The dimensions and location of a pinhole aperture between the object and gamma-ray detector are critical factors in the final imager's performance [Jaszczak, 1994].

There is, in general, a set of trade-offs between the size of the field of view, the magnification, the sensitivity, and the resolution that must be understood when an instrument is designed [Barrett, 1981]. The sensitivity of the system, the number of counts recorded in the detector for a unit quantity of radioactivity in the object, depends on the geometric efficiency of the pinhole as well as the quantum efficiency of the detector. (For this discussion, we consider the detector dimensions, number of resolvable elements, and quantum efficiency as fixed and focus on the role of the aperture.) The pinhole's geometric efficiency is given by the ratio between the solid angle subtended by the aperture's boundary and 4π steradians of isotropic emission. For a geometry where the pinhole radius r is small relative to the distance to the center of the field of view d, this can be approximated by the ratio of the area of the circle of radius r to the surface area of the sphere of radius b

$$E = \frac{r^2}{4b^2}. \tag{6.6}$$

Efficiency can, of course, be increased by using a larger pinhole, but only at the expense of introducing blur. This is easily seen in the construction of Fig. 6.5ii. A point at the center of the field of view projects through the pinhole as a circle with a diameter given by

$$R_{\text{pinhole}} = 2r(a+b)/a. \tag{6.7}$$

The effect of pinhole size on the resolution of the final three-dimensional reconstruction is not obvious, however, because iterative algorithms using measured point spread functions can at least partially compensate for pinhole blur. The measurement of calibration data will be discussed below and in Chapter 12 of this book.

The magnification in a pinhole system,

$$M = -a/b, \tag{6.8}$$

is easily understood from the construction in Fig. 6.5iii. While our examples consider activity at the center of the field of view, it should be noted that, if the object has dimensions that are not negligible to the center-to-pinhole distance, there can be a large difference between the magnifications of activity close to the pinhole and on the opposite side.

The field of view arises from the projection of the detector face back through the pinhole, undergoing a minimization by the inverse of the magnification (assuming $M > 1$). The FOV is, of course, actually a volume that is the result of rotating the detector projection through the orbit that will be used to acquire the tomographic data. While one might intuitively suspect that any activity outside the common FOV would confound the reconstruction process, iterative algorithms have been found to be somewhat tolerant of such a circumstance.

The final construction in Fig. 6.5v shows the approximate effect of the detector pixel size or otherwise determined smallest resolvable element on reconstructed resolution. Once again, the pixel is minified in the projection back through the pinhole (assuming that there is > 1 magnification in the forward direction). Detector resolution does immediately affect the tomographic reconstruction quality, and apart

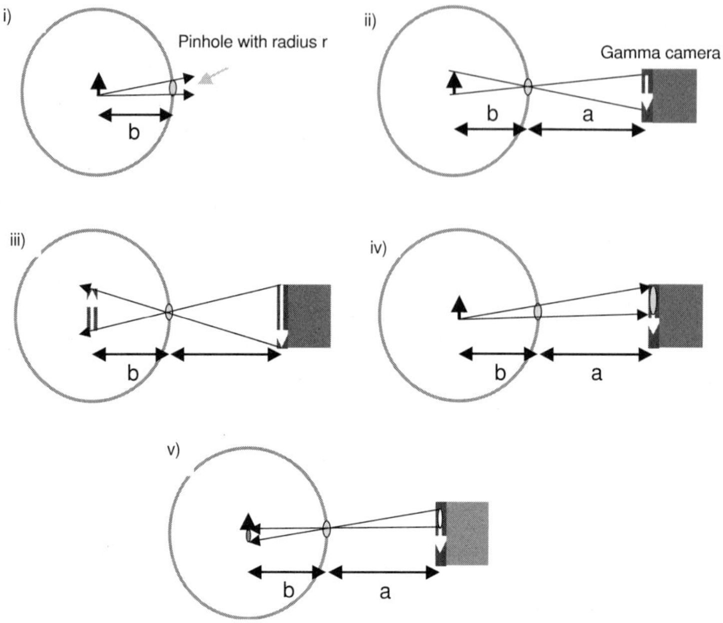

Figure 6.5. The geometric constructions for understanding i) efficiency, ii) magnification, iii) field of view, iv) pinhole blur, and v) detector resolution as it affects reconstructed resolution.

from the ability to stop gamma rays, there is no more important detector property than the space-bandwidth product — the total number of resolvable elements on the detector's face.

For pinhole-based imagers, a number of conclusions regarding the optical arrangement are readily drawn. It might seem that the magnification should be made as large as the required field of view and camera size permits. However, consideration must also be given to the obliquity; if the object to pinhole distance is very short, then vignetting by the pinhole and depth-of-interaction effects in the detector become problematic at the edges of the image. In fact, the principal conclusion that we wish to promote is that the imager design needs to consider the types of imaging experiments to be performed — and there will in general be a need for different pinhole sizes and locations for different imaging tasks.

2.5.1 Parallel hole collimators and their relatives. The parallel-hole collimator (PHC) is the classic image-forming aperture that is in use on most clinical SPECT systems. The idealized collimator allows a pixel or resolvable element to sense the activity in a tubular region that extends away from the detector without expanding in area. In practice, PHCs are of finite aspect ratio and always generate conical sensitivity functions (see Fig. 6.6) [Gunter, 1996]. The equations for efficiency and resolution as a function of distance from the face of the collimator as

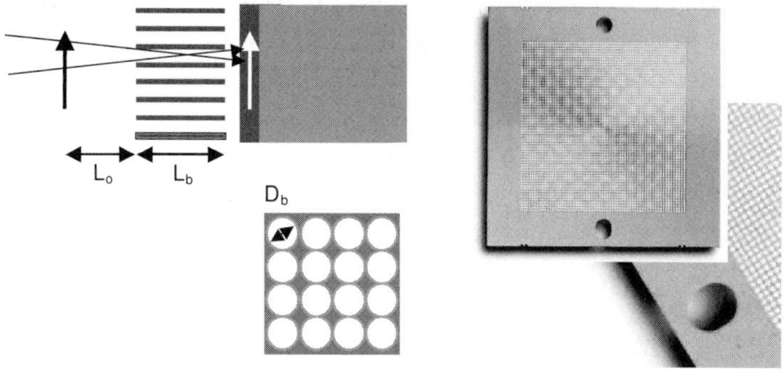

Figure 6.6. (a) The geometry of the parallel hole collimator. L_b is the bore length, D_b is the bore diameter, L_b/D_b is the aspect ratio, and F_{packing} is the ratio of the bore area to the unit cell area. (b) Laminated tungsten collimator produced by Tecomet of Woburn, MA.

derived from simple geometric arguments are given by:

$$E = \left(\frac{A_b}{4\pi L_b^2}\right) F_{\text{packing}}, \tag{6.9}$$

$$R \propto D_b \frac{(L_0 + L_b)}{L_b}. \tag{6.10}$$

The falloff in resolution with distance makes it imperative to image with the object as close to the collimator as possible.

The biggest challenge in using parallel-hole collimators for small-animal imaging has been the difficulty of fabricating optics with high resolution and high aspect ratio, yet with acceptable septal penetration (leakage of oblique rays through the walls between bores). New methods involving photolithographically etched and laminated tungsten have made it possible to produce very finely pitched structures of almost arbitrary thickness. Our laboratory's SpotImager makes use of a 7 mm thick lamination of approximately 100 sheets of tungsten, with 4096 280 micron by 280 micron square bores on a 380 micron by 380 micron pitch grid (Fig. 6.6b) [Balzer, 2002].

There are a number of variations on the standard parallel-hole collimator that can be of interest for special applications. For example, the bores can be made to converge or diverge in one or two dimensions, resulting in magnification or demagnification. The bores can also be made parallel, but at a slant relative to the detector face.

2.5.2 Coded apertures and other imaging elements. The coded aperture differs from the optics discussed above in one fundamental sense: light originating from a volume of activity in the object is allowed to reach the detector through more than one path. What is gained is sensitivity and for tomographic systems, angular sampling. The degree of multiplexing, the overlap of images, can vary. For simple objects with a few, well-defined concentrations of activity and diffuse backgrounds, substantial overlap is acceptable. If the object is complex, more counts are required to overcome the loss of information resulting from the uncertainty of which aperture each photon passed through.

Other aperture types have been demonstrated, including rotating slits and slats [Webb, 1993, Lodge, 1995], which point out that it is not necessary to form a set of recognizable planar images in order to perform tomographic reconstruction. Indeed, double listmode (see listmode data acquisition below) reconstructions can bypass the formation of any intermediate images entirely.

3. SPECT imager design

A small-animal SPECT imager can be designed, or an existing imager can be classified, by considering a short list of criteria:

- What is the camera type?
  - Are gamma rays detected via scintillators or by direct conversion?
  - How many pixels or resolvable elements are there?
  - What is the quantum efficiency, energy resolution, and count rate capability?
- How many cameras?
  - How many exposures are necessary to acquire a tomographic data set?
  - What, if anything, must move between exposures?
  - What is the optical arrangement?
  - What is the aperture type? Pinhole, collimator, or coded aperture?
  - What operating point has been selected for resolution, sensitivity, magnification, and field of view?
- How will the instrument be controlled and how will data be acquired into a PC or workstation?
  - How will data be stored? Bitmaps or listmode?
  - What methods will be employed for position estimation tasks? Will they be realized in hardware or software?
- Will the SPECT be augmented with any other imaging modalities, such as CT or optical bioluminescence?

Because this chapter is not about detectors, we defer discussion of camera types to Chapter 2 in this book. However, the question of how many cameras will be employed in the system is of great interest from the imager design standpoint. Systems with a single camera are basically of two types: those which rotate the imaging object in front of a stationary camera and those that move the camera through an orbit while the object (small animal) remains stationary.

Systems that rotate the animal have a number of appealing attributes. They lead to undoubtedly the simplest and most compact imager designs. Because the camera remains fixed, no electrical signals need to traverse slip rings or move in trailing cables. There is only one practical axis for the rotation: the vertical; rotation about any horizontal axis will result in animal movement, including organ shift. The animal can be oriented vertically or horizontally. The vertical orientation is not natural for rodentia, but makes for the most compact arrangements. As will be discussed later, fixed-camera orientation makes it possible to directly measure the system imaging matrix or point spread function (PSF). However, the matrix must be rotated mathematically during the reconstruction process to match each exposure. Because the collection of planar projections occurs one at a time, total acquisition times tend to be measured in minutes and tens of minutes.

SPECT imagers that translate one or a few cameras about the object have the benefit of permitting a normal, horizontal animal position and are the standard for clinical and commercial small-animal systems. However, high precision motions are required with typically heavy cameras (the cameras themselves may be light, but the shielding required to exclude background gamma rays is typically made of lead or tungsten alloys). Hence, careful counter weighting and substantial rotary bearings are needed. Acquisition times are again typically 10-30 minutes, and the direct measurement of an imaging matrix is not easily accomplished.

Multi-camera systems, specifically those that collect enough planar projections for full tomographic reconstruction without any motions, offer a number of advantages over one- and two-camera systems. The imager sensitivity scales linearly with the number of cameras, all data acquisition is parallel, and the system imaging matrix can be completely measured [Kastis, 1998]. The disadvantages are the added complexity and cost of operating all cameras simultaneously.

The importance of the parallel data acquisition should be emphasized. All nuclear medicine imaging procedures are, in principle, dynamic in nature. Not only is the tracer activity continuously decreasing, but the biological distribution is also changing as a result of metabolic and renal activity. In many cases, the most valuable scientific data to be derived from the imaging experiments are quantitative washout rates or peak accumulation values.

3.1 Calibration

Much of the success of the SPECT imagers developed in our laboratory depends on two levels of calibration measurements, as indicated in Fig. 6.7. The image-forming properties of each camera, the mean detector response function (MDRF), is measured by scanning a well-collimated source in a regular 2D grid across the camera face. The set of signals recorded as a function of position form a statistical basis for the inverse problem: maximum likelihood estimation of a position from a set of measurements. We also perform the direct measurement of the imaging matrix, the operator that maps radioactivity in a voxel into a set of observed signals.

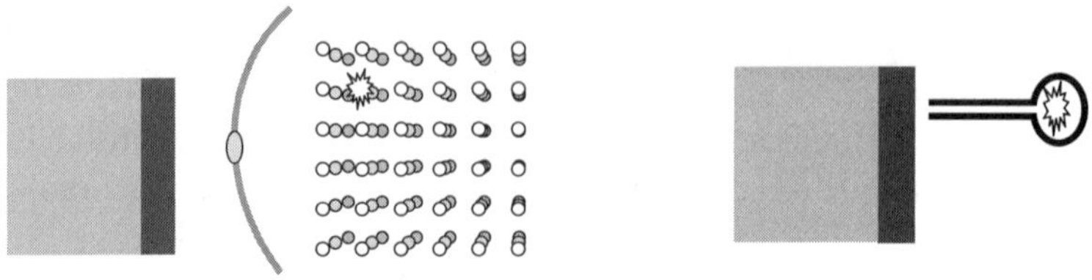

Figure 6.7. (a) The PSF measurement process. A point source is translated throughout the object volume on a 3D grid with all optical elements in place. (b) MDRF measurements are carried out on individual cameras using a collimated source and translating through a regular 2D grid.

The main advantages of full imager calibration is obvious: any imprecisions in pinhole locations, camera locations or orientation, inhomogeneity in camera sensitivities, and other optical factors are accounted for in the reconstruction process. In short, there is no better way to model the forward process than to simply go and measure it.

In order to measure a PSF, a robotic system is made to move a point source, approximated by a few (< 10) 100-micron radioactive chromatographic beads immobilized in a small dot of epoxy, throughout the object volume of the imaging system under calibration. Because the tracer is decaying throughout the scan, integration times are continually being adjusted upward to keep the total number of counts collected roughly constant. A scanned volume is typically a three-dimensional space with upwards of $60,000$ discrete locations; the process occupies approximately 24 hours of continuous measuring. The stage system for one of our larger imagers, FastSPECT II, is shown in Fig. 6.8. The theory and techniques of SPECT system calibration are discussed in detail in Chapter 12 of this book.

3.2 A survey of systems developed at CGRI

The Center for Gamma-ray Imaging (CGRI) develops SPECT and SPECT/CT systems based on both scintillator and semiconductor gamma-ray detectors. To illustrate a range of SPECT system designs, we will present a short survey of the imagers developed in our laboratory.

FastSPECT I is a 24-modular-scintillation-camera instrument originally designed as a human brain imager, but since converted into a dedicated small-animal imager for biomedical research. The research on position-estimation techniques and reconstruction algorithms that it spawned continues to influence the design of the newer multi-camera SPECT systems. Indeed, the instrument continues to be operated in support of in-house and collaborative research projects, and it produces millimeter resolution reconstructed images [Kastis, 1998].

Each modular camera has a scintillation crystal, a quartz light guide, and a 2×2 array of photomultiplier tubes [Milster, 1990]. Data are acquired via analog event

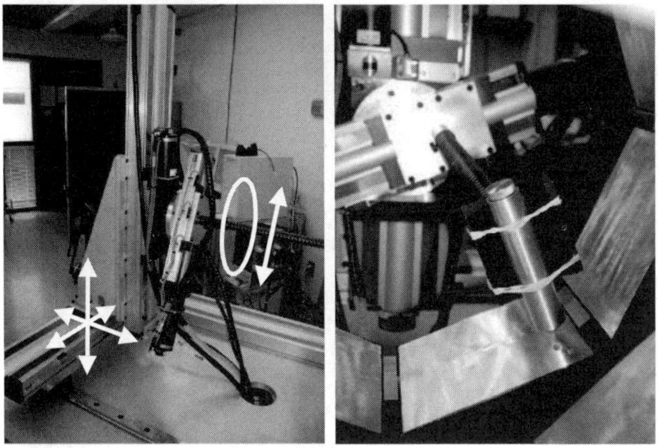

Figure 6.8. The FastSPECT II calibration stage. Three orthogonal translations, one rotation, and one supplementary translation make any scanning pattern feasible. Right: An *in situ* MDRF measurement in progress.

detection; when a PMT sum signal exceeds a preset threshold, a zero-crossing detector is enabled on the first derivative. When a peak is detected, individual sample and hold amplifiers are triggered that latch the peak amplitudes and present them to 8-bit flash A/D converters. Each 8-bit number is square-root compressed to 5 bits via a lookup table EPROM and then concatenated with the others to form a 20-bit word. This word is used as a lookup-table index to an array that contains the pre-computed, maximum-likelihood x, y, and energy-windowed estimates for every possible signal combination. The lookup table, which is downloaded into VME memory at execution time, is generated from an extensive calibration process that includes MDRF and PSF measurements. It can be computed in a number of ways to implement likelihood or energy windowing [Sain, 2001].

The imager, shown in Fig. 6.9a, is operated at a magnification of $\sim$3, with 24 1-mm pinholes machined directly into a lead aperture cylinder. The pinhole collection efficiency is approximately 2×10^{-4}, which yields a final point sensitivity of 6 counts per second (cps) per microCurie (μCi). The field of view is $3.0 \times 3.2 \times 3.2$ cm^3, and reconstructions are carried out on a 1 mm^3 voxel grid.

FastSPECT II, the follow-on instrument to FS I, has an enlarged camera design with a 3×3 array of PMTs and is shown in Fig. 6.9b [Furenlid, 2004]. Data are acquired via new listmode electronics (see below) and are not subject to any binning, compression, or other information loss. Position estimation is carried out in software in post-processing. The system has an inherent dynamic capability with every event timed to the nearest 30 nanosecond clock interval. The robotic stage, shown in Fig. 6.8, is improved over earlier versions to provide a rotation axis and secondary translation to permit *in situ* MDRF measurements.

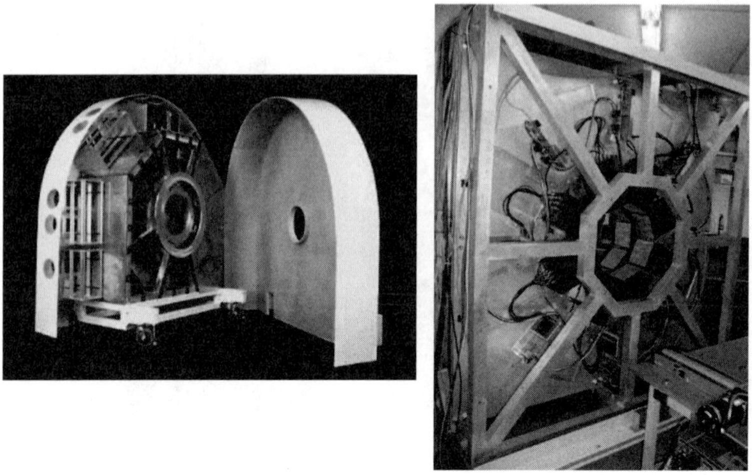

Figure 6.9. Above: FastSPECT I with 24 fixed 4 in^2 modular cameras. Right: FastSPECT II with 16 radially movable 4.5×4.5 in^2 gamma cameras.

FastSPECT II is built in and around a welded, 2" square cross-section, tubular aluminum skeleton. A pair of central plates with a small gap between them are mounted into this framework. The faces of the mounting plates have milled recesses for cameras and tapped mounting holes for electronics. The cameras are arranged as two rings of eight on opposite sides of the central plates, and each camera has an aluminum mounting bracket that is captured in one of the milled recesses. Drilled and tapped mounting holes provide a selection of three radial positions of increasing distance from the imager axis. The entire imager is shielded with a 1/8"-thick lead sheet laminated to a 1/8" thick powder-coated aluminum skin. The interior components can be accessed through two hinged doors for service or to change camera locations. The entire structure is built on a heavy-duty wheeled base that permits relocation of the imager if necessary. A cable routing maze is located at the top of the imager.

FastSPECT II does not have a fixed imaging geometry; camera positions and aperture locations can be adjusted to match the imaging problem at hand. The optical arrangement of FSII is shown in Fig. 6.10 along with a photograph of a cast aperture cylinder being installed in the imager bore. In the basic geometry suitable for small-animal imaging, the pinholes are placed along imaginary lines between the center of the field of view and each camera face. This provides a magnification of approximately $2.5\times$ for the default cylinder (two-inch radius) and closest camera position (6.5" from imager axis). The field of view then accommodates a 25-gram laboratory mouse, and the 16 pinholes combined provide a photon collection efficiency of $\sim .03\%$. Apertures/camera position combinations have been used with magnifications varying between 2.5 and 20, with pinhole inserts ranging from 0.1 to 1 mm in diameter. In the high magnification configuration, the field of view is less than 30 mm^3; the scientific problem it is designed for involves imaging bone metastases at known locations in murine femurs.

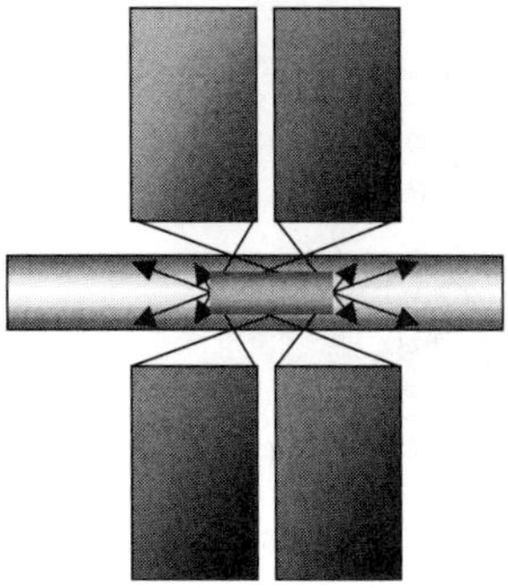

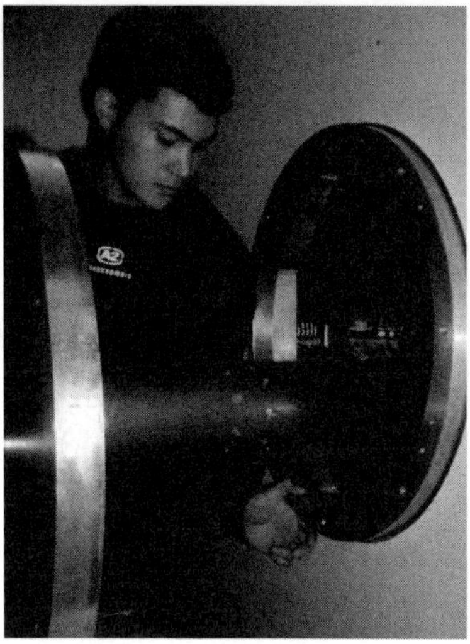

Figure 6.10. Left: The optical arrangement of FastSPECT II showing the shape of the field of view. Each camera is matched with a pinhole on the line between the center of the camera face and the center of the FOV. Right: An aperture with Au pinhole inserts being installed in the imager.

Data acquisition in FastSPECT starts with front-end list-mode event processors developed to support the nine-photomultiplier modular camera. Each event processor contains nine modular shaping amplifiers for analog signal conditioning, an array of nine free-running analog-to-digital converters with programmable gains, and a Lucent ORCA Field Programmable Gate Array (FPGA).

Event recognition is thus performed by the FPGA. Firmware was developed that implements a pipelined data-processing architecture. This technique, processing a stream of incoming data through a big shift register, compresses arbitrarily complex processing into a small number of effective clock cycles (at the expense of some latency). On each tick, a new data sample enters one end of the shift register, and an analyzed data sample exits the other. Thus, in our system, nine 12-bit data words are summed, analyzed for an event, and possibly packaged into a list-mode event packet in each 30-nanosecond clock cycle.

3.2.1 The SpotImager. SpotImagers, shown in Fig. 6.11, are compact gamma-ray cameras comprising an Arizona cadmium zinc telluride (CZT) hybrid and a matching laminated-tungsten parallel hole collimator of the kind shown in Fig. 6.6. The system is completed with a shielded, compact housing and a backend of support electronics and an acquisition computer. The SpotImager can be adapted to a variety of imaging applications [Balzer, 2002]. The detector housing consists of two parts: a nickel-plated tungsten head and an anodized aluminum handle. The imager head contains a single CZT detector, a water-cooled heat sink, a thermo-electric cooler, and readout electronics. The handle is equipped with attachment

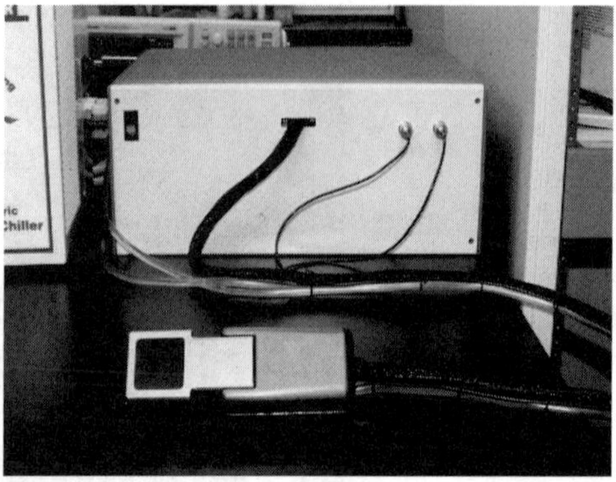

Figure 6.11. The SpotImager comprises a single 4096 pixel CZT detector, matching Tecomet collimator, and readout electronics in a shielded tungsten housing. External signal conditioning electronics, a water chiller, and data acquisition computer complete the system.

points to permit mounting to external supports, but it can also, in principle, be used as a hand-held imaging device (for a steady hand!). The entrance window, which sits above the collimator, is a thin Bakelite plate that prevents light from reaching the detector.

The imager head was manufactured from copper-tungsten alloy to provide shielding against radiation bypassing the collimator or pinhole. The tungsten alloy, with a minimum thickness of 5 mm, has a transmittance of 5×10^{-8} at 140 keV. An internal cable maze and use of tungsten screws completes the shielding.

The collimator used in the SpotImager has a 64×64 array of holes that match the pitch of the CZT detector's pixels [Kastis, 2000]. Approximately 90 tungsten layers give an overall thickness of 7 mm. The bore width is 260 microns on a center-to-center spacing of 380 microns. The collimator efficiency is 5×10^{-5}, and the spatial resolution has been measured at 450 microns for a source 4 mm from the collimator face. As with all parallel hole collimators, the resolution decreases with increasing distance, making this device principally suitable for applications where it can be held in close proximity to the imaging subject.

The collimator is aligned to the detector via an arrangement of set screws, springs, and ball plungers. The ball plungers provide an upward force on the collimator that holds it securely in place. The set screws and opposing springs are used to perform translations in two directions and rotation about the normal to the detector plane. By working with sources, the relative positioning of the collimator and detector are adjusted until Moire-type artifacts are removed.

Data acquisition in the initial SpotImagers is handled via a digital signal processing (DSP) board programmed with a custom application. LabView software interacts with this freestanding application to periodically download lists of events stored in memory. Images also can be acquired in a bitmap mode in which the entire image is stored on the DSP board. The LabView application is augmented with commands to control a simple rotary stage, which makes it possible to use a

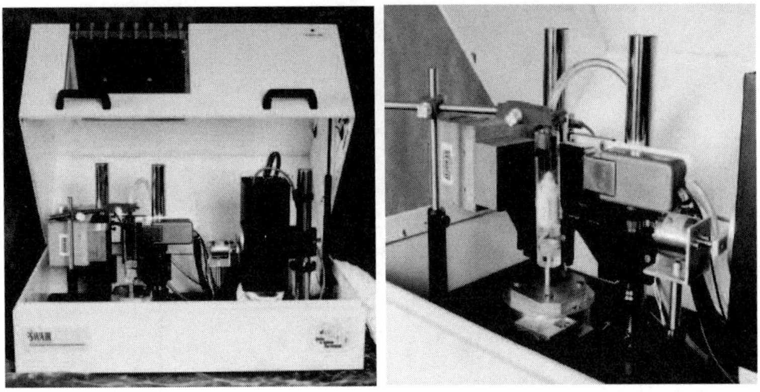

Figure 6.12. The CT/SPECT dual modality system combines a SpotImager with a transmission x-ray system. The imaging subject is rotated to collect angular samples.

SpotImager as a single camera SPECT system. In fact, this arrangement yielded the first tomographic images using the CZT arrays [Kastis, 2002, Wu, 2000].

3.2.2 The dual-modality system. SPECT is a functional imaging modality in that the radiotracer distribution is influenced primarily by biological and/or biochemical processes. This is in contrast with anatomical modalities, such as x-ray computed tomography, that image physical properties such as tissue density and mineral content. Hence, SPECT has been characterized as one of the technologies that can be employed in molecular imaging, namely the identification and localization of the presence of certain molecular species within living subjects. Indeed, it is becoming possible to design radiotracers with exquisite selectivity by mimicking the recognition techniques employed by the immune system.

A figure of merit for radiotracers is the ratio of uptake in the target tumor or organ of interest versus other "background" tissues such as muscle, liver, blood pool, etc. High ratios lead to high-contrast, high-quality images, but sometimes at the expense of adequate anatomical reference points to unambiguously assign regions of higher activity as corresponding to the site of investigation. This has led to the development of dual-modality instruments that combine coregistered functional and anatomical images for both clinical and research applications (see for example [Goode, 1999, Williams, 1999])

CGRI's first dual-modality system is a dedicated small-animal SPECT/CT that combines a SpotImager with a transmission x-ray system [Kastis, 2002a, Kastis, 2004]. In this system (Fig. 6.12), planar projections for tomographic reconstructions for both modalities are acquired by rotating a vertically oriented mouse or small rat about the vertical axis. Typical imaging experiments collect 180 step-and-shoot x-ray exposures followed by 30 gamma-ray exposures.

The x-ray camera is a CCD/phosphor screen detector manufactured by Dalsa-MedOptics. It consists of a Kodak KAF-1001E series 1024 $\times$ 1024 pixel CCD array that has an active area of 24.5 mm $\times$ 24.5 mm. The CCD is coupled via a

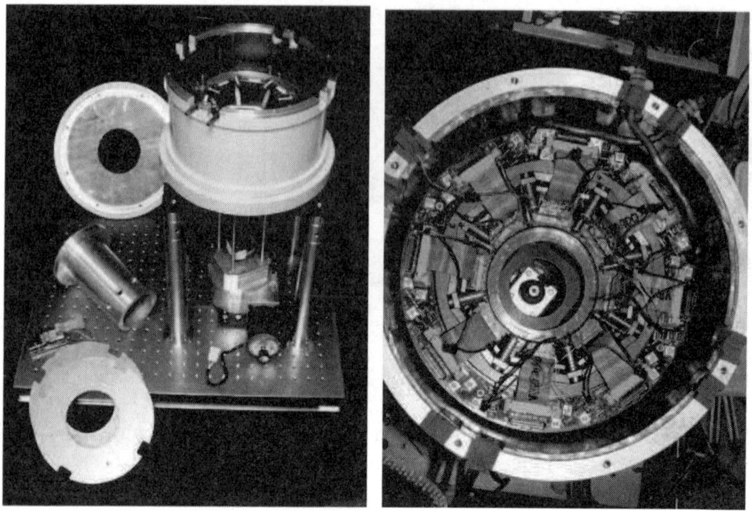

Figure 6.13. The SemiSPECT system combines 8 CZT detector modules in a dedicated mouse imager. Visible at left is the instrument on its optical table mount along with a cast aperture cylinder and shield pieces. At right is a view into the interior.

2:1 fiberoptic taper to a gadolinium oxysulfide phosphor screen that increases the active area to 50×50 mm^2. The camera is cooled to $-10°$C via a thermoelectric cooler. The x-ray tube is an Oxford Instruments XTF5000/75 with an 0.005-inch Be window. The same x-ray tube has been studied extensively in the microCAT system [Paulus, 1999]. X rays can be generated in the range of 4-50kVp with a maximum anode current of 1.5 mA.

3.2.3 SemiSPECT. The SemiSPECT imager (Fig. 6.13), comprising eight CZT hybrid detectors in a compact housing, brings together many years of effort in hybrid-detector production, electronics development, software authoring, and mechanical design.

The detector array consists of eight detector modules arranged in an octagonal geometry. Each hybrid detector and its daughterboard are part of a modular unit called a detector module [Crawford, 2003]. The module includes the thermoelectric cooler, a cold plate, thermal spacer, and base plate. In order to remove heat from the system, the detector array is mounted to a single, cylindrical heat exchanger using a spring loaded rail. The large copper heatsink has a milled recess about its exterior and is encircled by multiple loops of a copper tube coil that carries cooled liquid from an external chiller. The heatsink is mounted to the interior base of the housing that provides the imager's structural support, protection, and packaging. The housing also supports the shielding and provides feedthroughs for the electrical cabling and coolant lines.

The aperture assembly is made from an external frame into which we cast a cylinder of Cerrobend. The length of the aperture allows it to be placed into the system through the top cap of the housing and seated into retaining grooves. There are eight pinhole recesses machined into the structure into which gold pinhole inserts are mounted. Two apertures with different magnifications have been cast and a set of pinholes were produced with 0.5 mm openings.

We use a list-mode data acquisition scheme and the same backend electronics that are used with FSII to run SemiSPECT. In essence, the Arizona ASIC yields an output analogous to a rasterized video signal. That is, a two-dimensional pixel field is presented as a flattened, one-dimensional stream of analog values. At the beginning of each one millisecond integration frame, a trigger announces the beginning of a new data stream.

The challenge in designing a list-mode event processor to handle rasterized data was the need to identify and report 3×3 pixel neighborhoods rather than single pixels, in order to reduce false events triggered by noise and permit an improved recovery of energy resolution. Because the two-dimensional to one-dimensional data stream conversion results in the separation of pixels from neighboring rows, it is necessary to be able to look both forward and backward in time to recover a given neighborhood. This was accomplished by making the first task of the digital event processor (implemented as firmware in an FPGA) the storage of the data in a RAM element. By use of a circular pointer technique, the linear RAM is made to function as a nine-tap, 128-element shift register where a central pixel and its eight nearest neighbors are available for processing.

The additional requirements of stored baseline values (analogous to dark current measurements), event thresholds, and gain maps were each stored in separate small memories. Also implementing a fully pipelined processing algorithm (like the FastSPECT II processor), the event processor is able to sort through the incoming data, subtract baseline values, form a nine-term sum, compare that sum against a threshold, apply a veto map via the gain data, and create an event packet in a single 240 nanosecond clock cycle. The firmware also can be instructed to send an entire frame of data as a special packet. This is useful for measuring baseline (dark current) data and system noise.

4. Electrical signals from gamma-ray detectors

In both PMT and solid-state based detectors, the raw signal is a current pulse [Knoll, 1989]. When the sensor is a PMT, the shape of the pulse is dictated by the light-output timing characteristics of the scintillation crystal. The current amplification by the dynode stages in the PMT result in an mA-scale peak current that can be fed directly to a transimpedance stage based on a modern, low-noise operational amplifier with resistive feedback. On the other hand, the very small charge signals generated in direct conversion solid-state detectors must typically be amplified with very small capacitors (< 1 pF) and front-end transistors placed in close proximity to each pixel (hence the development of the bump-bonded readout ASIC). The timing characteristics are generally a result of the charge transport properties of the semiconductor material.

For event driven readouts, once signals have been amplified, there are several choices available for processing. One alternative is to continuously digitize immediately and use digital filtering techniques to reduce noise and detect events. Another alternative is to condition raw signals with analog filters, perform analog event detection, and then digitize the peak values. On the other hand, a hybrid approach can be adopted in which analog conditioning is used first, followed by continuous digitization, and then further digital processing and event detection. Each method has merits, and the choice is often dictated by whether it is feasible to have a separate A/D converter for each sensor or whether stored analog peak values for many sensors need to be multiplexed through a smaller number of A/D channels.

For integrating readouts that store signals accumulated over a framing time, such as CCDs or gated-integrator arrays, the data acquisition system typically sees a set of DC levels arriving at known times relative to a pixel clock. The signal stream is a linearized raster of the two-dimensional detector array, and the processing challenge is to recognize and extract events as they occur in each frame. This is certainly best accomplished via digital processing, in either DSPs or FPGAs.

5. Data acquisition architectures

There are essentially two choices available for accumulating data from a gamma-ray camera: list mode and image mode. In image-mode data acquisition, the signals associated with a gamma-ray photon are processed (with analog or digital techniques) to arrive at an x, y position. The x and y coordinates are treated as indices into a bitmap array stored in computer memory and, with each event, the corresponding array element is incremented. Because the bitmap occupies an addressable section of computer memory, the number of bits has typically been reduced from the raw measurements, i.e., the data have been binned. There are some advantages: the data have a fixed size and they can be instantly visualized.

In list-mode acquisition, data are maintained as an ordered list in which each entry corresponds to a detected gamma-ray photon. Each list entry contains all sensor data recorded at full precision along with other relevant parameters, such as the time the event occurred. The benefits of this approach are that new and arbitrarily sophisticated estimation algorithms can be applied to data at any time. There is no inherent information loss in the acquisition process, and image reconstructions can be performed using different attributes, such as intermediate images, fluence estimates, or even the raw data list. If times are recorded, list-mode acquisition also permits 4D reconstructions.

There is one principal drawback to list-mode acquisition: very large amounts of memory, both RAM and disk, are required to handle the accumulation of long lists of events. It is the recent rapid advance in processor speeds and storage capacity of inexpensive computers that makes list-mode acquisition a viable option.

5.1 List-mode data acquisition

The statistical advantages of list-mode data collection — the recording of the full set of observations associated with a data event as an entry in an ordered list —

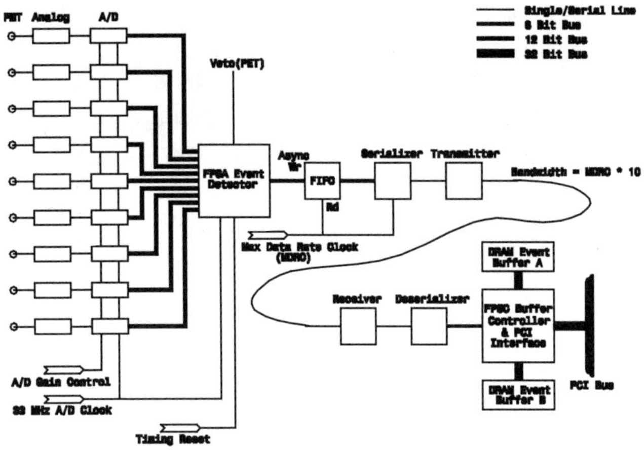

Figure 6.14. The list-mode data-acquisition architecture for a 9 PMT modular gamma camera.

have been demonstrated in prior work [Barrett, 1997, Parra, 1998]. In brief, methods applied to estimate individual photon properties, such as energy and position, always have access to the data observations at their full collected precision. CGRI's list-mode architecture, shown in Fig. 6.14, is based on the concept of dividing the data-acquisition task into a front end that resides in or close to a camera, a fast digital communications link, and an in-computer back end. The front end, which is detector-technology specific, digitizes signals and performs digital event recognition tasks. We call the front end of this system a list-mode event processor in recognition of its role in examining incoming digitized data streams for valid events and packaging up the measurements associated with an event in a byte packet, i.e., a list-mode data entry.

Communications are accomplished by taking advantage of the broad developments in networking technology. Thus, data are conveniently sent across to a back-end buffer via a network-based SERDES (serializer/deserializer) chipset that permits use of a standard category 5 cable. The particular technology adopted provides for autosynchronization, i.e., there is no need to cable along valid-data clocks of any kind.

The back-end maintains the list-mode data list, adding an entry to a buffer each time a valid event packet arrives from the front end. The particular virtues of this design are manifold: 1) event detection occurs early in the signal-processing chain, causing the data transmission bandwidth to depend only on the event rate and the number of measurements associated with a single photon event; 2) there is no need to bin or otherwise process the data in ways that reduce information content; 3) the same basic back-end hardware and software can support many different kinds of photon-counting imagers, leaving the much smaller task of designing new front ends when new instruments are contemplated; and 4) with each camera having its own dedicated high-speed data link, there are no limitations imposed by packet collisions, available communication bandwidth, or numbers of cameras in a single system.

The power of this approach is ably illustrated by the raw data rate in the FastSPECT II system. The 144 12-bit A/D converters running at 33 MHz produce an impressive 50 Gigabits of information per second that are continually digested by the list-mode electronics. In addition, the flexibility is demonstrated by SemiSPECT, whose data-acquisition electronics makes use of the identical data transmission and back-end hardware as FastSPECT II, despite having an entirely different detector technology.

6. Conclusions

A number of important lessons have been learned in the development of CGRI's current complement of imaging systems. The first is that small-animal SPECT imagers need flexible optical designs to be optimizable for different imaging problems. An instrument operating at a fixed point in terms of resolution, field of view, magnification, and sensitivity is analogous to a fixed-focus party favor camera. A second point is that careful calibration measurements can correct for minor manufacturing and material imperfections, and can dramatically improve imager performance.

List-mode data acquisition architectures have advantages, including the ability to support new camera technologies without having to reinvent software and data transmission links. Recent developments in computing power and storage device capacities make full list-mode acquisition completely feasible. The hardware developed for networking is ideal for adapting to the communications between front-end processors and back-end event buffers. Finally, stationary imager designs, such as the FastSPECT series, permit dynamic imaging applications and high throughput studies.

References

[Barrett, 1981] H. H. Barrett, W. Swindell, *Radiological Imaging: The Theory of Image Formation, Detection, and Processing Vol. 1 and 2,* Academic Press, New York, 1981.

[Barrett, 1997] H. H. Barrett, T. White, L. C. Parra, "List-mode Likelihood," *J. Opt. Soc. Am. A*, vol. 14, pp. 2914-2923, 1997.

[Balzer, 2002] S. J. Balzer, *A Portable Gamma-Ray Imager for Small Animal Studies*, Master's Thesis, University of Arizona, Tucson, Arizona, 2002.

[Crawford, 2003] M. Crawford, *Mechanical and Thermal Design and Analysis of a Small-Animal SPECT Imager,* Master's Thesis, University of Arizona, Tucson, Arizona, 2003.

[Furenlid, 2004] L. R. Furenlid, D. W. Wilson, Y. Chen, H. Kim, P. J. Pietraski, M. J. Crawford, H. H. Barrett, "FastSPECT II: A second-generation high-resolution dynamic SPECT imager," *IEEE Trans. Nucl. Sci.*, vol. 51, pp. 631-635, 2004.

[Goode, 1999] A. R. Goode, M. B. Williams, P. U. Simoni, V. Galbis-Reig, S. Majewski, A. G. Weisenberger, R. Wojcik, M. Stanton, W. Phillips, A. Stewart, "A system for dual modality breast imaging", *Conference Record of the 1999 IEEE Nuclear Science Symposium and Medical Imaging Conference*, Seattle, vol. 2, pp. 934-38, 1999.

[Gunter, 1996] D. L. Gunter, "Collimator characteristics and design," *Nuclear Medicine* eds R. E. Henkin, et al. St. Louis, MO, 1996.

[Hildebrandt, 2002] G. Hildebrandt, H. Bradazek, "Approaching real X-ray optics," *The Rigaku Journal,* vol. 17, pp. 13-22, 2000.

[Jaszczak, 1994] R. J. Jaszczak, J. Li, H. Wang, M. R. Zulutsky, R. E. Coleman "Pinhole collimation for ultra-high-resolution small-field-of-view SPECT," *Phys Med Biol*, vol. 39, pp. 425-437, 1994.

[Kastis, 1998] G. K. Kastis, H. B. Barber, H. H. Barrett, H. C. Gifford, I. W. Pang, D.D. Patton, J .D . Sain, G. Stevenson, D. W. Wilson, "Hight resolution SPECT imager for three-dimensional imaging of small animals," *Journal of Nuc. Med.*, vol. 39 (5 suppl), pp. 9P, 1998.

[Kastis, 2000] G. A. Kastis, H. B. Barber, H. H. Barrett, S. J. Balzer, D. Lu, D. G. Marks, G. Stevenson, J. M. Woolfenden, M. Appleby, J. Tueller, "Gamma-ray imaging using a CdZnTe pixel array and a high-resolution, parallel-hole collimator", *IEEE Trans. Nucl. Sci.*, vol 47, pp. 1923-27, 2000.

[Kastis, 2002] G. A. Kastis, M. Wu, S. J. Balzer, D. Wilson, L. Furenlid, G. Stevenson, H. H. Barrett, H. B. Barber, J. M. Woolfenden, P. Kelly, M. Appleby, "Tomographic small-animal imaging using a high-resolution semiconductor camera", *IEEE Trans. Nucl. Sci.*, vol. 49, pp. 172-75, 2002.

[Kastis, 2002a] G. A. Kastis, *Multi-modality Imaging of Small Animals,* Ph.D. Thesis, University of Arizona, Tucson, Arizona, 2002.

[Kastis, 2004] G. A. Kastis, L. R. Furenlid, D.W. Wilson, T. E. Peterson, H. B. Barber, H. H. Barrett, "Compact CT/SPECT small-animal imaging system," *IEEE Trans. Nucl. Sci.*, vol. 51, pp. 63-67, 2004.

[Knoll, 1989] G. F. Knoll, *Radiation Detection and Measurement,* John Wiley and Sons, New York, 1989.

[Lodge, 1995] M. A. Lodge, D. M. Binnie, M. A. Flower, S. Webb S. "The experimental evaluation of a prototype rotating slat collimator for planar gamma camera imaging," *Phys. Med. Biol.*, vol. 40, pp. 426-448, 1995.

[Milster, 1990] T. D. Milster, J. N. Aarsvold, H. H. Barrett, A. L. Landesman, L. S. Mar, D. D. Patton, T. J. Roney, R. K. Rowe, R. H. Seacat III, "A full-field modular gamma camera," *J. Nucl. Med.*, vol. 5, pp. 632-639, 1990.

[McMaster, 1969] W. H. McMaster, N. Kerr Del Granve, J. H. Mallett, J. H. Hubell, *Compilation of X-Ray Cross Sections*, National Technical Information Service, Springfield, Va., 1969.

[Parra, 1998] L. C. Parra, H. H. Barrett, "List-mode likelihood: EM Algorithm and image quality estimation demonstrated on 2-D PET," *IEEE Trans. Med. Imag.*, vol. 17, pp. 228-235, 1998.

[Paulus, 1999] M. J. Paulus, H. Sari-Sarraf, S. S. Gleason, M. Bobrek, J. S. Hicks, D. K. Johnson, J. K. Behel, L. H. Thompson, W. C. Allen, "A new x-ray computed tomography system for laboratory mouse imaging", *IEEE Trans. Nucl. Sci.*, vol. 46, pp 558-564, 1999.

[Sain, 2001] J. D. Sain, *Optical Modeling, Design Optimization, and Performance Analysis of a Gamma Camera for Detection of Breast Cancer*, Ph.D. Thesis, University of Arizona, Tucson, Arizona, 2001.

[Serlemitsos, 1988] P. J. Serlemitsos, "Conical foil X-ray mirrors: Performance and projections," *Applied Optics*, vol. 27, pp. 1533, 1988.

[Serlemitsos, 1996] P. J. Serlemitsos, Y. Soong, "Foil X-ray mirrors," *Astrophysics and Space Science*, vol. 239, pp. 177-196, 1996.

[Snigirev, 1996] A. Snigirev, V. Kohn, I. Snigireva, B. Lengeler, "A compound refractive lens for focusing high-energy X-rays," *Nature*, vol. 384, pp. 49-51, 1996.

[Webb, 1993] S. Webb, M. A. Flower, R. J. Ott. "Geometric efficiency of a rotating slit-collimator for improved planar gamma camera imaging," *Phys. Med. Biol.*, vol.38, pp. 627-638, 1993.

[Williams, 1999] M. B. Williams, V. Galbis-Reig, A. R. Goode, P. U. Simoni, S. Majewski, A. G. Weisenberger, R. Wojcik, W.Phillips, M. Stanton, "Multi-modality imaging of small animals", *RSNA Electronic Journal*, vol. 3, 1999.

[Wu, 2000] M. Wu, G. A. Kastis, S. J. Balzer, D. Wilson, H. B. Barber, H. H. Barrett, M. W. Dae, B. H. Hasegawa, "High resolution SPECT with a CdZnTe detector array and a scintillation camera," *Conference Record of the 2000 IEEE Nuclear Science Symposium and Medical Imaging Conference*, Lyon France, vol. 3, pp. 76-80, 2000.

Chapter 7

Computational Algorithms in Small-Animal Imaging

Donald W. Wilson*

1. Introduction

High-resolution small-animal imaging has seen recent advances on a number of fronts, with significant improvements coming in areas of detector technology, electronics, and collimation. Perhaps less recognized have been the accompanying software developments which have facilitated these hardware gains, including new algorithms that allow for better camera resolution, algorithms for faster reconstruction, algorithms for reconstructing data collected from irregular geometries, and modeling algorithms to improve reconstruction and to facilitate system design.

One reason that algorithms for small-animal imaging are sometimes overlooked is that, while clinical hardware must be specifically modified to optimize performance when imaging over a small field of view, algorithms are typically equivalent for both human and small-animal SPECT. For instance, reconstructed voxel size can simply be scaled when going from human to mouse imaging, and the same goals of fast and accurate algorithms are sought in both cases. In fact, most of the results presented below are general and could apply to any type of SPECT imaging. However, the nontraditional geometries specific to the small-animal problem as well as the rapid development of new detector types require more emphasis on the algorithm and warrant a fresh look at the algorithm and modeling problem.

In this section, we shall touch on various areas related to algorithms and modeling, giving examples taken from our work at the Center for Gamma-Ray Imaging (CGRI). We start with an overview of reconstruction algorithms. We show results from experiments exploring the effects of reconstruction-algorithm properties and parameters, including constraints and the reconstruction model. We then present studies using analytical and Monte Carlo modeling and conclude by demonstrating the importance of modeling in determining final system design.

2. Reconstruction

It is frequently said that, to understand an inverse problem such as tomographic reconstruction, one must first study the forward problem. This imaging (forward)

*Department of Radiology, The University of Arizona, Tucson, Arizona equation for a SPECT imaging system can be written in the linear form

$$\mathbf{g} = \mathcal{H}\boldsymbol{f} + \mathbf{n}, \tag{7.1}$$

where $\mathcal{H}$ is the continuous-to-discrete system operator, $\boldsymbol{f}$ is the continuous distribution of radioactive ions, and $\mathbf{n}$ is the noise. In this formulation, it should be noted that $\mathcal{H}$ contains in it not just the properties of the imaging system but also scatter and attenuation within the patient. Equation 7.1, up through such uncommon or unimportant phenomena as detector dead time and correlated noise in the electronics, is an exact representation of the SPECT imaging system.

Unfortunately, there exist no straightforward methods for solving the exact imaging equation, because $\mathcal{H}$ has rank of at most n (where n is the number of detector pixels), and an infinite n would be required to estimate a continuous $\boldsymbol{f}$. This issue is typically overcome by approximating the continuous $\boldsymbol{f}$ with a discrete $\mathbf{f}$, where the discretization is accomplished by voxelizing the object. The imaging equation is then written

$$\mathbf{g} = \mathbf{Hf} + \mathbf{n}. \tag{7.2}$$

It is this equation that tomography seeks to solve.

Reconstruction algorithms can be divided along a number of lines, but probably the most important division is between the filtered-backprojection-like algorithms and the iterative algorithms. Filtered backprojection (FB) is a modification of the Radon transform [Radon, 1917]. In his classic paper, Radon showed that a two-dimensional object could be perfectly reconstructed from a series of continuous measurements of the integrals through that object. This method was rediscovered by Bracewell in the field of solar astronomy [Bracewell, 1956] and by Cormack [Cormack, 1963, Cormack, 1964] in computerized tomography.

Motivating the FB algorithm begins by observing that simple backprojection of the projections of a point source leads to a $\frac{1}{r}$ blurring of the point in the reconstructed image. It is now well known that this $\frac{1}{r}$ blur can be removed by either multiplying the projection data by a ramp filter in the Fourier domain or taking the derivative of the data and then performing a Hilbert [Jain, 1989]. Because the Radon assumptions of continuous noise-free data are not realized in practice, and either a derivative or a ramp filter accentuate the high frequencies where noise power exists but little information is passed by the imaging system, low-pass filtering of the data is generally also required.

The main advantage of the filtered-backprojection-like algorithms is their speed. Performing projection/backprojection is usually the most time-consuming aspect of reconstruction, and FB requires only one backprojection. Its disadvantage is that it is difficult to incorporate complex properties of the imaging system ($\mathbf{H}$), although progress has been made in such areas as attenuation correction [Tretiak and Metz, 1980, Metz and Pan, 1995] and fanbeam/conebeam geometries [Feldkamp, 1984, Wang, 1993].

Iterative algorithms impose few restrictions on the form of $\mathbf{H}$. All attenuation, detector and collimator blur, and Compton scatter can be included in the system matrix, and by extension can be compensated for during the reconstruction process.

A number of iterative reconstruction have been proposed, including various flavors of the Algebraic Reconstruction Technique (ART) [Gordon, 1970, Kinahan, 1995], MAP-EM [Green, 1990], and ordered subsets expectation maximization [Hudson and Larkin, 1994]. However, in the following discussion, we shall focus on only two: maximum-likelihood expectation-maximization (ML-EM) [Dempster, 1977, Shepp and Vardi, 1982] and Landweber [Landweber, 1951].

The ML-EM algorithm can be written

$$\hat{f}_j^{(k+1)} = \frac{\hat{f}_j^{(k)}}{\sum_i h_{ij}} \sum_i h_{ij} \frac{g_i}{\hat{g}_i^{(k)}} \tag{7.3}$$

where $\hat{f}_j^{(k)}$ is the image estimate of voxel j after the k iterations, h_{ij}, an element of $\mathbf{H}$, represents the probability that a photon emitted from voxel j is detected by detector element i, and

$$\hat{g}_i^{(k)} = \sum_l h_{il} \hat{f}_l^{(k)} \tag{7.4}$$

is the estimated projection data after k iterations. Although originally derived on theoretical grounds, the method by which the algorithm works can be seen more qualitatively by studying Eq. 7.3. The estimated projection data, $\hat{\mathbf{g}}^{(k)}$, are estimated by projecting the current image estimate through $\mathbf{H}$, the $\hat{\mathbf{g}}^{(k)}$ is compared through division with the true g, and the backprojected result multiplicatively updates the current image estimate, $\hat{\mathbf{f}}^{(k)}$. When $\hat{\mathbf{g}}^{(k)} = \mathbf{g}$, the algorithm has converged.

A Landweber iteration has the form

$$\hat{f}_j^{(k+1)} = \hat{f}_j^{(k)} + \alpha \sum_i h_{ij}(g_i - \hat{g}_i^{(k)}) \tag{7.5}$$

where α is an acceleration factor that must be properly selected in order for the algorithm to converge. We see from Eq. 7.5 that Landweber iterations proceed by comparing through subtraction g and $\hat{\mathbf{g}}^{(k)}$, backprojecting, and additively updating.

Both ML-EM and Landweber allow for easy incorporation of any system model, $\mathbf{H}$. They differ in one aspect. Landweber is linear, and hence both positive and negative values can occur in $\hat{\mathbf{f}}^{(k)}$. ML-EM is nonlinear and, as long as $\mathbf{H}$ and $\hat{\mathbf{f}}^{(0)}$ have no negative values, $\hat{\mathbf{f}}^{(k)}$ will have none either. While this fact probably has little importance in most common imaging situations, we have found cases where it can greatly affect image quality, particularly what the projection data are poorly sampled. One example is given in the next section.

2.1 The effects of positivity on reconstructed images

Biopsy of lymph nodes is an important staging procedure for many cancers. Unfortunately, a complete lymphectomy can be both painful and debilitating. Techniques have recently been developed that seek to reduce these complications by biopsying only the first, or sentinel, node in the lymph chain, but the difficulty with this approach lies in finding the sentinel node. Nuclear-medicine approaches are frequently employed in the search, with a radiotracer injected into the tumor and a gamma camera used to follow the tracer's path through the lymphatic system until it reaches a node. This is a planar imaging procedure, and no information on the depth of the node is obtained.

Needle biopsy, rather than surgical biopsy, would further reduce surgical trauma. For this procedure to be successfully performed, however, the depth of the node must be known. Because nodes are relatively close to one's body surface, and because the tracer distribution is time dependent, it is generally believed that lymph-node tomography is not feasible with a conventional clinical system, and a more specialized system, able to estimate in 3D the location of the sentinel node, would be required.

There are generally only a few good "views" during a biopsy procedure, and one would prefer to make a 3D position estimate without moving the patient or camera. However, three-dimensional tomography typically requires that 2D data sets be obtained from many angular views. A number of sampling theorems have been advanced which state that views over at least 180° are needed for artifact-free imaging. However, all of these theorems are based on the premise that the reconstruction algorithm is linear, and it has been shown, using theoretical methods, that a positivity constraint can greatly reduce the number of possible poor solutions that arise from incomplete sampling information [Clarkson and Barrett, 1997, Clarkson and Barrett, 1998]. In this experiment, we set out to determine if positivity could play a role in the ability to reconstruct 3D lymph-node-like data collected from only one camera angle with a multiple-pinhole collimator.

We designed and constructed a system for 3D localization of a lymph node that employed one of our first-generation four-photomultiplier scintillation cameras. Gamma rays were imaged by a seven-pinhole collimator, and the magnification of the center of the field of view onto the camera face was one. No rotation of camera or phantom took place. The $\mathbf{H}$ matrix was generated by collecting data from a hot emitting point moved in 2-mm increments along the z axis at the center of the camera. We estimated the off-axis elements by assuming shift invariance in planes parallel to the detector face. The phantom consisted of three emitting sources separated by 5 mm. All three were in the (x, y) plane parallel to the face of the camera, and the central source had activity equal to twice the activity in each of the outside sources. There was no background activity. The projection data collected by the system are shown in Fig. 7.1.

We first reconstructed the data using linear Landweber (Eq. 7.5. We then added a nonlinear positivity constraint to Landweber by simply enforcing the condition that, after each iteration, any negative voxel value in $\hat{\mathbf{f}}^{(k)}$ is set to zero. The reconstructions after 100 linear Landweber iterations and 100 nonlinear positively-constrained Landweber iterations are given in Fig. 7.2. The slices represent different distances from the camera face (depth). It is clear that, without positivity, the algorithm is unable to arrive at a useful estimate of the object locations. However, Fig. 7.2(b) demonstrates that including positivity in the reconstruction algorithm allows excellent resolution in the (x, y) plane and reasonable z resolution. This

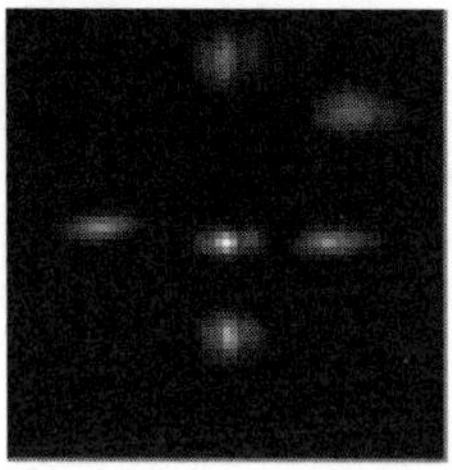

Figure 7.1. The projection data collected by the sentinel-node system.

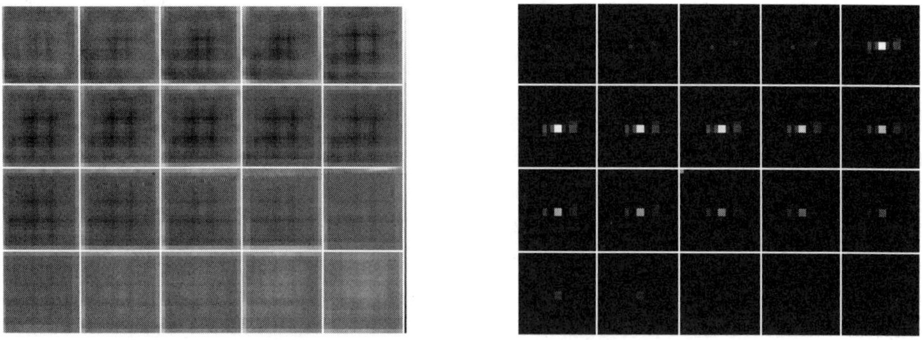

(a) (b)

Figure 7.2. The reconstructions using (a) linear Landweber iteration, and (b) Landweber iteration with a positivity constraint.

experiment, using real data, forcefully substantiated the theoretical conclusions reached in [Clarkson and Barrett, 1997, Clarkson and Barrett, 1998].

2.2 The effects of modeling errors

SPECT projection data are degraded by the physical effects of attenuation and Compton scatter within the patient and the blur produced by the resolution of the detector and collimator. If these effects are not compensated for, the resulting reconstructed images will be further degraded because the system model used by the reconstruction algorithm is not the same as the process that generated the data. This results in images with reduced resolution or with artifacts, and many studies have shown the benefits, in terms of image resolution and reduced artifacts, of properly modeling the imaging system in the reconstruction algorithm [Liang, 1992a, King and Farncombe, 2003, King, 1995, Jaszczak, 1981, Rosenthal, 1995]. Because iterative reconstruction methods such as ML-EM and Landweber iteration place few restrictions on the imaging-system model built into the algorithm, these are generally employed when compensation for physical effects is desired. It is well known that, with a correct model of the imaging process, with no statistical noise, and with enough iterations, these algorithms will arrive at an estimate that very closely resembles the original object. Unfortunately, an exact model of a

SPECT imaging system and data with no statistical noise is only truly realizable in computer simulations. Any real understanding of the properties of these algorithms requires that the consequences of statistical noise and improper models be understood. The effects of statistical noise in iterative SPECT reconstruction has been studied [Wilson and Tsui, 1993a, Barrett, 1994, Wilson, 1994]. The effects of modeling or not modeling scatter, detector response, and attenuation have also been studied [Liang, 1992a, Tsui, 1994, Welch, 1995, Beck, 1982, Liang, 1992b]. One area that has received less attention is the consequences of using an *incorrect* model of imaging-system properties.

When noise is present, the effects of compensation algorithms can be complicated. Roughly speaking, if the uncompensated image is blurred, then a compensation algorithm acts as a high-pass filter. If the system and the filter are shift invariant, the deterministic characteristics of the processed image are described by an overall modulation transfer function (MTF). Similarly, if the noise is stationary, the statistical properties can be described by the noise power spectrum (NPS). Of course, SPECT reconstructions are not shift-invariant, and the image noise is not stationary, but it is possible to define functions that describe locally the noise, resolution, and signal-to-noise properties. In this study, we employed three such quantities. The first is the local MTF_r (the Fourier transform of the image response to a point impulse at object position $\mathbf{r}$) [Wilson and Tsui, 1993b]. The second, is the Wigner spectrum (NPS_r) [Wigner, 1933], a measure of image noise correlations in the region about $\mathbf{r}$. The third is the local NEQ_r, the ratio of $\text{MTF}_r^2/\text{NPS}_r$ that serves as a local frequency-domain signal-to-noise ratio [Wilson and Tsui, 1993b].

Two phantoms were used during this portion of the study. The first, shown in Fig. 7.3, was a single slice from the Hoffman brain phantom [Hoffman, 1990]. The second was a uniformly emitting and attenuating 2D disk with an 8.5-cm radius, used to measure the noise and resolution properties of the reconstructed images. The measurements of the MTF_r were made by determining the differences in reconstructions of the disk phantom with and without a point source located 2.1 cm from the disk center with a contrast of 1% relative to the disk. The projection data were computer-generated with an analytical model of the system (the $\mathbf{H}$ matrix) that included the effects of attenuation and the finite resolution of a parallel-hole collimator with a bore length of 34 mm and a bore diameter of 1.4 mm. The incorrect $\mathbf{H}$ matrices used by the reconstruction algorithms were generated with imaging-system models that assumed bore diameters other than 1.4 mm.

Projection data from the Hoffman brain phantom were generated with 500,000 total projection counts over 64 projection angles. These data were then ML-EM reconstructed using $\mathbf{H}$ matrices that contained models assuming collimator blurs ranging from none to that resulting from a 2.0mm bore diameter. Figure 7.4 gives ML-EM estimates after 200 iterations with a model that assumed no collimator blur and blurring for 0.8-mm, 1.0-mm, 1.2-mm, 1.4-mm, 1.6-mm, 1.8-mm, and 2.0-mm bore diameters. It appears that, as the assumed collimator blur increases, the noise correlations also increase. This is a counterintuitive result, because compensation for a broader point spread function should sharpen the image, and one might in-

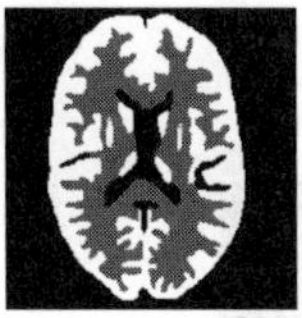

Figure 7.3. The slice of the Hoffman brain phantom used for study 2.2

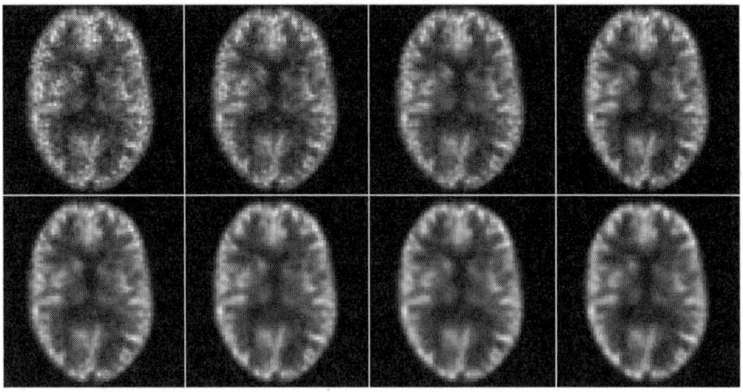

Figure 7.4. Reconstructions after 200 ML-EM iterations with no compensation and compensation assuming 0.8-mm, 1.0-mm, 1.2-mm 1.4-mm (correct), 1.6-mm, 1.8-mm, and 2.0-mm bore diameters.

stinctively believe it would sharpen the noise as well [Byrne, 1993]. Although it is difficult to visually estimate in a quantitative manner the resolution of the images reconstructed using the different system models, there are no obvious differences in resolution seen in Fig. 7.4. This is another counterintuitive result because for linear and shift-invariant systems, the resolution and noise should follow the same course.

These conclusions were based purely on qualitative visual analysis. In order to determine if they could stand up to more quantitative inspection, we turned to the local noise and resolution methods discussed previously. For this study, the uniformly emitting and attenuating disk served as the phantom. Noise-free projection data were generated for a collimator with a 1.4-mm bore diameter, and these noise-free data were ML-EM reconstructed using imaging-system models with assumed bore diameters of 0.8 mm, 1.4 mm, and 2.0 mm. The response to the point source was then Fourier transformed to generate the MTF_r. Figure 7.5 shows the MTF_r after 200 iterations for models assuming the three bore diameters, along with the radially averaged profiles through the MTF_r. It appears that the qualitative analysis was correct because no great differences in resolution are apparent among the different compensations, though some differences at lower frequencies are seen.

Poisson statistical noise was added at a count level of 500,000 counts, and 10,000 images were reconstructed using 200 iterations of ML-EM with the various correct and incorrect imaging-system models built in. The NPS_r was calculated for $\mathbf{r}$ again located 2.1cm from the center of the uniformly emitting disk and for compensation for collimators with bore diameters of 0.8 mm, 1.4 mm, and 2.0 mm. Images

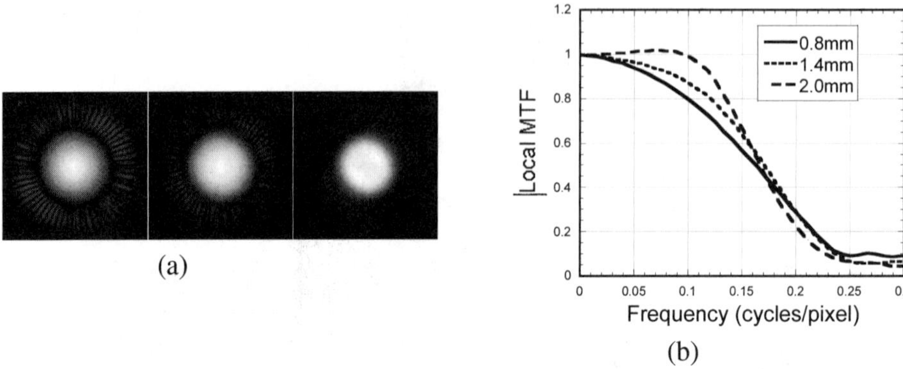

Figure 7.5. The MTF_r spectrum for compensations at 0.8 mm, 1.4 mm, and 2.0 mm.

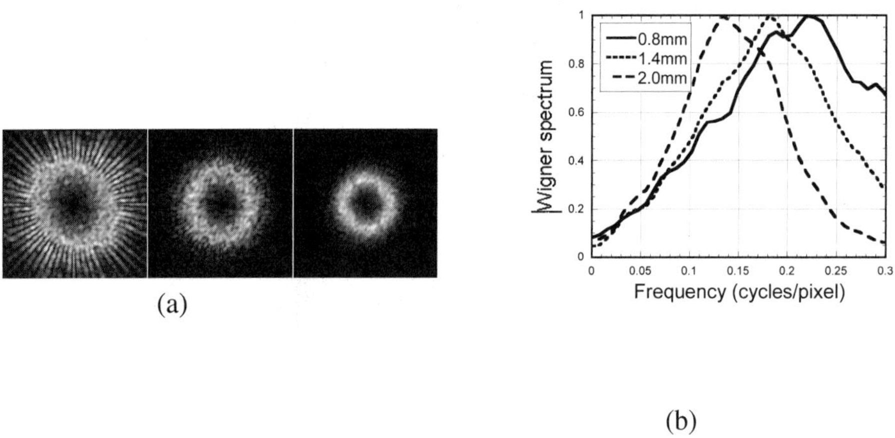

Figure 7.6. The NPS_r spectrum for compensations at 0.8 mm, 1.4 mm, and 2.0 mm.

of the NPS_r are given in Fig. 7.6, along with radially averaged profiles through the NPS_r. Again, the qualitative analysis appears correct. Fig. 7.6 shows large differences in the noise correlations among the different compensations, with the correlation length increasing as the assumed bore diameter increases.

From the previous results, where the noise power underwent large changes while the resolution remained relatively constant, we might expect large changes in the NEQ_r. However, Fig. 7.7, a radial average of the NEQ_r as a function of frequency, shows very little change. The differences at low frequencies are probably attributable to the fact that, at a small radius, there are fewer samples in the radial averaging, and hence greater estimation error for the NPS_r. The conclusion is that the large differences in the noise power occur where the MTR_r is essentially zero, though these high-frequency noise correlations have real impact on the qualitative properties of an image, as shown in Fig. 7.4.

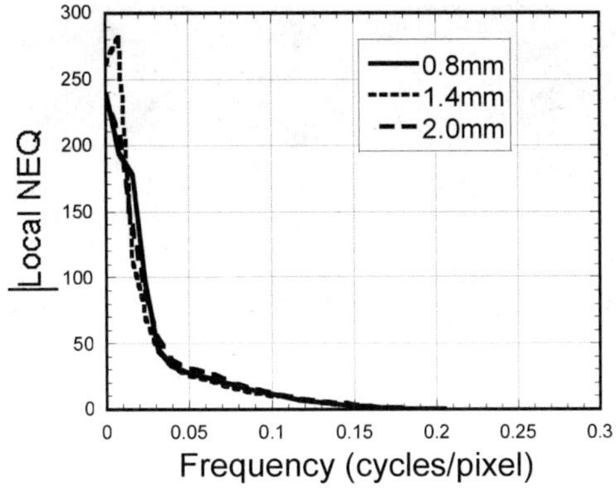

Figure 7.7. The NPS_r spectrum for compensations at 0.8 mm, 1.4 mm, and 2.0 mm.

2.3 Observer study: modeling error

We have shown that, although images possess very different qualitative properties they can be very similar in terms of the signal-to-noise ratio, NEQ_r. We next sought to determine if the difference in qualitative appearance (and correct or incorrect modeling of the original imaging system) had a strong affect on image quality in terms of a human observer's ability to perform a task. We generated images with a background consisting of randomly located Gaussian lumps, with the number of lumps Poisson distributed [Rolland and Barrett, 1992, Gallas and Barrett, 2003]. Poisson noise was then added at 100,000 total projection counts. The reconstructed lesion along with example reconstructed images with lesion are given in Fig. 7.8. A two-alternative-forced-choice study [Green and Swets, 1966, Metz, 1978, Burgess, 1995] was performed with five observers. Each observer was shown two images, one containing a lesion and the other without, and asked which he thought most likely to contain the lesion. There were five sets of images that all observers were tested on — with no compensation and with compensation assuming 1.0-mm, 1.2-mm, 1.4-mm (correct compensation), 1.6-mm, and 2.0-mm bore diameters. Each set included 50 training images and 200 test images, and the order the sets were shown was randomly selected for each observer. The results of the test, in terms of percent correct, are given in Fig. 7.9 and show very little difference in task performance among the different compensations. This study supports the signal-to-noise analysis, which implied there was little difference between images, rather than the original qualitative assessment of image quality.

2.3.1 Modeling error for pinhole apertures. Most of our new imaging systems call for single- or multiple-pinhole apertures. For this reason, we conducted

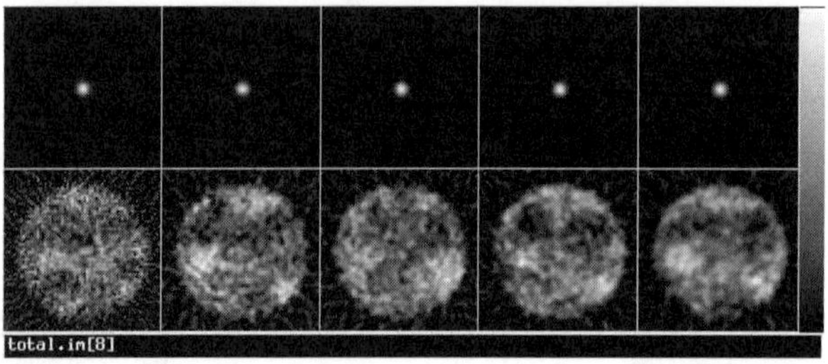

Figure 7.8. The lesion (top) and example reconstructed lumpy backgrounds with lesion (bottom) with compensation assuming bore diameter (left to right) of 0.0 mm, 1.2 mm, 1.4 mm, 1.6 mm, and 2.0 mm.

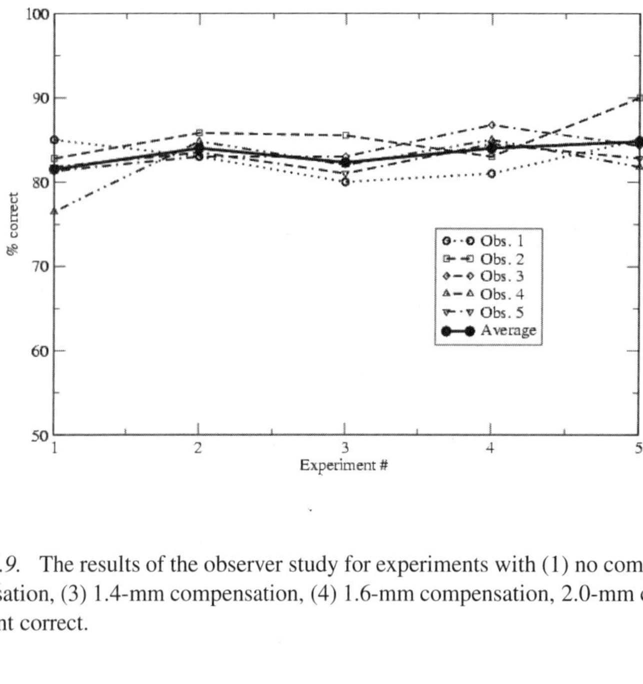

Figure 7.9. The results of the observer study for experiments with (1) no compensation, (2) 1.2-mm compensation, (3) 1.4-mm compensation, (4) 1.6-mm compensation, 2.0-mm compensation in terms of percent correct.

a preliminary study to determine if these aperture types are, like parallel-hole collimators, fairly robust in the face of incorrect modeling.

We performed this experiment using our computer simulation package for pinhole imaging systems. We simulated our 12 cm$\times$12 cm detectors with a resolution of 2.5 mm. Two detector models were assumed. The first had the detector infinitely thin (i.e., no depth of interaction effects occurred). The second model assumed that the detector had a 5mm thickness and that the probability of interaction of a 140 KeV photon in the NaI scintillator followed Beer's law. Example projections from a single source through a circular array of pinholes, with the geometry selected such that the photon beams struck the detector at approximately 45°, is given in

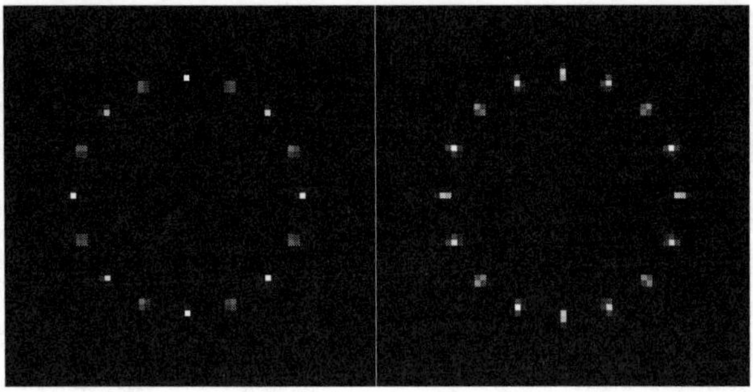

Figure 7.10. The response to a circular set of photon beams striking a detector at a 45° angle with (a) no depth of interaction modeled, and (b) depth of interaction modeled.

Fig.7.10. Little apparent difference seems to arise from depth of interaction with a 5 mm crystal.

The digital phantom used in this study was the Hoffman brain phantom. Although only one slice of the reconstructions will be shown for comparison, full 3D reconstruction was performed. The first aperture examined had a single 1.0 mm pinhole. We generated projection data from 64 projection angles using the model with a 5.0-mm detector thickness. We then reconstructed the data using ML-EM both with and without a model for detector thickness. The results are given in Fig. 7.11 for noise-free projection data and projection data with noise equivalent to 960 seconds, 96 seconds, and 9.6 seconds of imaging time. A small artifact appears near the center of the images with the incorrect detector model, but otherwise the images are nearly indistinguishable. The second aperture consisted of 64 1.0mm pinholes jittered regularly about a regular array. The other imaging parameters were the same as in the single-pinhole case. The results are given in Fig. 7.12, with the imaging times the same as in the previous experiment. Unlike the single-pinhole case, severe artifacts are seen in the images reconstructed with an incorrect depth-of-interaction model.

At CGRI, we typically do not use an analytical computer model of the imaging system in our reconstruction algorithm. Rather, we carefully calibrate our systems using a point-like source moved about the field of view on a very fine grid. Thus, we have been relatively impervious to issues like the one just demonstrated, because our reconstruction algorithms inherently have all of the imaging-system physics built in. However, as we push toward finer and finer resolution, the calibration process will become far more burdensome. At the same time, a number of these higher-resolution systems call for multiple pinholes. This study indicates that we must maintain care with the reconstruction models for these systems, either with very accurate computer models or by careful interpolation of coarse-grid calibration data.

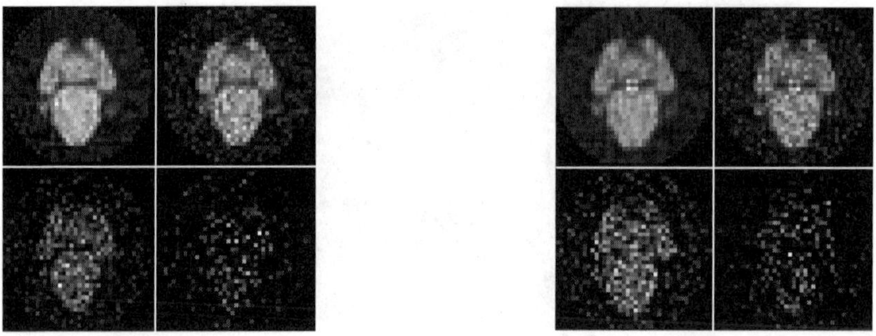

(a) (b)

Figure 7.11. A slice from the reconstruction of the single-pinhole data with noise-free data and 960 seconds, 96 seconds, and 9.6 seconds of imaging time at (a) depth of interaction correctly modeled, and (b) depth of interaction not modeled.

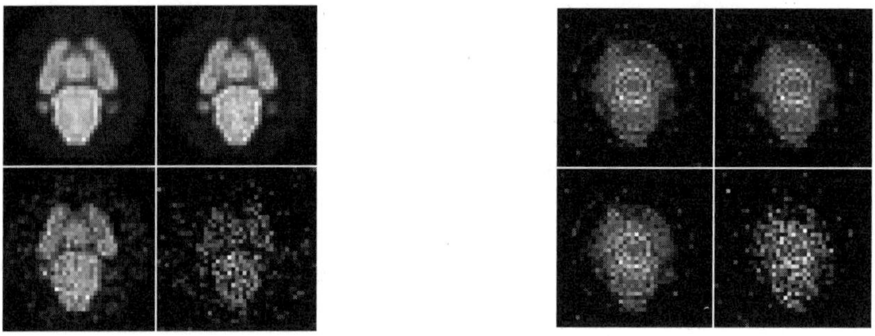

(a) (b)

Figure 7.12. A slice from the reconstruction of the multiple-pinhole data with noise free data and 960 seconds, 96 seconds and 9.6 seconds of imaging time and (a) depth of interaction correctly modeled and (b) depth of interaction not modeled.

3. System modeling

While it is expected that new detector technology will lead to better imaging systems, it also present new challenges. Traditional collimator and system designs may not be well suited for high-resolution cameras. Systems that take advantage of high-detector resolution must be developed, which requires establishing initial design parameters and optimizing the final system design. In order to maximize the advantages of the detectors, it is necessary to understand the relationship between detector properties and imaging-system performance.

Although part of this understanding can come via theoretical studies, the precise connection will ultimately be determined by experimental methods. Some of the experiments may be conducted in the laboratory, but laboratory experiments are time consuming and necessarily require the construction of the imaging system prior to testing. For this reason, the initial system design parameters are typically determined using computer models. An example of a system first conceived in simulation, and optimized largely in simulation, is given in Section 3.1. The multi-modular multi-resolution (M^3R) SPECT imager described is relatively simple, but offers a deceptively large number of design choices. These include the magnifications, pinhole number, and pinhole placement for each of the four aperture/camera modules. The system construction, calibration, and data collection would prohibit direct testing of more than a few designs. With a computer simulation, however, thousands of designs can be thoroughly analyzed in the time it would take to study one real configuration.

In order to optimize an imaging system, the first order of business must be to define "optimum," and the definition must encompass both the task for which the image is intended and the statistics of the imaging process. This component of the optimization formulation is discussed more fully in Chapter 5, and that should serve as reference as to how to use modeling for system optimization.

3.1 The M^3R imaging system

We previously advanced the synthetic collimator as a means of achieving high sensitivity without the typically accompanying loss of resolution [Wilson, 2000]. The original synthetic-collimator concept relied on movement of the aperture and/or detector to reduce the effects of multiplexing. In this study, we examined a small-animal SPECT imaging system, termed the Multi-Modular Multi-Resolution (M^3R) imager, that could potentially achieve the same advantages without actively changing pinhole-detector distances. We studied, in simulation, different pinhole sizes and pinhole numbers as well as different magnifications. We concluded by collecting preliminary data from a very simplified version of M^3R.

The proposed system consists of four modular scintillation cameras with multiple pinhole collimators focusing the photons onto each camera face. The cameras are the same as those employed by our FastSPECT II system [Furenlid, in press], but the M^3R system design offers advantages in terms of simplicity, cost, footprint, and weight. The preliminary experiments were carried out with analytic computer simulations using code developed in our laboratory. The geometry of the simulated system is sketched in Fig. 7.13. The camera was assumed to have a resolution of 2 mm. Attenuation and scatter were not included in the model.

The mouse brain phantom used in this study is presented in Fig. 7.14. This phantom, available at mbl.org (unassociated with our group), was produced by fixing the animal's brain, sectioning it into 30-μm slices, staining it with cresyl violet, and optically imaging it [Rosen, 2000]. A cylindrical background source, with an activity/unit volume of 10% of the average activity in the brain, surrounded the brain. For this study, we assumed a total activity in the phantom of 2 mCi and varied the collection time. Seventy percent of the 140 KeV photons were assumed captured by the scintillation crystal. The total phantom size was 24.6 mm$\times$24.6 mm$\times$24.6 mm. The size of the voxels used to generate the projections was 0.2, mm while the data were reconstructed onto a 0.6-mm grid – thus approximating the true continuous-to-discrete projection process versus discrete-to-discrete reconstruction that is inherent in all tomographic imaging. Reconstruction was performed

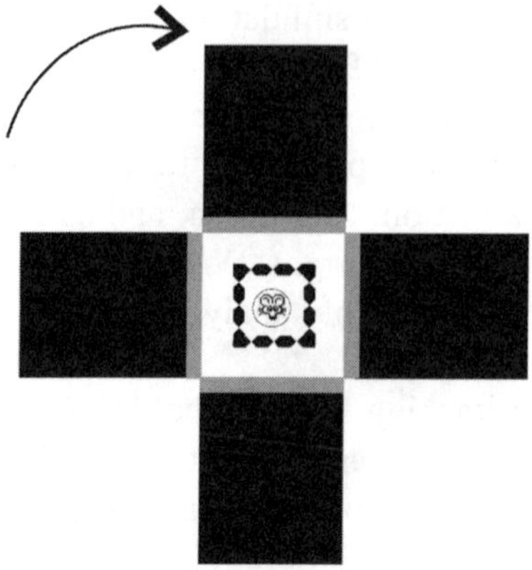

Figure 7.13. A sketch of the M^3R system.

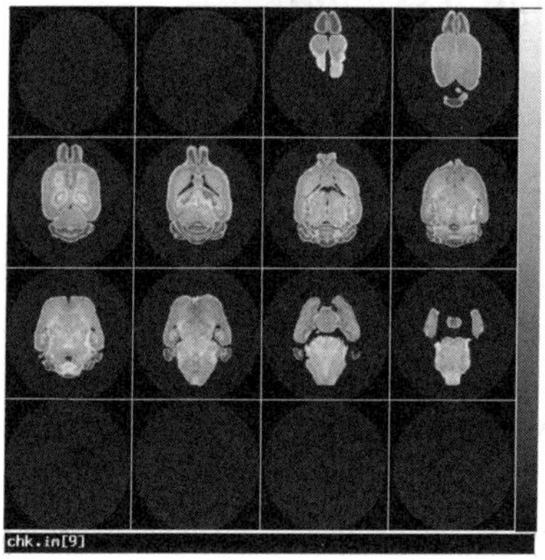

Figure 7.14. The mouse-brain phantom used in this study.

using the ordered-subsets expectation-maximization (OS-EM) algorithm. Opposite projections served as two-projection subsets.

The first experiment involved studying the effects of pinhole size on the properties of reconstructed images for a single-pinhole aperture. The pinhole-to-center-of-rotation (COR) distance was 16 mm, giving a 3.75 magnification of the COR onto the camera, and data were collected over 64 projection angles. We compared single-pinhole apertures with 1.0 mm and 2.0 mm pinhole sizes. Data were collect at both 960 and 96 second acquisition times. Figures 7.15 and 7.16 show one slice from the 3D reconstruction at 4, 7, 10, 15, 20, 30, 50, 70, and 100 iterations, with Fig. 7.15 at 960 seconds and Fig. 7.16 at 96 seconds.

A number of qualitative observations can be made from these figures. First, we see that larger pinholes reduce resolution in the lower-noise case, but that data taken with the smaller pinholes degrade more quickly with reduced imaging time. We also see that what appears to be a good iteration stopping point changes for both pinhole size and imaging time. Neither is a surprising result, but the latter fact underscores the need for using a quantitative measure of image quality. One fortunate effect

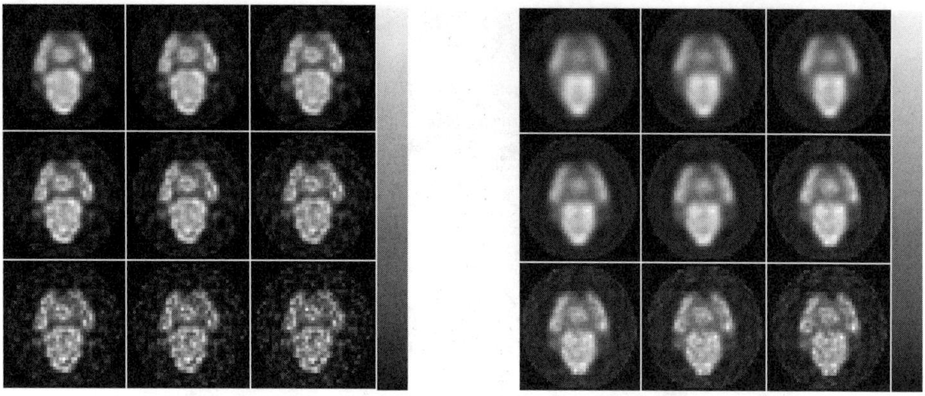

(a) (b)

Figure 7.15. One slice from 3D reconstructed images after 4, 7, 10, 15, 20, 30, 50, 70, and 100 iterations with 960 second imaging time and an aperture consisting of a single pinhole of diameter (a) 1.0 mm and (b) 2.0 mm.

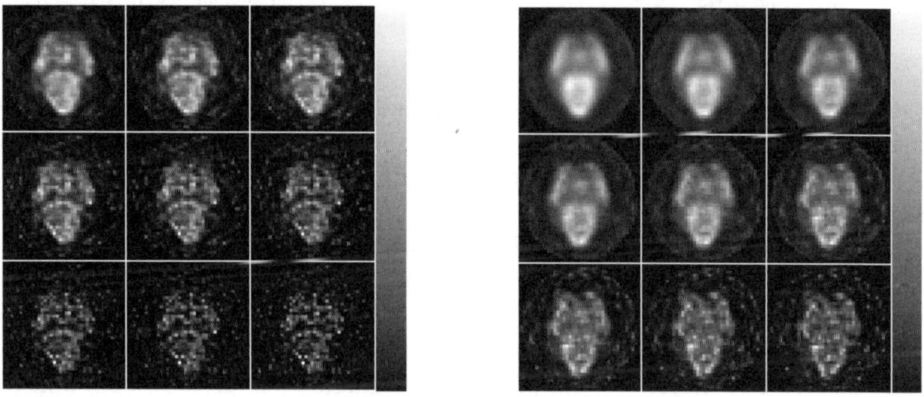

(a) (b)

Figure 7.16. One slice from 3D reconstructed images after 4, 7, 10, 15, 20, 30, 50, 70, and 100 iterations with 96 second imaging time and an aperture consisting of a single pinhole of diameter (a) 1.0 mm and (b) 2.0 mm.

seen in Figs. 7.15 and 7.16 is that image properties appear to be fairly constant over a broad range of iterations in the region of the qualitatively "best" stopping point. Thus, after studying all stopping points, we can hope that presenting only one image will give an idea of the reconstructed image properties. For the rest of this study, we shall make comparisons using only one such stopping point.

We next explored the possibility of multiple-pinhole configurations on each of the four cameras. In this study, we compared two different multiple-pinhole apertures – an aperture with 36 1.5-mm pinholes (25-mm pinhole-COR distance) and an aperture with 36 0.75-mm pinholes (20-mm pinhole-COR distance). We also included results from a hybrid system with two cameras using the first aperture

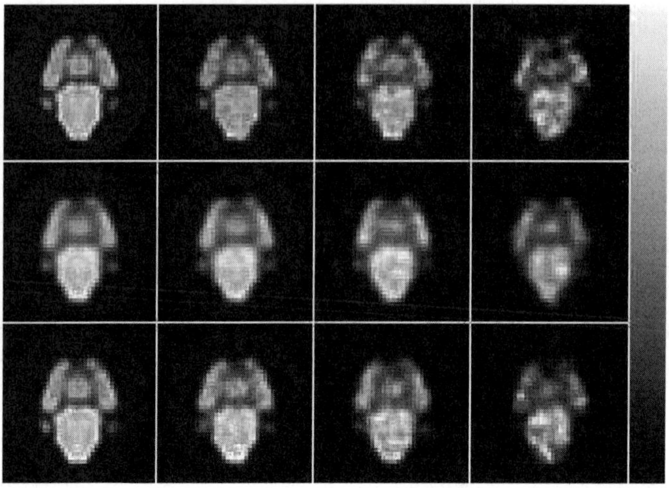

Figure 7.17. Comparison between images reconstructed from the M^3R system with (top to bottom) (1) 36 0.75 mm pinholes, (2) 36 1.5 mm pinholes, and (3) a combination of apertures (1) and (2). Imaging times (left to right) were (1) noise free, (2) 960 seconds, (3) 96 seconds, and (4) 9.6 seconds.

(36 1.5-mm pinholes) and two using the second (36 0.75-mm pinholes). For the multiple-pinhole apertures, data were taken from only 16 camera angles. Results are given in Fig. 7.17 for noise-free projection data, and data were collected for 960 seconds, 96 seconds, and 9.6 seconds.

A conclusion drawn from Fig. 7.17 when compared to Fig. 7.16 is that the multiple-pinhole apertures appear to offer superior performance at shorter imaging times. Less conclusive are comparisons between the different multiple-pinhole configurations. Eventually, we expect to use a system with combined resolutions and sensitivities, but because our proposed imaging system presents such a large number of options in the full design space, we leave optimization to the more rigorous methods discussed in Chapter 5.

As a preliminary test of this type of small modular-camera-based imager, we constructed a mock-up system using one modular camera with a single 1.0-mm pinhole aperture. Magnification of the center of rotation onto the camera face was approximately 2:1, and the calibration PSF was collected on an 0.7-mm grid. The phantom, shown in Fig. 7.18, consisted of a set of micro-hematocrit tubes with an internal diameter of approximately 1.1 mm and an external diameter of approximately 1.5 mm. We filled 6 of the 40 tubes (those sealed with the white critoseal shown in Fig. 7.18) with a total of less than 0.5 milliCuries of ^{99m}Tc pertechnetate. The sealed tubes most proximal to each other had a center-to-center separation of $\sim$2.5 mm and activity-to-activity separation of $\sim$1.4 mm.

Data were collected by rotating the phantom 64 times and imaging for 3 seconds at each projection angle. Because we collected the calibration PSF from only one angle, interpolation was necessary. For this data set, we used a simple nearest-neighbor approach, which is certainly a suboptimal interpolation scheme. We were

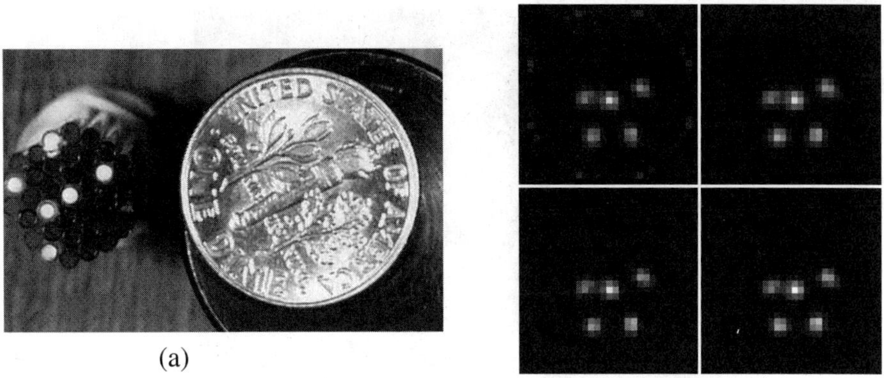

(a) (b)

Figure 7.18. (a) The micro-hematocrit-tube phantom used for the study, and (b) four slices from the 3D reconstructed image.

still able to get an excellent ML-EM reconstructed image, 4 slices of which are shown in Fig. 7.18. All of the tubes are easily differentiated, even the 2 separated by less than 1.5 mm (one of the 6 tubes was out of the field of view).

We concluded from these simulation and data-collection studies that the M^{3}R system can be a simple, inexpensive, and sound alternative to the more complicated and expensive small-animal SPECT systems available today, and that performance could well dramatically improve with the development of more complicated aperture systems, better interpolation schemes, and more sophisticated methods for exploring aperture-design space through objective assessment of image quality.

3.2 Preliminary simulations for a silicon-strip detector

In Chapter 20, Dr. Todd Peterson presents his work on an extremely high resolution detector based on double-sided silicon-strip technology. This system attracted our interest, as we had shown that the synthetic collimator offers advantages over traditional parallel-hole and pinhole collimators for both 2D and 3D reconstructions, particularly when a high-resolution detector is employed [Wilson, 2000]. While the synthetic collimator and silicon-strip detector seemed a perfect match, before proceeding with this technology, and before our collaborator could request funding, we needed to establish that this type of system would perform properly. We employed computer modeling to make this determination.

A preliminary study with computer simulations was carried out to evaluate the feasibility of the proposed imaging system. Data were collected using the synthetic-collimator paradigm, with multiple pinholes and multiple pinhole-detector distances. In this study, the pinhole to center-of-phantom distance remained at 22 mm, and data were collected at pinhole-to-detector distances of 5 mm, 20 mm, and 30 mm. There was no rotational motion of the object or detector.

Two-millimeter slices from the digital "mouse" phantom used for this experiment are shown in Fig. 7.19. The objects in the phantom were a sphere of 2.5-mm radius

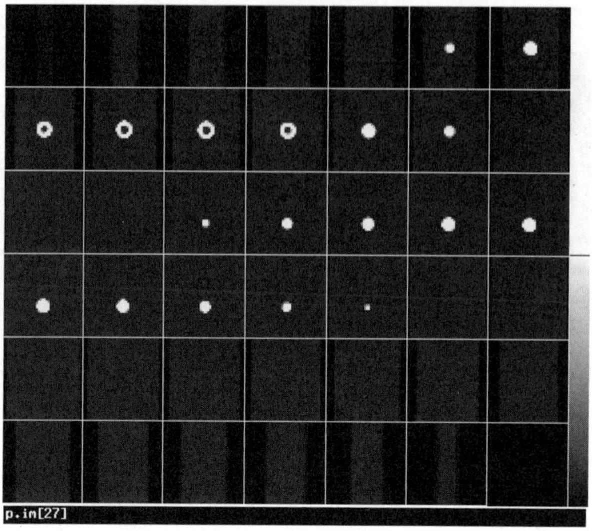

Figure 7.19. (a) The "mouse" phantom used for the imaging simulation, shown in 2-mm slices.

containing a 1.5-mm hollow center (simulating a tumor with necrotic center) and a bright ellipsoid of length 6 mm and diameter 4 mm. The mouse body was modeled as a 12.5-mm radius cylinder of water with a background specific activity of 5% relative to the objects. In order to simulate out-of-field activity, the cylinder was extended beyond the field of view shown in Fig. 7.19, with the out-of-field length equal to the in-field length and radiotracer concentration equal to half the specific activity of the in-field portion. The detector had 320×320 pixels with a pixel size of 200 microns. The collimator had 400 0.2-mm pinholes. Scatter and attenuation were not included in the model. An imaging time of 10 seconds with a total phantom activity of 1 millicurie and a detector sensitivity of 0.33% was assumed. The projections are shown in Fig. 7.20.

Two data sets were reconstructed. The first had data with only a 20-mm pinhole-to-detector distance. The second set had three projections — one each from 5-mm, 20-mm, and 30-mm pinhole-to-detector distances. The imaging times were normalized assuming one detector that was either stationary (in the single-projection case) or in motion (in the three-projection case) during the 10-second data-collection window. The results are given in Fig. 7.21. Figure 7.21(a) gives the reconstruction from only the 20-mm pinhole-detector distance. It shows some fairly severe artifacts, presumably from the multiplexing seen in Fig. 7.20. Figure 7.21(b) shows the reconstruction of data taken from all three pinhole-detector distances. It is seen that the artifacts have been removed and that the system has produced a high-quality tomographic image.

Because good-quality images were generated despite the short imaging times, we concluded that this was a very feasible system that offers the possibility of exquisite resolution. Dr. Peterson submitted a proposal to the National Institute of

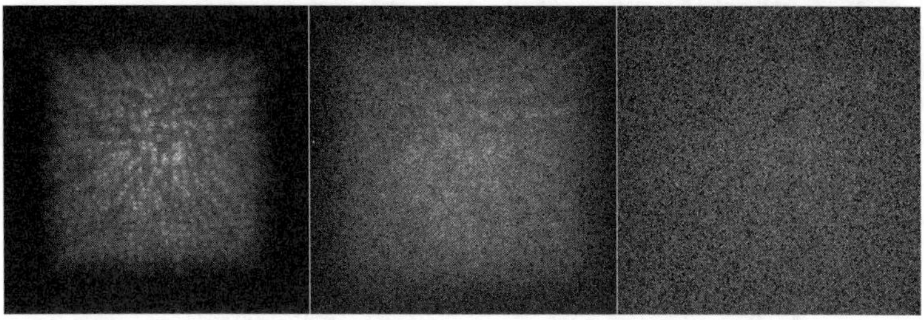

Figure 7.20. The projection data with pinhole-detector distances of 5.0 mm (left) 20 mm (center) and 30 mm (right).

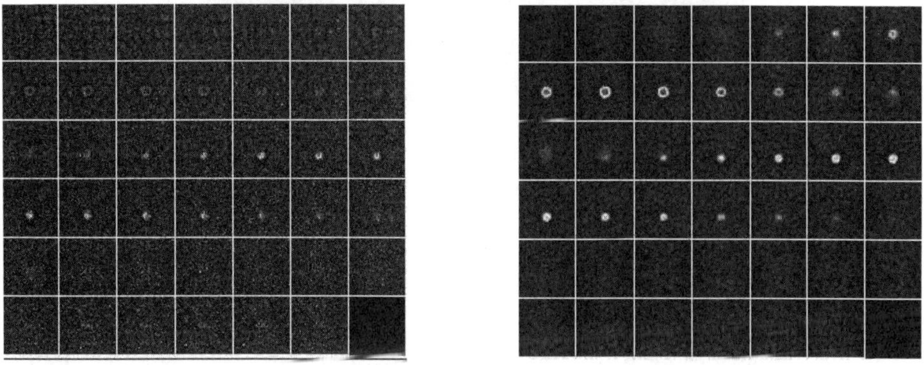

(a) (b)

Figure 7.21. The reconstructed images with (a) only the 20-mm data and (b) with all of the 5-mm, 20-mm, and 30-mm data.

Biomedical Imaging and Bioengineering to build such a system, and the proposal was subsequently funded.

3.3 Monte Carlo modeling of a modular scintillation camera

The previous experiments were conducted using analytical models, but Monte Carlo techniques also can be employed. The analytical methods usually have advantages in computational speed, and the results they generate are noise free. Because noise-free data are frequently desired for the system-optimization techniques presented in Chapter 5, we often choose analytical rather than Monte Carlo models. However, it is difficult to incorporate complex physics into the analytical methods and, for this reason, Monte Carlo approaches play an important role in computer imaging-system modeling.

We have developed a Monte Carlo optical-transport model for our scintillation cameras that includes all of the effects of the reflection, refraction, and diffusive scatter that the various applied surface treatments can impart on an optical photon at the individual camera interfaces. Any of the camera properties can be freely varied so that any reasonable design can be modeled. We simulated one of our 12 cm $\times$ 12

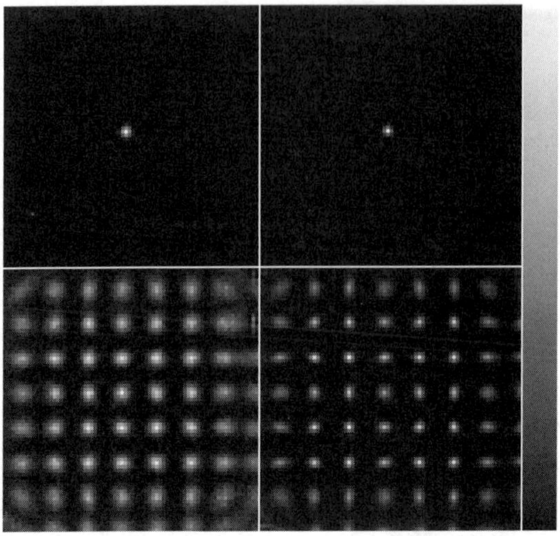

Figure 7.22. Top: a Monte Carlo estimated point response for a camera with a 15mm light guide and 8mm light guide; bottom: real point arrays for cameras with 15mm and 8mm light guides.

cm nine-PMT modular cameras with an NaI(Tl) scintillator and a fused quartz light guide, In the study presented below, the camera had a 5-mm scintillation crystal, optical-photon-absorbing walls, and a Lambertian-reflecting front window. In this study, we varied the light-guide thickness in order to determine if our current choice of 15 mm was, in fact, optimal.

We explored light-guide thicknesses between 5 mm and 20 mm and compared the cameras in terms of width of the position estimate of photons arriving in a thin beam directed normal to the camera surface. The results for 15 mm and 8 mm are given in Fig 7.22, where it is clearly seen that the model predicts that our 15-mm light guide is inferior to the thinner one.

Based on these results, we designed our next camera with an 8-mm light guide. We compared it, in terms of resolution, with the old 15-mm light-guide camera. The experiment was performed in the same manner as the Monte Carlo simulation. A 1-mm-bore-diameter collimator was used to illuminate the crystals with a beam normal to the scintillator surface (in this case, at multiple positions). Estimates of the position of interaction for the photons were then performed using a maximum-likelihood approach. The results are given in Fig. 7.22. The resolution of the 8-mm light-guide camera appears clearly superior to the one with the thicker light guide, as was predicted by the simulation. This study demonstrates the power of Monte Carlo methods and the importance of modeling an imaging system prior to construction.

4. Conclusions

We have introduced two reconstruction algorithms used in small-animal SPECT, briefly discussed their manner of operation, and showed some of their properties. We demonstrated that, for poorly sampled data, a positivity constraint can have profound effects on the resulting tomographic images. We also studied the consequences of modeling error on the quality of reconstructed images. Using detector response as an example, we showed that different models can greatly affect the qualitative properties of an image, but that the differences are far less significant when measured using the noise-equivalent quanta or the signal-to-noise of a human observer performing a lesion-detection task. We demonstrated that, for multiple-pinhole systems, modeling errors can lead to serious problems in the reconstructed images.

We also illustrated the importance of computer modeling in the development of an imaging system. We followed the course of a four-camera SPECT system from its origin in a computer model to fruition and showed how simulations can be further used to optimize it. Finally, we presented a Monte Carlo model experiment which indicated that current design parameters for our scintillation cameras were suboptimal, and we demonstrated with real cameras that the model's predictions were correct.

References

[Barrett, 1994] H. H. Barrett, D. W. Wilson, and B. M. W. Tsui. "Noise properties of the EM algorithm: 1. Theory," *Phys. Med. Biol.*, vol. 39, pp. 833-846, 1994.

[Beck, 1982] J. W. Beck, R. J. Jaszczak, R. E. Coleman, C. F. Starmer, and L. W. Nolte. "Analysis of SPECT including scatter and attenuation using sophisticated Monte Carlo modeling methods," *IEEE Trans. Nucl. Sci.*, vol. 29, pp. 506-511, 1982.

[Bracewell, 1956] R. N. Bracewell. "Strip integration in astronomy," *Aust. J. Phys.*, vol. 9, pp. 198-217, 1956.

[Burgess, 1995] A. E. Burgess. "Comparison of receiver operating characteristic and forced choice observer performance measurement methods," *Med. Phys.*, vol. 22, pp. 643-655, 1995.

[Byrne, 1993] C. L. Byrne. "Iterative image reconstruction algorithms based on cross-entropy minimization," *IEEE Trans. Imag. Proc.*, vol. 9, pp. 96-103, March 1993.

[Clarkson and Barrett, 1997] E. Clarkson and H. H. Barrett. "A bound on null functions for digital imaging systems with positivity constraint," *Optics Letters*, vol. 814-815, pp. 649-658, 1997.

[Clarkson and Barrett, 1998] E. Clarkson and H. H. Barrett. "Bounds on null functions of linear digital imaging systems," *J. Opt. Soc. Am. A*, vol. 15, pp. 1355-1360, 1998.

[Cormack, 1963] A. M. Cormack. "Representation of a function by its line integrals, with some radiologyical applications," *J. Appl. Phys.*, vol. 34, pp. 2722-2727, 1963.

[Cormack, 1964] A. M. Cormack. "Representation of a function by its line integrals, with some radiologyical applications," *J. Appl. Phys.*, vol. 35, pp. 2908-2913, 1964.

[Dempster, 1977] A. D. Dempster, N. M. Laird, and D. B. Rubin. "Maximum likelihood from incomplete data via the EM algorithm," *J. Royal Stat. Soc.*, vol. 39, pp. 1-38, 1977.

[Feldkamp, 1984] L. A. Feldkamp, L. C. Davis, and J. W. Kress. "Practical cone-beam algorithm," *J. Opt. Soc. Amer. A*, vol. 1, pp. 612-619, 1984.

[Furenlid, in press] L. R. Furenlid, D. W. Wilson, P. J. Pietraski, H. K. Kim, Y. Chen, and H. H. Barrett. "FastSPECT II: A second-generation high-resolution dynamic SPECT imager," *IEEE Trans. Nucl. Sci.*, in press.

[Gallas and Barrett, 2003] B. D. Gallas and H. H. Barrett. "Validating the use of channels to estimate the ideal linear observer," *Journal of the Optical Society of America: A*, vol. 20, pp. 1725-1738, 2003.

[Gordon, 1970] R. Gordon, R. Bender, and G. T. Herman. "Algebraic reconstruction techniques (ART) for 3-dimensional electron microscopy and x-ray photography," *J. Theoretical Biology*, vol. 29, pp. 471-481, 1970.

[Green and Swets, 1966] D. M. Green and J. A. Swets. *Signal detection theory and psycophysics*. Wiley, 1966.

[Green, 1990] P. J. Green. "Bayesian reconstructions from emission tomography data using a modified em algorithm," *IEEE Trans. Med. Imag.*, vol. 9, pp. 84-93, 1990.

[Hoffman, 1990] E. J. Hoffman, P. D. Cutler, W. M. Digby, and J. C. Mazziotta. "2-D phantom to simulate cerebral blood flow and metabolic images for pet," *IEEE Trans. Nucl. Sci.*, vol. 37, pp. 616-620, 1990.

[Hudson and Larkin, 1994] H. M. Hudson and R. S. Larkin. "Accelerated image-reconstruction using ordered subsets of projection data," *IEEE Trans. Med. Imag.*, vol. 13, pp. 601-609, 1994.

[Jain, 1989] A. K. Jain. *Fundamentals of Digital Image Processing*. Prentice Hall, 1989.

[Jaszczak, 1981] R. J. Jaszczak, R. E. Coleman, and F. R. Whitehead. "Physical factors affecting quantitative measurements using camera-based single photon-emission computed-tomography (SPECT)," *IEEE Trans. Nucl. Sci.*, vol. 28, pp. 69-80, 1981.

[Kinahan, 1995] P. E. Kinahan, S. Matej, J. S. Karp, G. T. Herman, and R. M. Lewitt. "A comparison of transform and iterative reconstruction techniques for a volume-imaging PET scanner with a large axial acceptance angle," *IEEE Trans. Nucl. Sci.*, vol. 42, pp. 2281-2287, 1995.

[King and Farncombe, 2003] M. King and T. Farncombe. "An overview of attenuation and scatter correction of planar and SPECT data for dosimetry studies," *Cancer biotherapy and radiopharmaceuticals*, vol. 18, pp. 181-190, 2003.

[King, 1995] M. A. King, B. M. W. Tsui, and T. S. Pan. "Attenuation compensation for cardiac single-photon emission computed tomographic imaging 1. Impact of attenuation and methods of estimating attenuation maps," *Journal of Nuclear Cardiology*, vol. 2, pp. 513-524, 1995.

[Landweber, 1951] L. Landweber. "An iterative formula for Fredholm integral equations of the first kind," *Amer. J. Math.*, vol. 73, pp. 615-624, 1951.

[Liang, 1992a] Z. Liang, T. G. Turkington, D. R. Gilland, R. J. Jaszczak, and R. E. Coleman. "Simultaneous compensation for attenuation, scatter and detector response for SPECT reconstruction in 3 dimensions," *Phys. Med. Biol.*, vol. 37, pp. 587-603, 1992a.

[Liang, 1992b] Z. Liang, T. G. Turkington, D. R. Gilland, R. J. Jaszczak, and R. E. Coleman. "Simultaneous compensation for attenuation, scatter and detector response for SPECT reconstruction in 3 dimensions," *Physics in Medicine and Biology*, vol. 37, pp. 587-603, 1992b.

[Metz, 1978] C. E. Metz. "Basic principles of ROC analysis," *Seminars in Nuclear Medicine*, vol. 7, pp. 283-298, 1978.

[Metz and Pan, 1995] C. E. Metz and X. C. Pan. "A unified analysis of exact methods of inverting the 2D exponential radon transform, with implications for noise control in SPECT," *IEEE Trans. Med. Imag.*, vol. 14, pp. 643-658, 1995.

[Radon, 1917] J. Radon. "On the determination of functions from their integrals along certain manifolds (translated)," *Ber. Verbhandl. Sachs. Akad. Wiss. Leipzig Math-Phys. K1*, vol. 69, pp. 262-277, 1917.

[Rolland and Barrett, 1992] J. P. Rolland and H. H. Barrett. "Effect of random background inhomogeneity on observer detection performance," *J. Opt. Soc. Am. A*, vol. 9, pp. 649-658, 1992.

[Rosen, 2000] G. D. Rosen, A. G. Williams, J. A. Capra, M. T. Connolly, B. Cruz, L. Lu, D. C. Airey, K. Kullcarni, and R. W. Williams. The mouse brain library@www.mbl.org. 2000.

[Rosenthal, 1995] M. S. Rosenthal, J. Cullom, W. Hawkins, S. C. Moore, B. M. W. Tsui, and M. Yester. "Quantitative SPECT imaging – a review and recommendations by the focus committee of the Society of Nuclear Medicine Computer and Instrumentation Council," *J. Nucl. Med.*, vol. 36, pp. 1489-1513, 1995.

[Shepp and Vardi, 1982] L. Shepp and Y. Vardi. "Maximum likelihood reconstruction for emission tomography," *IEEE Trans. Med. Imag.*, vol. 1, pp. 113-122, 1982.

[Tretiak and Metz, 1980] O. Tretiak and C. Metz. "The exponnential radon-transform," *Siam. J. Appl. Math.*, vol. 39, pp. 341-354, 1980.

[Tsui, 1994] B. M. W. Tsui, E. C. Frey, X. Zhao, D. S. Lalush, R. E. Johnston, and W. H. McCartney. "The importance and implementation of accurate 3D compensation methods for quantitative SPECT," *Phys. Med. Biol.*, vol. 39, pp. 509-530, March 1994.

[Wang, 1993] G. Wang, T. H. Lin, P. C. Cheng, and D. M. Shinozaki. "A general cone-beam reconstruction algorithm," *IEEE Trans. Med. Imag.*, vol. 12, pp. 486-496, 1993.

[Welch, 1995] A. Welch, G. T. Gullberg, P. E. Christian, F. L. Datz, and T. Morgan. "A transmission-map based scatter correction technique for SPECT in inhomogeneous-media," *Medical Physics*, vol. 22, pp. 1627-1635, 1995.

[Wigner, 1933] E. P. Wigner. "On the quantum correction for thermodynamic equilibrium," *Physics Review*, vol. 40, pp. 749-759, 1933.

[Wilson, 2000] D. W. Wilson, H. H. Barrett, and E. W. Clarkson. "Reconstruction of two- and three-dimensional images from synthetic-collimator data," *IEEE Trans. Med. Imag.*, vol. 19, pp. 412-422, 2000.

[Wilson, 1994] D. W. Wilson, H. H. Barrett, and B. M. W. Tsui. "Noise properties of the EM algorithm: 2. Monte Carlo simulations," *IEEE Trans. Med. Imag.*, vol. 13, pp. 601-609, 1994.

[Wilson and Tsui, 1993a] D. W. Wilson and B. M. W. Tsui. "Noise properties of filtered backprojection and ML-EM reconstructed emission tomographic images," *IEEE Trans. Nucl. Sci.*, vol. 40, pp. 1198-1203, 1993a.

[Wilson and Tsui, 1993b] D. W. Wilson and B. M. W. Tsui. "Spatial resolution and quantitation properties of fb and ML-EM reconstructed emission tomographic images," *Proceedings of the IEEE Medical Imaging Conference*, pp. 1189-1193, 1993b.

Chapter 8

Reconstruction Algorithm with Resolution Deconvolution in a Small-Animal PET Imager

Edward N. Tsyganov, Alexander I. Zinchenko, Nikolai V. Slavine, Pietro P. Antich, Serguei Y. Seliounine, Orhan K. Oz, Padmakar V. Kulkarni, Matthew A. Lewis, Ralph P. Mason and Robert W. Parkey*

1. Experimental setup

A small-animal PET imaging device has been developed at the University of Texas Southwestern Medical Center at Dallas using scintillating 1-mm round BCF-10 fibers and small admixture of CsF microcrystals between the fibers [Antich, 1990, Atac, 1991, Fernando, 1996]. The fiber core is polystyrene $(C_8H_8)_n$ doped with butyl-PBD and dPOPOP. The fibers are clad in a non-scintillating lucite cladding. The scintillation mechanism can be either from the excitation of π-electrons in the butyl-PBD benzene ring in the fiber or from excitation within the microcrystals. In both cases, the emitted light is compatible with the optimal spectral response of standard photomultiplier cathodes. For a 511 keV photon in plastic, the photo-absorption is small, and Compton scatter interactions are dominant. The scattered electrons give up their energy well within a fiber diameter, but wave-shifting produces light in proximal fibers. The current imager uses the 2-fold coincident detection of a single event in 2 orthogonal fibers of 1-mm diameter to detect the location and the energy transferred at a point within the detector. Two sets of fibers each 60 cm in length and 1 mm in diameter were used to construct two alternating, mutually orthogonal sets of 14 planar arrays of 135 fibers each. In this detector, the planar fiber arrays are arranged along two alternating mutually orthogonal (X and Y) axes and are stacked along a third (Z). Scintillating light from the fibers is detected by two (X and Y directions) Hamamatsu R-2486 Position Sensitive Photomultiplier Tubes (PSPMT). A single-ended readout scheme is used, where the X,Z and Y,Z interaction positions in a detector are determined from coincident detection in the two PSPMT. The precision of the detection of the interaction point depends upon PSPMT performance and software filters.

The current Data Acquisition (DAQ) system is based on a multi-standard platform: a custom backplane for the Analog-to-Digital Convertor (ADC) modules and

*The University of Texas Southwestern Medical Center, Dallas, Texas

a PXI (the Compact PCI standard from National Instruments) enclosure for the data readout from the ADCs. Two interface modules (PXI-6508 for slow control and PXI-6533 for the fast data transfer) are included in this enclosure. The current data transfer rate is about 6 MB/s ($\sim$40 K events per second), but we expect a final data transfer rate of 40 MB/s.

For PET imaging, two planar detectors are required. Each planar detector is positioned to measure one of the two 511 keV annihilation photons. By requiring a coincidence between the two detectors (i.e. 4 PSPMT), the position of an electron-positron interaction can be reconstructed. The two detectors can be rotated around the central axis to approximate a truncated cylindrical detector. The performance of the system is shown in Table 1. The object spatial resolution is unchanged across the entire field of view, while the sensitivity varies between 40% and 100% of the central maximum over a 10×10 cm^2 field of view.

The data in Table 1 show that the system has both high resolution and sensitivity and achieves a level of performance comparable to that of other current animal imaging systems [Antich, 1990]. These results are significant considering the construction from non-standard materials, the novel design, and the fact that only two of the four detectors necessary for closed 2π geometry have been completed at this time. Noise reduction avails itself of the very fast scintillation time of plastic (1-2 ns), which permits a narrow coincidence window. Software algorithms have also been implemented to further reduce noise on the data themselves.

Table 8.1. Performance characteristics of the system.

Detector type	Scintillating optical fibers and CsF microcrystals in Teflon matrix
Detector dimensions (mm)	$135 \times 135 \times 28$ (3780 fibers)
Detection and digital channels	4 position-sensitive PMTs 128 channels
Equivalent TCD radius	Variable, 15 to 45 cm
Spatial resolution without system modeling	<2 mm (isotropic in entire volume)
Spatial resolution with system modeling	<0.6 mm (isotropic in entire volume)
Point source sensitivity (ID=12 cm)	490 cps/μCi
Sensitivity (ID=30 cm)	4600 cps/μCi/ml (NEMA phantom)
Scatter fraction	20% for a lucite phantom of 6-cm diameter

2. List-mode EM algorithm with convolution model

In order to fully exploit the advantages offered by the experimental apparatus, an appropriate image reconstruction method should be used. The method should also offer reasonable processing time and manageable data volumes for practical applications.

One of the most attractive approaches appears to be the recently developed list-mode EM algorithm [Andrew, 1998]. The algorithm was developed from the standard projection-data based ML-EM (Maximum Likelihood-Expectation Maximization) algorithm [Shepp and Vardi, 1982] and is given by:

$$n_j^{k+1} = \frac{n_j^k}{\sum\limits_{i=1}^{I} a_{ij}} \sum_{i=1}^{M} a_{ij} \frac{1}{q_i^k} \quad \text{with} \quad q_i^k = \sum_{j=1}^{J} a_{ij} n_j^k, \tag{8.1}$$

where q_i^k is the expected integral count in line of response (LOR) i if the intensity was n_j^k (at the kth iteration), a_{ij} is the probability of an emission from voxel j being detected along LOR i, M is the number of measured events, and I is the number of all possible system LORs. J is the number of voxels in the image. The algorithm takes into account the fact that the measured list-mode data are implicitly 1 for each acquired LOR.

Depending on the number of events, direct iterative reconstruction from list-mode data can be burdensome and computationally expensive. If the data are abundant, the MLEM algorithm can be extended to incorporate subsets (one-pass list-mode OPL-EM) [Andrew, 2002]:

$$n_j^{k+1} = \frac{n_j^k}{\sum\limits_{i=1}^{I} a_{ij}} \sum_{i \in S^k} a_{ij} \frac{1}{q_i^k} \tag{8.2}$$

where only a subset S^k of the M total LORs is used in each update. Each subset S^k (k=1,..K) contains equal numbers of list-mode events.

In the simplest approach, the element a_{ij} of the probability matrix is taken as the intersection length of LOR i with voxel j. However, in this case, all resolution effects (positron range, photon non-collinearity and intrinsic detector resolution) are neglected. To account for these effects, which can be measured and considered known, the following approach can be used. The matrix of probabilities $A = (a_{ij})_{I \times J}$ can be factorized as:

$$A = WXH \tag{8.3}$$

The matrix $H = (h_{j'j})_{J \times J}$ accounts for finite resolution effects, $X = (x_{ij})_{I \times J}$ is the matrix of intersection lengths as mentioned above, and the diagonal matrix $W = (w_{ii})_{I \times I}$ takes into account geometric sensitivity variations. Then, the expected count is expressed as:

$$q_i^k = w_{ii} \sum_{j=1}^{J} x_{ij} \sum_{b=1}^{J} h_{jb} n_b^k \tag{8.4}$$

and the list-mode EM algorithm becomes:

$$n_j^{k+1} = \frac{n_j^k}{\sum\limits_{b=1}^{J} h_{bj} \sum\limits_{i=1}^{I} w_{ii} x_{ib}} \sum_{b=1}^{J} h_{bj} \sum_{i \in S^k} x_{ib} \frac{1}{\sum\limits_{p=1}^{J} x_{ip} \sum\limits_{v=1}^{J} h_{pv} n_v^k} \tag{8.5}$$

The expression (8.5) can be rewritten in vector form:

$$\mathbf{n^{k+1}} = \mathbf{n^k} \times \mathbf{s} \times \mathbf{c^k}, \tag{8.6}$$

where $\times$ denotes an element-by-element multiplication of vectors, $\mathbf{n}^{k+1}$ and $\mathbf{n}^k$ contain the new and old image estimates, and $\mathbf{s}$ contains the sensitivity correction factors. $\mathbf{c}^k$ contains the multiplicative image correction values given by:

$$\mathbf{c}^k = H^T \left[\sum_{i \in S^k} \mathbf{BP_i} \left(\frac{1}{\mathrm{FP_i}(H\mathbf{n^k})} \right) \right], \tag{8.7}$$

where $\mathrm{FP_i}$ is an operator which forward projects vector $H\mathbf{n^k}$ along LOR i to give a scalar value, and $\mathbf{BP_i}$ is an operator which back projects a scalar value along LOR i into a 3D image.

If the system can be considered as shift-invariant, the blurring component H can be taken as a shift-invariant kernel $\boldsymbol{\rho}$. Then, the one-pass list-mode EM algorithm becomes:

$$\mathbf{n^{k+1}} = \mathbf{n^k} \times \mathbf{s} \times \left(\left[\sum_{i \in S^k} \mathbf{BP_i} \left(\frac{1}{\mathrm{FP_i}(\mathbf{n^k} \otimes \boldsymbol{\rho})} \right) \right] \otimes \boldsymbol{\rho} \right) \tag{8.8}$$

Thus, the algorithm OPL-EM has 2 parameters: the resolution kernel $\boldsymbol{\rho}$, which can be taken as a Gaussian function, and the number of subsets (equal to the number of image updates) to use K.

Incorporation of the system model into the EM procedure proposed in [Andrew, 2002] is a mathematically elegant deconvolution mechanism taking into account the spatial resolution due to finite detector accuracy, positron range in tissue, etc. As will be seen below, this step is of primary importance for our utilization of the algorithm. To emphasize this fact and distinguish the approach from the "conventional" MLEM method with only the matrix of intersection lengths taken into account, we call it the Expectation Maximization with Deconvolution (EMD).

3. Results for simple phantoms

Fig. 8.1 shows the reconstructed image for a simulated phantom consisting of two point-like sources separated by 2-mm distance in X, where the coordinate system of the image was aligned with that of the detectors. The detector resolution was taken to be Gaussian with sigma of 2 mm, and only the data for one rotation angle of the detectors were considered. The "conventional" list-mode MLEM is

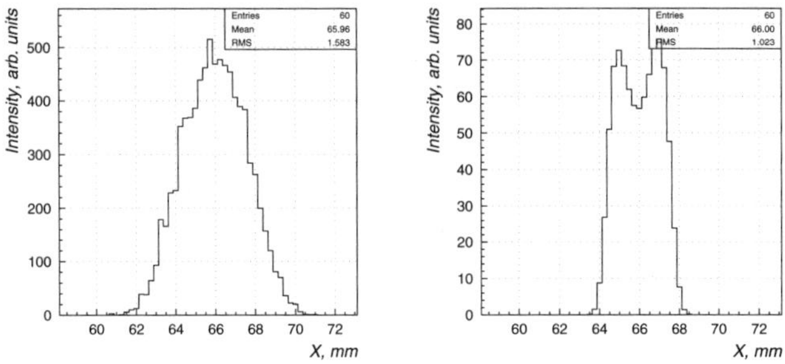

Figure 8.1. Reconstruction of a 2-point simulated phantom with 2-mm separation between sources. Left: conventional MLEM, 10 image updates; right: EMD, 250 image updates. Voxel size $0.25 \times 0.25 \times 0.25$ mm^3. Note that conventional MLEM does not improve the quality of image after 10 iterations, while EMD continues to improve the quality, and more iterations are needed.

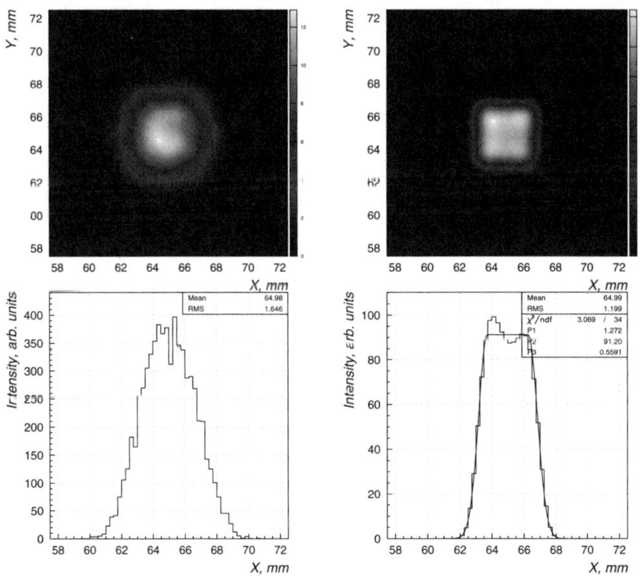

Figure 8.2. Reconstruction of a simulated "box" phantom. Left: "conventional" EM, 10 image updates; right: EMD, 150 updates. Upper row shows X-Y image slices at true Z. Lower row shows X-projection (along Y) at true Z. Line shows results of the fit by a function with a flat top and Gaussian edges (with $\sigma = 0.56$ mm).

unable to separate the sources, whereas EMD with a Gaussian resolution kernel with σ=1.4 mm, corresponding to the transverse spatial resolution in the median plane of the detector, achieves the separation.

Fig. 8.2 shows reconstructed images for a simulated box-shaped active volume with dimensions of $4\times4\times1$ mm^3. One hundred and fifty updates of EMD were performed.

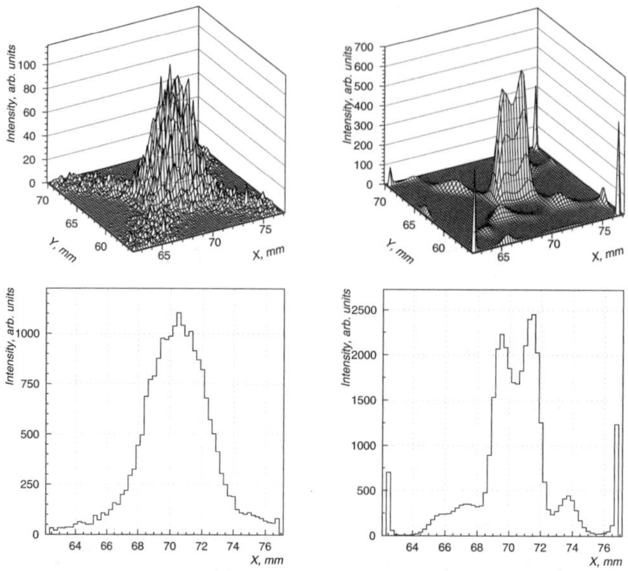

Figure 8.3. Reconstruction of a 2-point ^{22}Na phantom with 2-mm separation between sources. Upper row: slices at true Z: left - "conventional" MLEM, 10 image updates; right - EMD, 600 image updates. Lower row: X-distributions: left - conventional MLEM, right - EMD.

Reconstruction results for two real ^{22}Na "point-like" sources (physical diameter <1 mm) are shown in Fig. 8.3. Here, the image coordinate system was rotated by 45° in the detector plane in order to suppress the effect of non-Gaussian tails, whose treatment will be discussed in the next section. Only the data for one rotation angle of the detectors were used (500,000 list-mode events). EMD does improve the source separation, but significant artifacts appear because the Gaussian kernel does not describe the system model sufficiently well.

Similar results for two-line FDG sources are shown in Fig. 8.4 for relatively low statistics (200,000 list-mode events). The inner diameter of the tube of the source was 1.05 mm, and the outer diameter was 1.2 mm. Separation of the data (50%-50%) was made numerically.

Fig. 8.5 shows the reconstructed image of a rod phantom, made of a 60-mm diameter lucite cylinder containing four $^{18}F^{-}$-filled holes. Hole diameters are 1.5 mm, and the distances between their centers are 2.5 mm, 3.5 mm, and 4.5 mm (right to left). Eight million events for 8 angular positions of the detectors around the Y-axis were acquired and processed. Due to photon scattering effects, the resolution for the lucite phantom is not as good as for phantoms in air.

Just for reference, Fig. 8.6 characterizes the spatial resolution of our system after system modeling. The image of the ^{18}F line phantom is also presented in this figure. FWHM resolution is 0.63 mm.

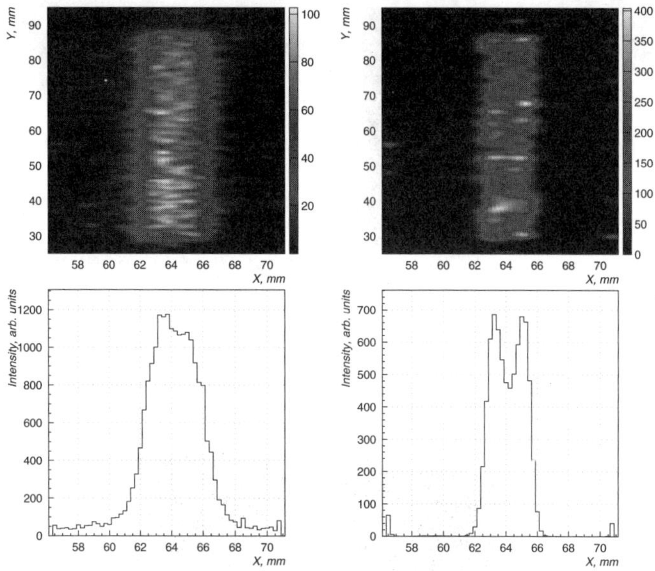

Figure 8.4. FDG two-line phantom with 2 mm center to center separation between the lines, reconstructed after 10 iterations of the conventional MLEM (left) and 600 iterations of EMD (right). Top: X-Y view for true Z, bottom: X projection. Additional Gaussian smearing with σ=0.4 mm was applied for X-Y views.

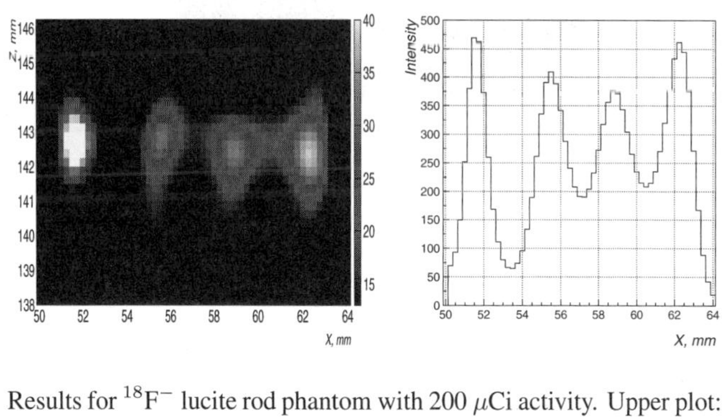

Figure 8.5. Results for $^{18}F^-$ lucite rod phantom with 200 μCi activity. Upper plot: X-Z distribution of activity, lower plot: X-distribution of the activity. Seven hundred iterations of EMD with Gaussian kernel σ=1.1 mm, voxel size $0.25 \times 0.25 \times 0.25$ mm^3.

After introduction of system modeling (deconvolution of smearing effects from an image), we obtained superb images of small animals. Fig. 8.7 shows an 0.7-mm slice of a cocaine-addiction rat with FDG. High activity in the front part of the cerebral hemispheres is obvious. Fig. 8.8 presents projections of the rat brain where a tumor was implanted in a median fissure. Fig. 8.9 presents a mouse bone activity under $^{18}F^-$.

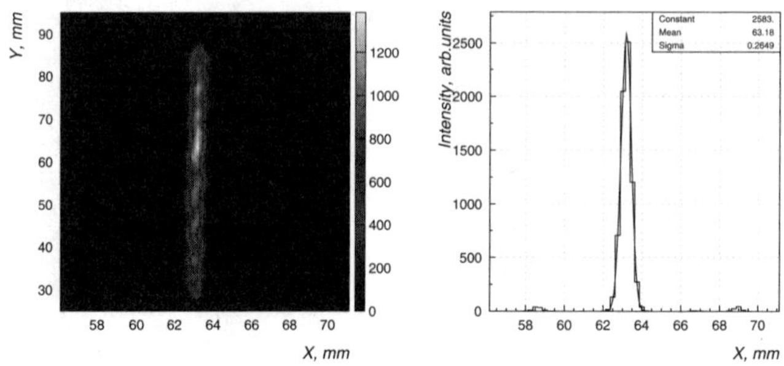

Figure 8.6. FDG one-line phantom after 600 updates of EMD; left: X-Y-view; right: X-projection for Y=50-70 mm.

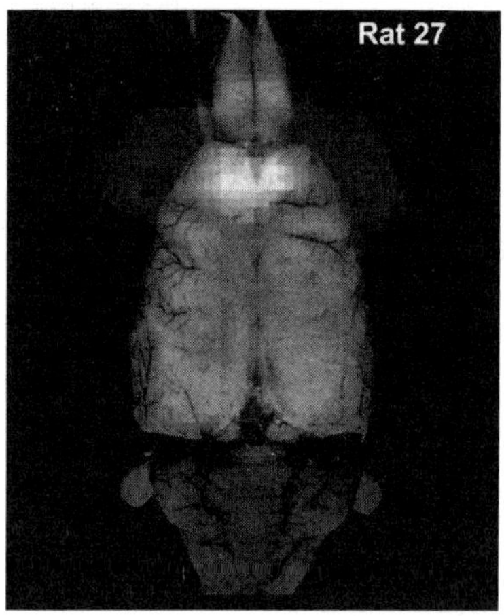

Figure 8.7. Cocaine-addicted rat, brain slice 0.7 mm, FDG.

4. Double Compton scattering model

As seen in the previous section, making use of a simplified resolution kernel for the reconstruction results in the appearance of artifacts. To improve the image quality, a more accurate system model should be considered.

As can be seen in Fig. 8.10, the point spread function of our small animal PET device shows visible deviations from the Gaussian shape. These deviations are caused by a non-negligible fraction of double Compton scattering events in the active material of the detectors, resulting in position analyzing.

For those events, selection of signals from the second scattering results in faulty reconstruction of photon lines and can be seen as a "cross-like" pattern for a point-like source. However, it is possible to include this effect into the system model of the EMD reconstruction algorithm. This can be illustrated by the results of the point-like source image reconstruction. If only the peak of the distribution is included in

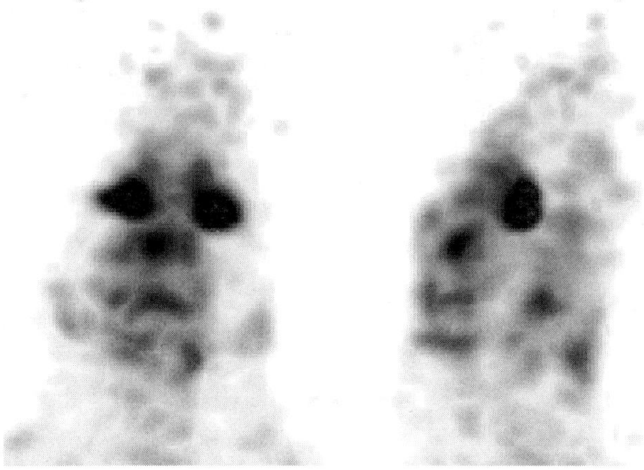

Figure 8.8. Image of a tumor implanted in a rat brain using FDG. Left: coronal view; right: side view.

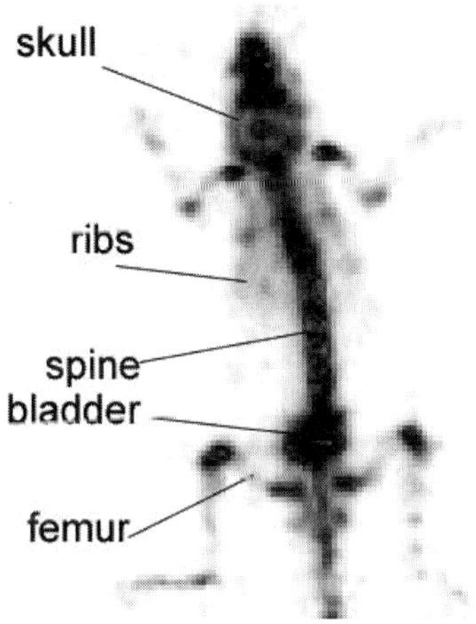

Figure 8.9. An image taken using $^{18}F^-$.

the convolution kernel of the method, the reconstructed image shows significant tails (Fig. 8.10). If the whole distribution is described, the image becomes significantly cleaner (Fig. 8.11).

The exact form of the kernel k was found by fitting to the distribution in Fig. 8.10 an expression, which included three parts: the central peak k_{peak} describing the detector resolution, the "cross" k_{comp} due to double Compton scattering, and the background k_{bkgr} due to random coincidences and coincidences of the annihilation photon and a photon from γ-decay of ^{22}Na:

$$k = k_{peak} + c_{comp}k_{comp} + c_{bkgr}k_{bkgr} \tag{8.9}$$

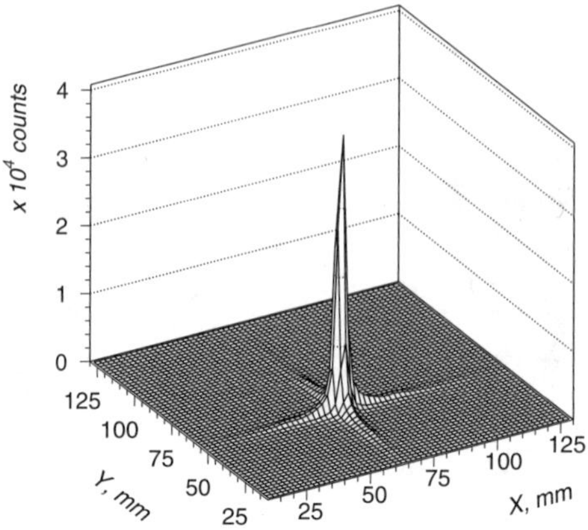

Figure 8.10. Projected X-Y-view of the point-like source at true Z for one rotation angle of detectors.

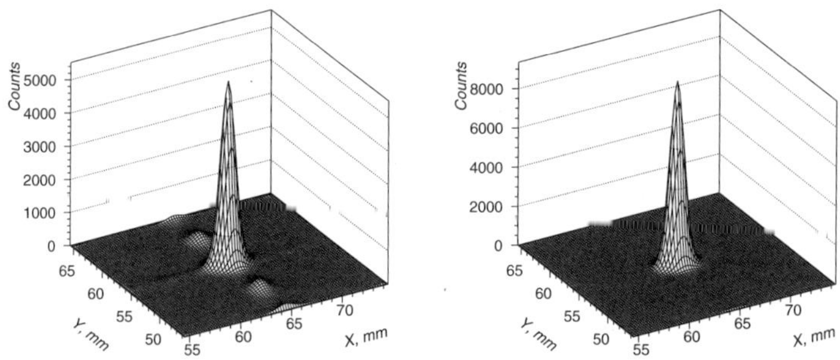

Figure 8.11. Reconstructed X-Y-view of the point-like source. Left: with Gaussian kernel with σ = 1.35 mm; right: kernel is chosen to fit the distribution in Fig. 8.10. Fifty iterations of the EMD method with voxel size of $0.25 \times 0.25 \times 0.25$ mm^3.

with

$$k_{peak} = \exp\left[-0.5\left\{\left(\frac{r}{\sigma_r}\right)^2 + \left(\frac{y}{\sigma_y}\right)^2\right\}\right], \tag{8.10}$$

$$
\begin{aligned}
k_{comp} &= \exp\left[-\frac{r}{\lambda_r}\right]\left(1 + a_r\frac{r}{\lambda_r} + b_r\left(\frac{r}{\lambda_r}\right)^2\right) \\
&\times \exp\left[-0.5\left(\frac{y}{\sigma_y}\right)^2\right] \\
&+ \exp\left[-\frac{|y|}{\lambda_y}\right]\left(1 + a_y\frac{|y|}{\lambda_y} + b_y\left(\frac{y}{\lambda_y}\right)^2\right) \\
&\times \exp\left[-0.5\left(\frac{r}{\sigma_r}\right)^2\right] \qquad (8.11)
\end{aligned}
$$

and

$$k_{bkgr} = \exp\left[-\rho\right](1 + a_\rho \rho + b_\rho \rho^2), \qquad (8.12)$$

where

$$\rho = \sqrt{(r/\lambda'_r)^2 + (y/\lambda'_y)^2}. \qquad (8.13)$$

Thus, the peak is described by a double Gaussian function (in radial r and axial y directions), the double Compton scattering term by an exponentially decaying expression in one direction (modified by a second-degree polynomial), and a Gaussian in the other direction, while the background is described by a modified exponentially decaying function.

5. Application of EM algorithm for image deblurring

The results presented above show that the EMD method can be successfully used for image reconstruction. However, introduction of two array convolutions for each image update increases the processing time as compared to "conventional MLEM," even if the "one-pass" mode is implemented.

In order to overcome the problem, an image deblurring procedure was used to improve the image reconstructed after several iterations of "conventional" MLEM. Here, the reconstructed image is taken as the observation, the reconstructed point-like source gives parameters of the reconstruction kernel, and an iterative procedure similar to that described above is applied:

$$\mathbf{n}^{\mathbf{k}+1} = \mathbf{n}^{\mathbf{k}} \times \left\{ \left(\frac{\mathbf{n}^{MLEM}}{\mathbf{n}^{\mathbf{k}} \otimes \boldsymbol{\rho}} \right) \otimes \boldsymbol{\rho} \right\}, \qquad (8.14)$$

where $\mathbf{n}^{MLEM}$ is the image obtained after "conventional" MLEM. Because looping over all recorded lines is not needed, processing speed was improved (factors of 4-5 were observed for the studied phantoms with relatively low statistics).

Comparison of the reconstruction results from an *in vivo* animal imaging is shown in Fig. 8.12, where a rat's beating heart is shown. Results are also shown in Figs. 8.13 and 8.14 for ^{22}Na 2-point and FDG 2-line phantoms with 2-mm separation between sources.

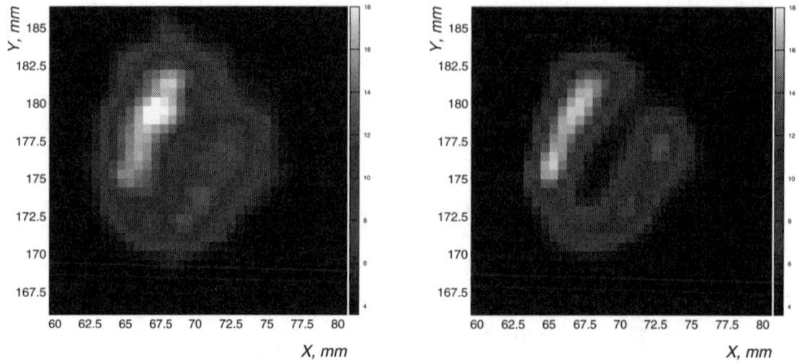

Figure 8.12. Coronal slice of a rat's heart *in vivo*, FDG 1.2 mCi. Top: after 16 updates of MLEM and Gaussian filter with σ=0.6 mm; bottom: after 16 updates of MLEM and 10 iterations of the deblurring procedure. The data are from a whole-body ^{18}FDG rat scan with 13 million events recorded. Voxel size $0.6 \times 0.6 \times 0.6$ mm^3.

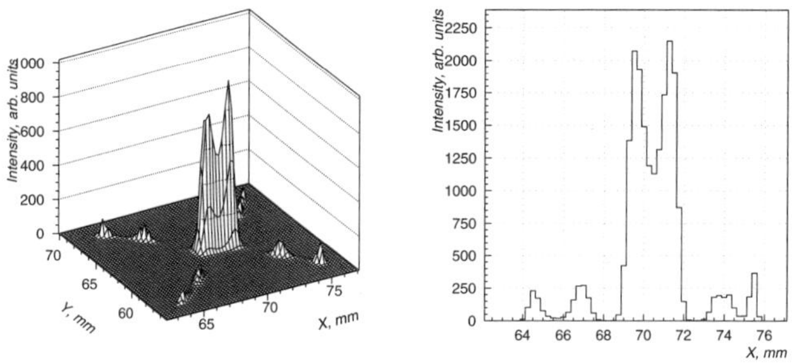

Figure 8.13. ^{22}Na two-point phantom with 2-mm separation between sources after 300 iterations of the deblurring procedure. Left: XY view for true Z; right: X-projection.

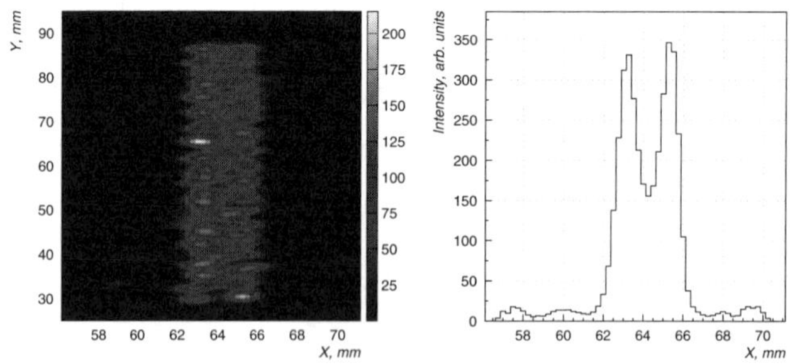

Figure 8.14. FDG two-line phantom after 100 iterations of the deblurring procedure. Left: X-Y view for true Z (after additional Gaussian smearing with σ=0.4 mm); right: X-projection.

6. Conclusions

The presented results show that the list-mode EMD method produces higher quality images when proper account is taken of the finite resolution effects through incorporation of the extended system model into the EM procedure.

Additionally, the proposed EM deblurring procedure can be used to improve the image quality after the "conventional" EM reconstruction on a much shorter time scale than EMD.

Acknowledgments

We are grateful to Drs. G. Arbique, A. Constantinescu, and R. McColl for their valuable help. Addiction studies are under way with supervision by Dr. J. Bibb and Mr. D. Benavides. Brain tumor studies were carried out by Drs. C. Giller and T. Psarros. The work was supported in part by the Cancer Imaging Program (an NCI Pre-ICMIC) P20 CA 86354.

References

[Andrew, 1998] J. Andrew, J. Reader et. al., "Fast accurate iterative reconstruction for low-statistics volume imaging", *Phys.Med.Biol.*, vol. 43, pp. 835-846, 1998.

[Andrew, 2002] J. Andrew, J. Reader et al., "One-Pass List-Mode EM Algorithm for High Resolution 3D PET Image Reconstruction into Large Arrays", *IEEE Transactions on Nuclear Science*, vol. 49(3), pp. 693, 2002.

[Antich, 1990] PP Antich, M Atac, RC Chaney, et al, "Development of a high resolution scintillating fiber gamma ray telescope", *Nucl. Instr. and Meth. in Physics Research*, vol. A297, pp. 514, 1990.

[Atac, 1991] M. Atac, R. Chaney, D. Chrisman, D. Cline,E. Fenyves,J. Park, and P.P Antich, "Development of a High Resolution Scintillating Fiber Gamma Ray Telescope", *IEEE Transactions on Nuclear Science*, vol. 38(2), pp. 568-573, 1991.

[Fernando, 1996] JL. Fernando, "High resolution positron emission tomography imaging with plastic scintillating fibers: application to a small animal imager", Ph.D. in Radiological Sciences, Southwestern Graduate School of Biomedical Sciences, The University of Texas Southwestern Medical Center at Dallas, 1996.

[Shepp and Vardi, 1982] L. A. Shepp and Y. Vardi, "Maximum likelihood reconstruction for emission tomography", *IEEE Trans. Med. Im.*, vol.1, pp.113-122, 1982.

Chapter 9

Estimates of Axial and Transaxial Resolution for One-, Two-, and Three-Camera Helical Pinhole SPECT

Scott D. Metzler and Ronald J. Jaszczak*

1. Introduction

There is ongoing work to improve the sensitivity and resolution of pinhole collimation for small-animal studies [Moore, 1991, Strand, 1994, Weber, 1994, Jaszczak, 1994, Ishizu, 1995, Tsui, 2001, Beekman, 2001, Metzler, 2001, Beekman, 2002a, Beekman, 2002b, Metzler, 2002, Ogowa, 1998, Kastis, 2002, Acton, 2002]. One method is the reduction of radius of rotation [Mortimer, 1954].

Circular orbits of pinhole collimators give incomplete data [Tuy, 1983, Smith, 1985]. The data completeness worsens as ROR decreases, which is where resolution and sensitivity increase [Metzler, 2001]. Helical orbits are one method for improving data completeness.

When helical orbits are used, the symmetry of the acquisition, compared with circular orbits, is broken. This leads one to question what is the spatial dependence of resolution. This spatial dependence is not unique to helical orbits, but helical orbits do not have the axial mirror symmetry for resolution that is present for circular orbits.

We discuss a method for determining the axial and transaxial resolutions as a function of position.

2. Experimental acquisition

Experimental data were acquired for a disk phantom and a cold-rod phantom. To simulate one-, two-, and three-collimator operation using a single collimator, orbits were acquired with that single collimator using several different starting positions: 0° (one-camera), 0° and 180° (two-camera), and 0°, 120°, and 240° (three-camera). The total scan time was reduced for multiple-camera operation so that the same total number of counts were expected regardless of the number of collimators in use.

The data were reconstructed using an iterative algorithm that modeled penetrative sensitivity and point-spread [Metzler, 2001, Metzler, 2002]. The grid size

*S. D. Metzler, Duke University Medical Center, Department of Radiology, Durham, North Carolina; R. J. Jaszczak, Duke University, Department of Biomedical Engineering, Durham, North Carolina

was 120x120x100 0.5-mm-edge voxels. The reconstruction used 5 iterations of OSEM [Hudson, 1994] and did not compensate for attenuation or scatter.

3. Estimating experimental resolution

Experimental resolution was estimated in two orthogonal directions: axial and transaxial. Both components were measured as a function of axial and radial position. Axial position is measured along the axis of rotation from the center of the helix or helices; it is a signed quantity. Radial position is measured from the axis of rotation; it is a non-negative quantity.

Axial resolution was measured using a disk phantom. The phantom consisted of disks alternating between active (hot) and inactive (cold). The phantom was filled with a homogeneous solution of ^{99m}Tc-pertechnetate so that all hot areas had the same activity concentration. To determine axial resolution as a function of axial position, a local profile of 11 axials bins was selected for a particular transaxial location. Those 11 bins were fit to a Gaussian-convolved impulse function (Section 4). The result of that fit was averaged with the other fit results for that same axial location; the result is an axial resolution that is averaged over a transaxial slice. The center of the profile was used as the axial location for that resolution. The rationale for choosing 11 bins is that the thickness of a cold disk is 4.3 mm = 8.6 bins and that of a hot disk is 4.0 mm = 8.0 bins. Therefore, 11 bins will give at least one transition from hot to cold (or vice versa), but no more than two transitions. To determine axial resolution as a function of radial position, a small radial interval from r to $r + \Delta r$ was selected, and averaging was performed along the axial direction.

Transaxial resolution was measured using a cold-rod phantom. The phantom consisted of six sectors, each of which had multiple rods with the same diameter: 1.0 mm, 1.6 mm, 2.4 mm, 3.2 mm, 4.0 mm, and 4.8 mm. The phantom was filled with a homogeneous solution of ^{99m}Tc-pertechnetate so that all hot areas had the same activity concentration. To determine transaxial resolution as a function of axial position, profiles through the 3.2-mm rods were determined for each axial slice. Each profile contained rods at several different radial positions. Each contiguous 11-bin region of the profile was fit to a Gaussian-convolved impulse function (Section 4). The center of each region was considered to be the radial position for that resolution measurement. The resulting set of fits was averaged over the radial position to determine the average resolution as a function of position; it was averaged over the axial position to determine the average resolution as a function of radial position.

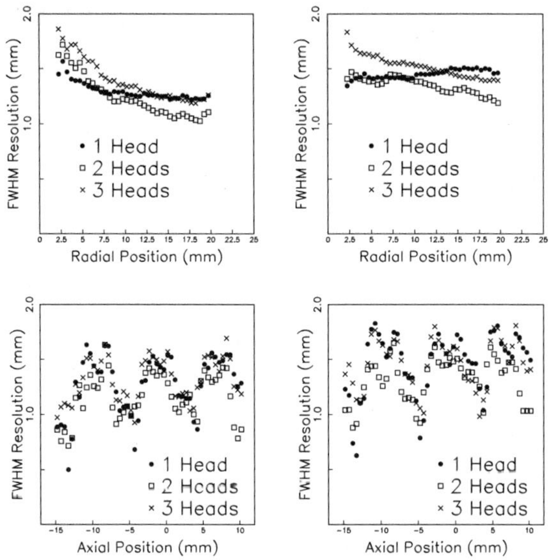

Figure 9.1. Axial resolution as a function of radial (top) and axial position (bottom). The resolutions were measured for an ROR of 34 mm (left) and 50 mm (right).

4. Fitting a Gaussian-convolved impulse function

The phantoms used in this study have alternating regions of hot and cold. With perfect resolution, a profile could be modeled as:

$$f(x) = \begin{cases} a & |x - x_0| \geq \frac{d}{2} \\ b & |x - x_0| < \frac{d}{2} \end{cases}. \tag{9.1}$$

This is a peak (valley) of width d centered at x_0. To account for experimental resolution, the expected profile may be modeled as:

$$\tilde{f}(x) = \frac{1}{\sqrt{2\pi}\sigma} \int_{-\infty}^{\infty} dx' f(x') e^{-\frac{(x-x')^2}{2\sigma^2}} = a + \frac{b-a}{2} \left[\text{erf}(C_2) - \text{erf}(C_1)\right], \tag{9.2}$$

where σ is the standard deviation of the Gaussian distribution and

$$C_1 = \frac{-\frac{d}{2} + x_0 - x}{\sqrt{2}\sigma}; C_2 = \frac{\frac{d}{2} + x_0 - x}{\sqrt{2}\sigma}. \tag{9.3}$$

The fit was performed by binning Eq. 9.2 into the same number of bins as the profile. The binning was performed by integrating over the bin to account for binning effects. Ten such binned functions were formed with 0.1 bin offsets between them. The binned functions were jointly minimized with respect to σ, x_0, a, and b using a least-squared metric.

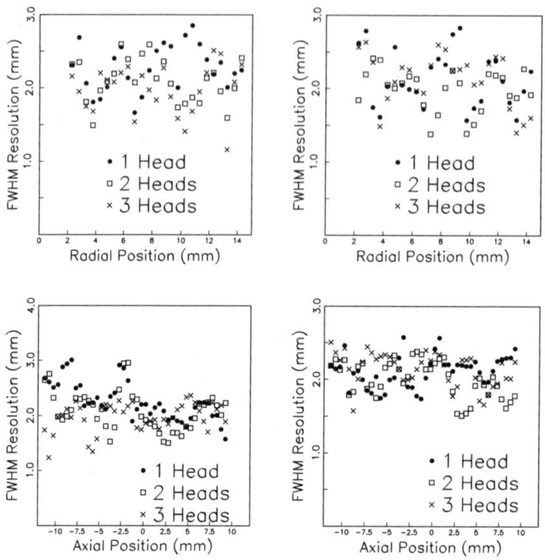

Figure 9.2. Transaxial resolution as a function of radial (top) and axial position (bottom). The resolutions was measured for an ROR for 34 mm (left) and 50 mm (right).

5. Results

Figure 9.1 shows the measured axial resolution as a function of radial (top) and axial position (bottom). The resolution was measured for an ROR of 34 mm (left) and 50 mm (right). Figure 9.2 shows the measured transaxial resolution as a function of radial (top) and axial position (bottom). The resolution was measured for an ROR or 34 mm (left) and 50 mm (right).

6. Summary

The method for measuring axial resolution seems to give stable results. The method for measuring transaxial resolution seems less robust. Because the transaxial method uses only a single set of rods, many fewer fits are used in the average. As the number of cameras increases, both efficiency and resolution improve.

7. Acknowledgments

This work was supported by the National Institute for Biomedical Imaging and Bioengineering of the National Institutes of Health under Grants R21-EB-001543 and R01-EB-01910. Experimental data were acquired using shared instrumentation funded by the National Center for Research Resources of the National Institutes of Health under Grant Number S10 RR15697.

References

[Acton, 2002] P.D. Acton, S.R. Choi, K. Plössl, H.F. Kung, "Quantification of Dopamine Transporters in the Mouse Brain Using Ultra-high Resolution Single-photon Emission Tomography," *Eur. J. Nucl. Med.*, vol. 29(5), pp. 691-698, 2002.

[Beekman, 2001] F.J. Beekman, D.P. McElroy, F. Berger,E.J. Hoffman, and S.R. Cherry, "Sub-millimeter resolution I-125 *in vivo* imaging in mice using micro-pinholes," *J. Nucl. Med.*, vol. 42(5)(Suppl.), pp. 204, 2001.

[Beekman, 2002a] F.J. Beekman, D.P. McElroy, F. Berger, S.S. Gambhir, E.J. Hoffman, and S.R. Cherry, "Towards *in vivo* Nuclear Microscopy: I-125 Imaging in Mice using Micro-pinholes," *Eur J. Nucl. Med.*, vol. 29(7), pp. 933-938, 2002.

[Beekman, 2002b] M. Gieles, H.W.A.M de Jong and F.J. Beekman, "Accelerated Monte Carlo simulation of micro-pinhole imaging using Kernel Forced Detection," *Phys. Med. Biol.*, vol. 47(11), pp. 1853-1867, 2002.

[Jaszczak, 1994] R.J. Jaszczak, J. Li, H. Wang, M.R. Zalutsky, and R.E. Coleman, "Pinhole collimation for ultra-high-resolution, small-field-of-view SPECT," *Phys. Med. Biol.*, vol. 39, pp. 425-437, 1994.

[Hudson, 1994] H.M. Hudson and R.S. Larkin, "Accelerated Image Reconstruction Using Ordered Subsets of Projection Data," *IEEE Trans. Med. Imag.*, vol. 13(4), pp. 601-609, 1994.

[Ishizu, 1995] K. Ishizu, T. Mukai, Y. Yonekura, M. Pagani, T. Fujita, Y. Magata, S. Nishizawa, N. Tamaki, H. Shibasaki, and J. Konishi, "Ultra-high Resolution SPECT System Using Four Pinhole Collimators for Small Animal Studies," *J. Nucl. Med.*, vol. 36(12), pp. 2282-2287, 1995.

[Kastis, 2002] G.A. Kastis *et al.*, "Tomographic Small-animal Imaging Using a High-resolution Semiconductor Camera," *IEEE Trans. Nucl. Sci.*, vol. 49, pp. 172-175, 2002.

[Metzler, 2001] S.D. Metzler, J.E. Bowsher, M.F. Smith, and R.J. Jaszczak, "Analytic Determination of Pinhole Sensitivity with Penetration," *IEEE Trans. Med. Img.*, vol. 20(8), pp. 730-741, 2001.

[Metzler, 2002] S.D. Metzler, J.E. Bowsher, K.L. Greer, and R.J. Jaszczak, "Analytic Determination of the Pinhole Collimator's Point-Spread Function and RMS Resolution with Penetration," *IEEE Trans. Med. Img.*, 2002.

[Metzler, 2003] S.D. Metzler, K.L. Greer, and R.J. Jaszczak, "Helical Pinhole SPECT for Small-Animal Imaging: A Method for Addressing Sampling Completeness," *IEEE Trans. Nucl. Sci.*, vol. 50(5), pp. 1575-1583, 2003.

[Moore, 1991] R.H. Moore, H. Ohtani, B.A. Khaw, and H.W. Strauss, "High Resolution Pinhole Sequence Imaging of Small Laboratory Animals," *Cancer*, vol. 32(5), p. 987, 1991.

[Mortimer, 1954] R.K. Mortimer, H.O. Anger, and C.A. Tobias, "The Gamma Ray Pinhole Camera with Image Amplifier," Convention Record of the Institute or Radio Engineers, Part 9 - Medical and Nuclear Electronics, pp. 2-5, 1954.

[Ogowa, 1998] K. Ogawa, T. Kawade, K. Nakamura, A. Kubo, T. Ichihara, "Ultra High Resolution Pinhole SPECT for Small Animal Study," *IEEE Trans. Nucl. Sci.*, vol. 45, pp. 3122-3126, 1998.

[Smith, 1985] B.D. Smith, "Image Reconstruction from Cone-Beam Projections: Necessary and Sufficient Conditions and Reconstruction Methods," *IEEE Trans. Med. Imag.*, vol. MI-4(1), pp. 14-25, 1985.

[Strand, 1994] S-E. Strand, M. Ivanovic, K. Erlandsson, D. Franceschi, T. Burton, K. Sjogren, and D.A. Weber, "Small Animal Imaging with Pinhole Single-Photon Emission Computed Tomography," *Cancer*, vol. 73(3), pp. 981-984, 1994.

[Tsui, 2001] B.M.W. Tsui, Y. Wang, E.C. Frey, and D.E. Wessell, "Application of Ultra High-Resolution Pinhole SPECT System Based on a Conventional Camera for Small Animal Imaging," *J. Nucl. Med.*, vol. 42(5), pp. 54P-55P, 2001.

[Tuy, 1983] H.K. Tuy, "An Inversion Formula for Cone-Beam Reconstruction," *SIAM J. Appl. Math.*, vol. 43(3), pp. 546-552, 1983.

[Weber, 1994] D.A. Weber, M. Ivanovic, D. Franceschi, S-E. Strand, K. Erlandsson, M. Franceschi, H.L. Atkins, J.A. Coderre, H. Susskind, T. Button, and K. Ljunggren, "Pinhole SPECT: An Approach to *in vivo* High Resolution SPECT Imaging in Small Laboratory Animals," *J. Nucl. Med.*, vol. 35(2), pp. 342-348, 1994.

Chapter 10

Pinhole Aperture Design for Small-Animal Imaging

Chih-Min Hu, Jyh-Cheng Chen, and Ren-Shyan Liu*

1. Introduction

Pinhole collimation is one of the techniques available for SPECT imaging. The usage of transgenic mice has evolved and has become more and more popular. Functions of genes are studied by over-expression of a certain protein in the transgenic mice or by the lack of expression of a certain protein in the knock-out mice. For the small animal functional imaging, an ultra-high-resolution functional imaging technique is required. Improvement of nuclear imaging spatial resolution enables the preclinical and clinical imaging methods in which monoclonal antibodies, receptor-specific molecules, peptides, and other new radio-pharmaceuticals are used [Weber, 1999]. Live-animal functional imaging is desirable in comparison to anatomical study for its versatility for series study at different time point and built-in controls. In order to apply SPECT on live animals, especially transgenic mice, a clinical gamma camera is adopted using a special pinhole aperture to enhance spatial resolution [Simmons, 1988].

2. Theory

System spatial resolution of a gamma camera system is [Habraken, 2001],

$$R_t = \left[R_g^2 + R_i^2 + R_s^2\right]^{1/2}, \tag{10.1}$$

where R_g is the collimator or geometrical resolution, R_i is the intrinsic detector resolution, and R_s is the scatter resolution which is often negligible for mouse imaging. Pinhole-collimator resolution is given by:

$$R_o = \left[R_g^2 + (z/l)^2 R_i^2\right]^{1/2}, \tag{10.2}$$

where

$$R_g = a_e(l + z)/l, \tag{10.3}$$

*C. M. Hu, J. C. Chen, National Yang-Ming University, Institute of Radiological Sciences, Taipei, Taiwan; R. S. Liu, National Yang-Ming University, Taipei Veterans General Hospital, Taipei, Taiwan

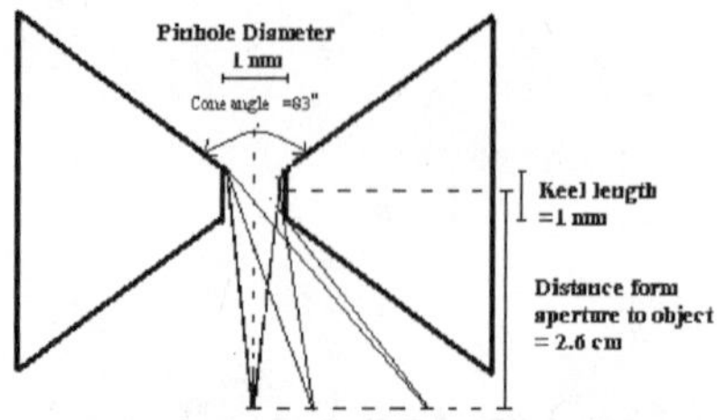

Figure 10.1. A keel-edge pinhole aperture.

z is the distance from the object to the aperture, and l is the distance from the aperture to the detector surface. With the perpendicular distance from aperture to detector surface l and the perpendicular distance from object to aperture z, the theoretical magnification factor M is defined as the ratio l/z. In Eqn. (10.3), a_e is the effective pinhole diameter given by:

$$a_e = \left[a(a + 2\mu^{-1}\tan(\alpha/2))\right]^{1/2}, \tag{10.4}$$

where a is the pinhole diameter, μ is the attenuation coefficient of the aperture, and α is the cone angle of the pinhole collimator.

3. Materials and methods

A keel-edge aperture is designed. The aperture diameter and the length of the keel are both 1mm, and the cone angle is 83° as shown in Figure 10.1. To test the resolution of this design, an Elscint Apex 409 ECT gamma camera with an Elscint high-energy pinhole colllmator is used. A mouse weighing 30 g was anesthetized with phenobarbital and injected with 740 MBq of ^{99m}Tc-MDP in 200 μL.

As stated above, the theoretical magnification factor $M = l/z$. With the perpendicular distance from aperture to detector surface l being 28.5 cm, and the perpendicular distance from object to aperture z being 2.6 cm, the theoretical magnification factor M is $28.5/2.6 = 10.96$.

The actual magnification factor is measured by pixel size with the parallel-hole collimator, system pixel size, over that with the pinhole collimator. The measured magnification factor is then compared to the theoretical magnification factor. System pixel sizes with the parallel-hole collimator and the pinhole collimator were measured using point sources on a preset distance of drops of ^{99m}Tc. For measuring the system pixel size of the parallel-hole collimator, the ^{99m}Tc drops were spotted as follows [Figure 10.2].

The pixel numbers were measured between spots, and the distances between spots divided by respective pixel numbers gives the pixel sizes. The mean of the three pixel sizes is used as the system pixel size of the parallel-hole collimator.

To measure the system pixel sizes of the pinhole collimator, the ^{99m}Tc drops were spotted as follows [Figure 10.3]. The pixel numbers were measured between spots, and the distances between spots divided by respective pixel numbers gives

Figure 10.2. System pixel size measurement.

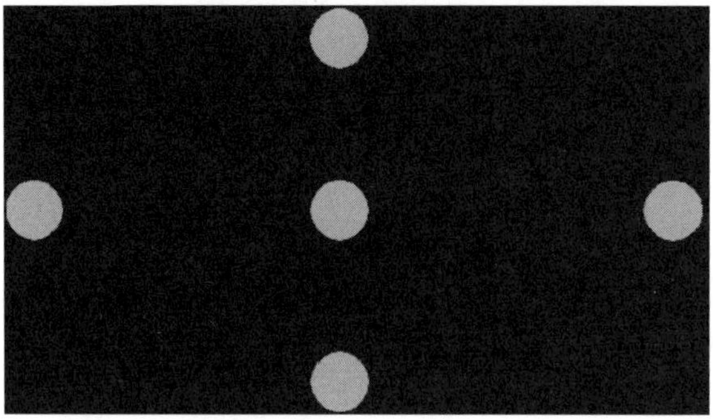

Figure 10.3. Pinhole pixel size measurement.

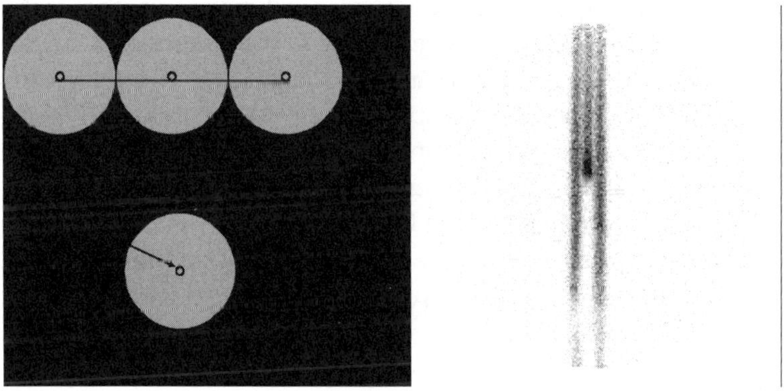

Figure 10.4. (a) A set of three capillaries; (b) images of these three capillaries.

the pixel sizes. The mean of the four pixel sizes is used as system pixel size of the pinhole collimator.

A resolution test was performed by imaging a set of three capillaries with the pinhole collimator. The interior diameter of the capillaries is 0.2 mm, and the outer diameter is 1.1 mm [Figure 10.4(a)]. If the image of the three capillaries can be separated, the resolution of the system is better than 1.1 mm.

4. Results

System pixel size of the parallel-hole collimator is measured to be 0.1653 cm at a matrix size of 256×256. System pixel size of the pinhole collimator is measured to be 0.0149 cm at a matrix size of 256×256. The actual magnification factor M

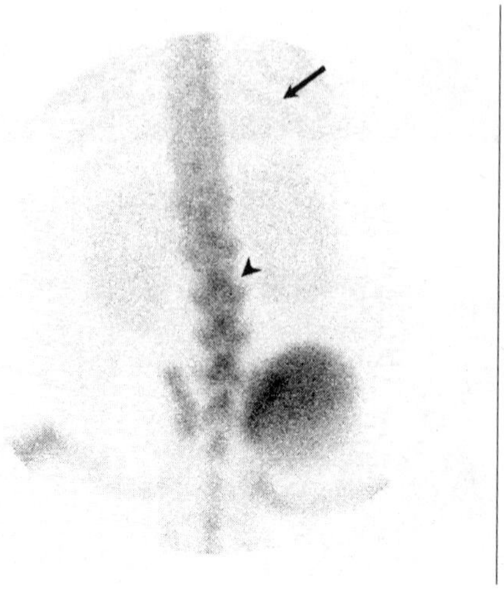

Figure 10.5. Mouse skeletal system.

defined as system pixel size of the parallel-hole collimator over that of the pinhole is $0.1653/0.0149 = 11.09$, which is very close to the predicted value of 10.96. A capillary resolution test is performed, and the image of a set of three capillaries is obtained. In the image, these three capillaries are well separated [Figure 10.4(b)] With 1.1-mm outer diameter of each capillary, we observe that the 1.-mm resolution is achieved by this design of pinhole aperture. The equivalent FWHM of this system is 1.049 mm calculated from measured FWHM divided by magnification factor M. The planar image of a mouse skeletal system is presented in Figure 10.5. The resolution of the image enables the clear visualization of individual ribs (arrow) and vertebra (arrow head).

5. Discussion

The keel-edge aperture is advantageous because it keeps the geometric resolution R_g close to the aperture diameter in the copper-tungsten alloy. Application of keel edge on high-energy photons, such as ^{131}I, will sacrifice the system field of view because longer keel results in cone angle of incident photons reduced [Tsui, 2001]. Although ultra-high resolution with sub-mm resolution is possible by reducing the pinhole aperture diameter to a few hundred microns, the sensitivity will be decreased dramatically at the same time. The sensitivity problem might be solved by use of a multi-pinhole collimator [Schramm, 2003] or a coded aperture architecture [Smith, 1985].

6. Conclusions

Capillary tests show that the resolution of pinhole aperture with 1 mm in diameter and 1 mm of keel length is less than 1.1 mm. The planar moue skeletal image reveals the mouse ribs and vertebra in details. Thus, the system resolution is adequate for small-animal imaging.

References

[Habraken, 2001] J. B. A. Habraken, et al., "Evaluation of High-Resolution Pinhole SPECT Using a Small Rotating Animal," *J Nucl Med*, vol. 42, pp. 1863-1869, 2001.

[Schramm, 2003] N. Schramm, et. al., "Multi-Pinhole SPECT for Small Animal Research," Pinhole Aperture Design for Small-Animal Imagingwww.fz-juelich.de, 2003.

[Simmons, 1988] G. H. Simmons, "The Scintillation Camera", New York, SNM, 1988.

[Smith, 1985] W. E. Smith, R. G. Paxman, H. H. Barrett, "Application of Simulated Annealing To Coded-Aperture Design And Tomographic Reconstruction," *IEEE Trans Nucl Sci*, vol. NS-32, pp. 758-761, 1985.

[Tsui, 2001] B. M. W. Tsui, T. Wang, E. C. Frey, and D. E. Wessell, "Application of an Ultra High-Resolution Pinhole SPECT System Based On a Conventional Camera For Small Animal Imaging," *Radiology Research Symposium*, 2001.

[Weber, 1999] D. A. Weber and M. Ivanovic, "Ultra-high-resolution imaging of small animals: Implications for preclinical and research studies," *J Nucl Cardiol*, vol. 6, pp. 332-344, 1999.

Chapter 11

Comparison of CsI(Ti) and Scintillating Plastic in a Multi-Pinhole/CCD-Based Gamma Camera for Small-Animal Low-Energy SPECT

Edmond Richer, Matthew A. Lewis, Billy Smith, Xiufeng Li, Serguei Seliounine, Ralph P. Mason, and Peter P. Antich*

1. Introduction

SPECT with submillimeter resolution (μSPECT) is needed for small-animal imaging and differs from clinical SPECT – a rich and well-established methodology of nuclear medicine – in that its focus is on the specific requirements of high-resolution imaging over small distances with matching sensitivity, requiring differences in collimator schemes and image reconstruction methods specialized for that task. Current efforts toward this goal have focused on adapting established technologies from clinical to animal imaging. Currently available devices have resolution in the range of 1-3 mm and adequate sensitivity, but we believe that these parameters should be improved to facilitate molecular imaging. Prototypes are being developed [Ogawa, 1997, Ogawa, 1998, MacDonald, 2001, McElroy, 2001, Schramm, 2001] in response to a rising level of interest by pharmaceutical companies and molecular biologists [Russo, 1998].

Nevertheless, a significant factor for penetration of μSPECT into general usage remains the cost and ease of use of a system with adequate resolution for studies in mice and rats. In the case of small animal imaging, pinhole collimator and a closed detector-object configuration can be used with SPECT. This presents the advantage to minimize the time for data collection, allowing a superior detector sensitivity at high-spatial resolution by using multiple pinholes and crystals. A pinhole size of 0.5 mm would provide the sub-millimeter resolution required to study small animals such as mice.

2. CCD-based gamma camera

With the goal of achieving high resolution with appropriate sensitivity for use in small-animal studies, we have developed a multi-pinhole gamma camera based on

*University of Texas Southwestern Medical Center, Dallas, Texas

thallium-doped cesium iodide [CsI(Tl)] crystals and wavelength-matched charge-coupled devices (CCDs).

A Scientific Imaging Technologies Inc (SITe SIA502AB1 CCD), a 512×512 pixels, non-color, back-illuminated, full-frame image sensor was selected due to its excellent sensitivity (greater than 85 % quantum efficiency from 400 nm to 750 nm). The pixel size is 24 x 24 μm, providing a large well capacity of 350,000 e^-. Coupled with a good sensitivity (2.6 μV/e^-), low dark current (20 pA/cm^2 at 20°C), and low readout noise (5 e^-), this provides a dynamic range of 70,000, more than a full 16 bits.

The CCD is be incorporated into a self-contained, cooled camera, equipped with electronic circuitry and optics. The principal method for noise suppression with CCD technology is cooling the chip itself. In our proposed implementation, the CCD camera employs a five-stage thermoelectric cooling element equipped with a controller circuit that keeps the operational temperature of the CCD at -40°C. An external heat exchange unit eliminates the generated heat. The net effect will be a substantial reduction of the dark noise generated inside the CCD, and thus better image quality and longer possible exposures. The internal chamber of the camera is kept under vacuum to allow better cooling and to eliminate ice crystals formation on the sensitive element.

The light exposure is controlled using a mechanical shutter. The shutter allows for short exposure times, down to 5 msec, which are not attainable when an electronic shutter is employed. In addition, the mechanical shutter prevents light from affecting the CCD during the readout phase, thus eliminating the smear effect observed in full-frame CCD cameras without a shutter. To widen the dynamic range, the CCD readout employs a 16-bit A/D conversion chip equipped with a low-noise preamplifier and correlated double-sampling circuitry. This architecture provides a high dynamic range combined with very low readout noise. Finally, a flexible pixel binning scheme is implemented allowing for a better signal-to-noise ratio in the extremely low light level conditions that are expected with higher resolution imaging. Optical coupling of the CCD to the scintillating crystal is implemented using an off-the-shelf low reflectance optical lens.

We selected CsI(Tl) as the scintillator rather than the more traditional gamma camera scintillator, NaI(Tl). NaI(Tl) has a scintillation wavelength of maximum emission at 415 nm, ideally matched to the efficiency profile of photomultiplier tubes (PMTs), which have typical quantum efficiencies of 20%. CsI(Tl), on the other hand, has a maximum emission at 550 nm, which is well into the region where solid-state detectors are dominant. While most scintillator property tables list CsI(Tl) as having 45% the photoelectron yield as compared to NaI(Tl), this comparison is deceptive because it holds true only for PMTs; using CCDs, the light yield of CsI is 53% higher than NaI. Further advantages are sturdier mechanical properties, limited hygroscopicity, and higher density. This last factor will allow thinner scintillators with the same capture efficiency.

Two potential drawbacks exist for this gamma camera design, intrinsic to the scintillator and the detector. First, CsI(Tl) is a slow scintillator (900 ns versus 230 ns

Figure 11.1. 100 μm I-125 line source displaced 0.5 mm across the crystal face.

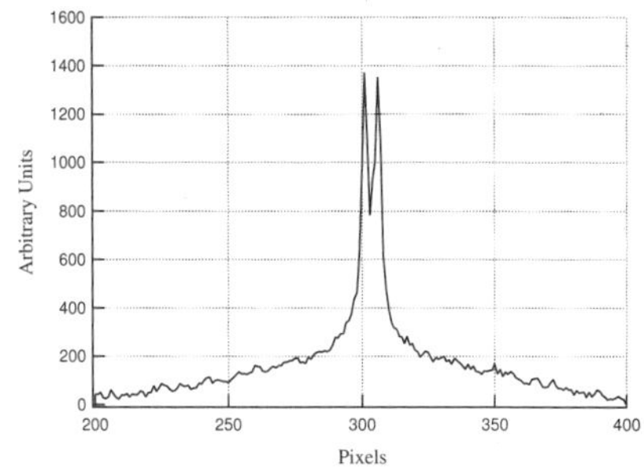

Figure 11.2. Profile of the line source displaced 0.5 mm across the crystal face.

for NaI(Tl)). However, this is not a problem because timing and triggering is not needed because the CCD is an integrating device, and subsequently an exposure will contain the recorded detection of many high energy photons. Second, and more importantly, energy discrimination is not possible. Two facts make its application to mouse imaging possible and free of excessive scatter contributions. First, our major applications of the proposed μSPECT is to I-125 imaging, in which case the existence of a K-edge at 32.2 keV for the crystal is sufficient to accept the 35 keV gamma emitted by this nuclide and reject lower energy noise. Second, the completed system is not intended for use in humans, where gamma rays have an appreciable probability of scatter before exiting the body, but for a small animal, so that scatter rejection is less important and can be accounted for with absorption corrections.

The intrinsic resolution of the gamma detector was determined using a 100-μm slit collimator displaced across the surface of the scintillating crystal using a micrometric positioning device. Figure 11.1 shows the image from an I-125 line source displaced 0.5 mm across the crystal face. The corresponding profile is presented in Fig. 11.2. The intrinsic resolution of the camera was determined to be below 0.4 mm (see [Antich, 2003]). Considering a field a view of 50 mm, suitable for an animal the size of a mouse, the number of pixels required to record an image in a non-magnifying geometry is less than 128. Comparing with the much higher resolution of the CCD (512×512 pixels), one concludes that a set of up to 16 pinhole projections can be acquired on a single CCD image.

Thus, in our design, collimation is provided by a 3×3 array of pinholes that provide some field-of-view overlap in the transverse plane, but are non-degenerate in the longitudinal axis of the animal. A schematic rendering of the geometry of this setup and an actual multiple-pinhole image is shown in Figs. 11.3 and 11.4.

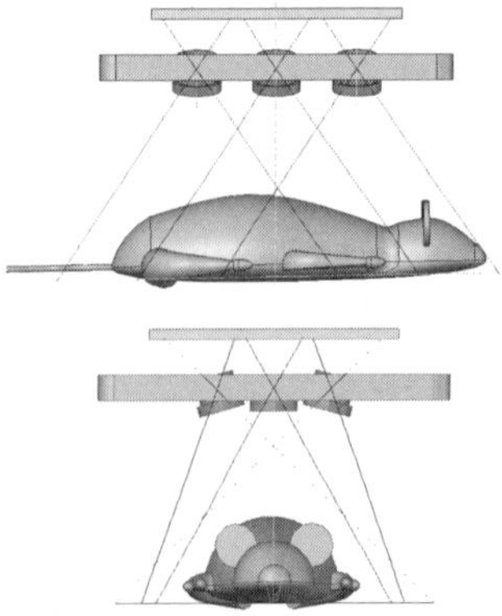

Figure 11.3. Field of view of pinhole collimators.

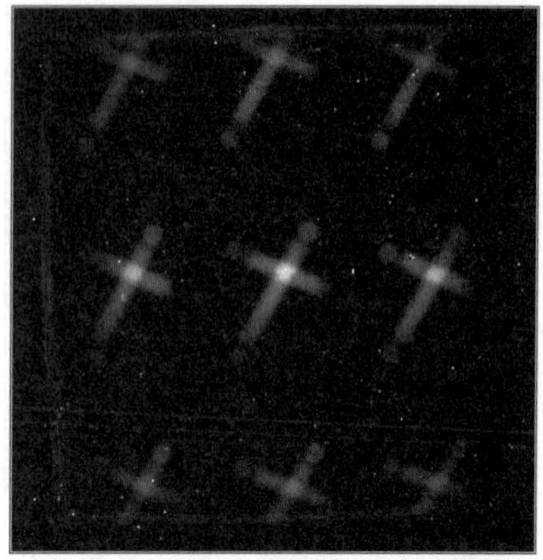

Figure 11.4. Convergent 9-pinhole (1.5 mm) collimator, 2 400 μCi (14.8 MBq) line sources, 30-minute acquisition.

3. Plastic scintillators

For imaging with low-energy iodine-125 labeled agents (<35.5 keV), we further consider scintillating plastic as an alternative to CsI(Tl). Plastic scintillators have the advantage of being mechanically sturdier than crystals, have less hygroscopicity, and more importantly can be shaped in any desired shape and dimension. Moreover, the light emission can be tuned to the optimum wavelength sensitivity of the CCDs using waveshifting doping materials. A potential drawback is their lower densities, which require thicker scintillators to achieve a good detector cross-section with negative effects on resolution.

In order to determine the efficiency of the plastic scintillators, we compared the light output produced by an 125-I line source (400 μCi) in direct contact with a 5.6 mm BC-408 scintillator (Bicron, Inc.) and a 2-mm CiI(Tl) crystal. The light output normalized to the thickness shows a factor of 237 in favor of the CsI(Tl) crystal.

A set of PVT-based scintillators containing different microcrystals in two concentrations were also tested with the results presented in Table 11.1. The concentration is given in mg of microcrystal material per g of PVT, and the light output is in arbitrary light units per minute of exposure (ALU/min) as obtained from the CCD camera. The light output normalized to the scintillator material thickness is also presented. All tested microcrystals significantly improved the efficiency of the scintillator, with LSO in 100 mg/g concentration showing spectacular results, increasing the thickness of normalized light output almost 600 times compared to the PVT alone. Comparing the PVT containing LSO with the CsI(Tl) crystal, we observed that, while the total light output is larger for the crystal by a factor of 2.26, the normalized light output is higher for the PVT containing LSO by a factor of 1.58.

Table 11.1. Comparison of plastic scintillators light output with different microcrystals.

Microcrystal Material	*Microcrystal Concentration*	*Thickness [mm]*	*Light Output [ALU/min]*	*Normalized Light Output*
ErSO	50	0.5	375	750
ErSO	100	0.5	625	1,250
YbSO	50	0.35	525	1,500
YbSO	100	0.35	888	2,537
LSO	50	0.35	10,125	28,929
LSO	100	0.35	16,065	45,900
None	0	5.6	431	77

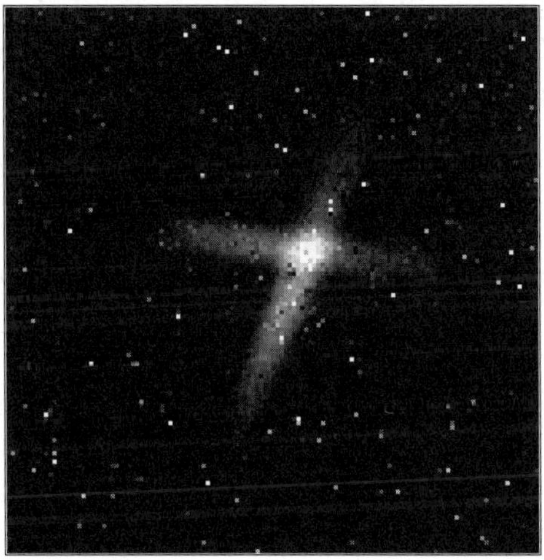

Figure 11.5. Pinhole (1.5 mm) collimator, 2 400 μCi (14.8 MBq) line sources, 30-minute acquisition.

The intrinsic resolution of the scintillating plastic LSO/CCD-coupled gamma camera was determined by the same method to be $<$0.5 mm, comparable to our previously reported results for the CsI(Tl)-based detector. An image of 2 400 μCi (14.8 MBq) line sources, obtained using LSO 100 mg/g scintillator and a 1.5-mm pinhole collimator, is presented in Fig. 11.5.

A potential problem with the natural radioactive background of ^{176}Lu in LSO has been identified with single photon imaging [Huber, 2002]. However, because the natural background radiation spectrum is primarily above 300 keV, the thin section of the doped plastic scintillator will minimize unwanted noise from this source.

4. Conclusions and future work

We have made considerable progress in designing and constructing devices which will allow us to quantitatively compare different designs and technologies for high-resolution, high-sensitivity μSPECT. In future studies, we will optimize the plastic scintillator thickness and the microcrystal concentration with respect to the resolution and sensitivity.

Challenges also remain in the development of the image reconstruction algorithms suitable for multiple-pinhole CCD-based μSPECT cameras.

Acknowledgments

Partial funding for this work was provided by NCI P20 CA 86354.

References

[Antich, 2003] P. P. Antich, M. A. Lewis, E. Richer, P. V. Kulkarni, B. Smith, B., R. P. Mason, "A novel multi-pinhole/CCD-coupled CsI(Tl) crystal gamma camera for fully 3D μSPECT / μCT small-animal imaging," In *Proceedings of the 50th Annual Meeting of Society of Nuclear Medicine*, 2003.

[Huber, 2002] J. S Huber, W. W. Moses, W. F. Jones, C. C. Watson, "Effect of ^{176}Lu background on singles transmission for LSO-based PET cameras." *Phys. Med. Biol.*, vol. 47, pp. 1–7, 2002.

[MacDonald, 2001] L. R. MacDonald, B. E. Patt, J. S. Iwanczyk, B. M. W. Tsui, Y. Wang, E. C. Frey, D. E. Wessell, P. D. Acton, H. F. Kung, "Pinhole SPECT of mice using the LumaGEM gamma camera," *IEEE Transactions on Nuclear Science*, vol. 48(3), pp. 830–836, 2001.

[McElroy, 2001] D. P. McElroy, L. R. MacDonald, F. J. Beekman, Y. Wang, B. E. Patt, J. S. Iwanczyk, B. M. W. Tsui, E. J. Hoffman, "Evaluation of A-SPECT: A desktop pinhole SPECT system for small animal imaging," In *IEEE Nuclear Science Symposium Conference Record*, vol. 3, pp. 1835–1839, 2001.

[Ogawa, 1997] K. Ogawa, T. Kawade, K. Nakamura, A. Kubo, T. Ichihara, "Ultra high resolution pinhole SPECT," In *IEEE Nuclear Science Symposium and Medical Imaging Conference*, vol. 2, pp. 1600–1604, 1997.

[Ogawa, 1998] K. Ogawa, T. Kawade, K. Nakamura, A. Kubo, T. Ichihara, "Ultra high resolution pinhole SPECT for small animal study," *IEEE Transactions on Nuclear Science*, vol. 45(6), pp. 3122–3126, 1998.

[Russo, 1998] E. Russo, "Going micro: Imaging devices to benefit both mouse and biologist," *The Scientist*, vol. 12(21), pp. 1, 1998.

[Schramm, 2001] N. Schramm, A. Wirrwar, H. Halling, "Development of a multi-pinhole detector for high-sensitivity SPECT imaging," In *IEEE Nuclear Science Symposium*, vol. 3, pp. 1585–1586, 2001.

Chapter 12

Calibration of Scintillation Cameras and Pinhole SPECT Imaging Systems

Yi-Chun Chen, Lars R. Furenlid, Donald W. Wilson, and Harrison H. Barrett*

1. Introduction

Linear digital-imaging systems are most accurately described as mappings from an object, which is a function of continuous variables, to a discrete set of measurements. When the object is approximated by a discrete vector (e.g., a linear combination of some expansion functions), the image-forming mechanism can be formulated as:

$$\boldsymbol{g} = \boldsymbol{H}\boldsymbol{f} \tag{12.1}$$

where $\boldsymbol{f}$ denotes the object vector, $\boldsymbol{g}$ is the image vector, and $\boldsymbol{H}$ represents the system matrix that transforms the object into the image being detected. Because iterative reconstruction typically requires that a model of the imaging system be built into the algorithm, accurate knowledge of $\boldsymbol{H}$ is essential for object reconstruction. The $\boldsymbol{H}$ matrix can be obtained by many methods, including purely theoretical analysis, simulation, experimental calibration, or some combination of these methods. In any case, it is preferable to assure that all of the system physics are contained in the matrix.

2. Background

The $\boldsymbol{H}$ matrix specific to pinhole SPECT imaging is influenced by properties of the object (scatter and attenuation), the image-forming system (e.g., pinholes), and the detector. A thorough understanding of these effects could provide the analytical composition of $\boldsymbol{H}$. More detailed discussions on this subject can be found in Barrett and Myers [2004].

A 3D object $f(\boldsymbol{r})$ can be approximated by a vector and discretized using voxel functions as:

$$f_a(\boldsymbol{r}) = \sum_{n=1}^{N} \theta_n \phi_n(\boldsymbol{r}), \tag{12.2}$$

*The University of Arizona, Department of Radiology, Tucson, Arizona

where the subscript a denotes an approximation, $\boldsymbol{n}$ is a 3D index to indicate the location in the object space, and $\phi_{\boldsymbol{n}}(\boldsymbol{r})$ is a voxel function, which is uniform within a cube centered on point $\boldsymbol{r}_{\boldsymbol{n}}$. The elements of $\mathcal{H}$ can then be expressed as:

$$H_{\boldsymbol{mn}} = \int_{\infty} d^3r \, h_{\boldsymbol{m}}(\boldsymbol{r}) \phi_{\boldsymbol{n}}(\boldsymbol{r}), \tag{12.3}$$

where $\boldsymbol{m}$ is a 3D multi-index to specify the 2D location on the detector face and the projection angle, and $h_{\boldsymbol{m}}(\boldsymbol{r})$ represents the system sensitivity function. Eqn. (12.3) shows that a column of H matrix is the image of $\phi_{\boldsymbol{n}}(\boldsymbol{r})$ for all projection directions. Furthermore, when properly normalized, $H_{\boldsymbol{mn}}$ can be viewed as the probability that a photon emitted from voxel $\boldsymbol{n}$ is detected in bin $\boldsymbol{m}$. Because the scattered and unscattered events are mutually exclusive, $\boldsymbol{H}$ can be decomposed into two parts as:

$$\boldsymbol{H} = \boldsymbol{H}^{(\mathrm{sc})} + \boldsymbol{H}^{(\mathrm{un})}, \tag{12.4}$$

where the superscripts (sc) and (un) denote scattered and unscattered, respectively. Both matrices are $M \times N$, where M is the number of detector pixels multiplied by the number of projection angles, and N is the number of voxels. Only the unscattered part is discussed herein. The unscattered part of $\boldsymbol{H}$ can be further decomposed as:

$$\boldsymbol{H}^{(\mathrm{un})} = \boldsymbol{H}^{(\mathrm{det})} \left[\boldsymbol{H}^{(\mathrm{geom})} \odot \boldsymbol{A} \right], \tag{12.5}$$

where $\boldsymbol{H}^{(\mathrm{det})}$ denotes the influence of detectors on the $\boldsymbol{H}$ matrix, $H^{(\mathrm{geom})}$ represents the straight-line propagation from the voxel location to the detector element without scatter or attentation, $\boldsymbol{A}$ indicates the attenuation along the propagation path, and $\odot$ denotes an element by element product. The sizes of $\boldsymbol{H}^{(\mathrm{det})}$, $\boldsymbol{H}^{(\mathrm{geom})}$, and $\boldsymbol{A}$ are $M \times M$, $M \times N$, and $M \times N$, respectively. If the attenuation factor is slowly varying over a scale comparable to the spatial resolution of the detector, the following approximation is tenable [Barrett and Myers, 2004]:

$$\boldsymbol{H}^{(\mathrm{un})} \approx \left[\boldsymbol{H}^{(\mathrm{det})} \boldsymbol{H}^{(\mathrm{geom})} \right] \odot \mathrm{A}. \tag{12.6}$$

The advantage of this form is that the product $\boldsymbol{H}^{(\mathrm{det})} \boldsymbol{H}^{(\mathrm{geom})}$ depends on the system, while $\boldsymbol{A}$ depends only on the particular object being imaged. The product $\boldsymbol{H}^{(\mathrm{det})} \boldsymbol{H}^{(\mathrm{geom})}$ can be obtained empirically by measuring the system response in air and will be introduced in the next section.

3. Experiment construction and data processing

Experimental calibration methods for the system-specific components of $\boldsymbol{H}$, $\boldsymbol{H}^{(\mathrm{det})}$, and $\boldsymbol{H}^{(\mathrm{geom})}$ are described using the calibration of the FastSPECT II system as an example. FastSPECT II is an animal SPECT system developed at the University of Arizona and has 16 scintillation cameras with a single-pinhole aperture associated with each camera.

3.1 MDRF acquisition for non-pixelized detectors

To characterize the detector response, a collimated ^{99m}Tc source is scanned in a 2D grid pattern across the detector face. This measurement is performed with the cameras mounted in the imager but no pinholes or collimator in place. Each scintillation camera is composed of 5-mm thick NaI crystal, 15-mm thick quartz light guide, and 3×3 array of 1.5" diameter photomultiplier tubes (PMTs). The radioactive beam is oriented normal to the camera face, and the diameter of the collimated beam is designed to be smaller than the spatial resolution of the scintillation detector. A Cerrobend[1] cast tube carrying a radioactivity-filled syringe cap (see Fig. 12.1) provides a collimated beam of gamma rays with beam size of 0.84 mm at zero distance and 0.056 radians divergence. The source count rate is designed to be more than 30 times that of the environmental radiation. A scan size of 78×78 points is performed to cover the crystal width of 115 mm, and the grid spacing is 1.5 mm that is comparable to the intrinsic resolution of the scintillation detector.

This measurement yields samples from the mean detector response function (MDRF) of the scintillation camera. Figure 12.1 shows an *in situ* MDRF acquisition of a scintillation camera in the FastSPECT II system. Histograms of the signals obtained from each PMT are plotted with energy windowing applied [Sain, 2001], and the sample mean is calculated. Figure 12.2 shows the tube arrangement and the mean response of all nine tubes as a function of the collimated source location. A normalized 1D slice of the 2D MDRF along a diagonal line across the camera face is shown in Fig. 12.3. The MDRF is used to construct a maximum-likelihood position estimator [Milster, 1990]. When a radiation event is detected, an estimate of the interacting location and energy can be found using the strength of the nine PMT outputs and this position estimator. More details about the position estimation can be found in chapter 3 of this volume.

3.2 $\boldsymbol{H}$ matrix acquisition

As described in Section 2, the object can be decomposed as a set of voxels. A ^{99m}Tc point source was made to mimic the voxel function $\phi_n(\boldsymbol{r})$. Several resin chromatography beads were used to absorb radioactivity and glued together in an epoxy ball smaller than 1-mm diameter.

With the imager fully assembled (i.e., pinholes in place), a radioactive point source is stepped on a 3D grid through the object space. The radioactivity of the point source is around 20 mCi, and the sensitivity of FastSPECT II is 10 counts/μCi. Our most recent calibration for FastSPECT II contained 64,000 calibration points with a grid spacing of 1mm and took 24 hours to finish. As shown in Eqn. (12.3), one column of $\boldsymbol{H}$ is the images of the point source $\phi_n(\boldsymbol{r})$ for all projection directions. The recorded response of the scintillation cameras as a function of the point-source location is processed into projection images using the MDRF position estimator. Figure 12.4 shows one column of $\boldsymbol{H}$, the images of the point source for all 16 projection directions.

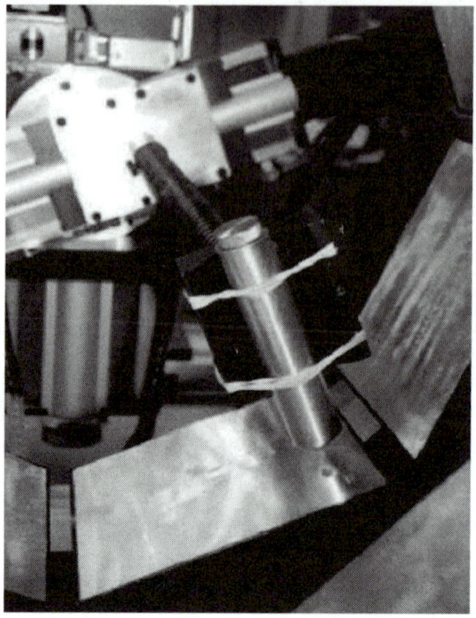

Figure 12.1. *In situ* acquisition of an MDRF for a scintillation camera.

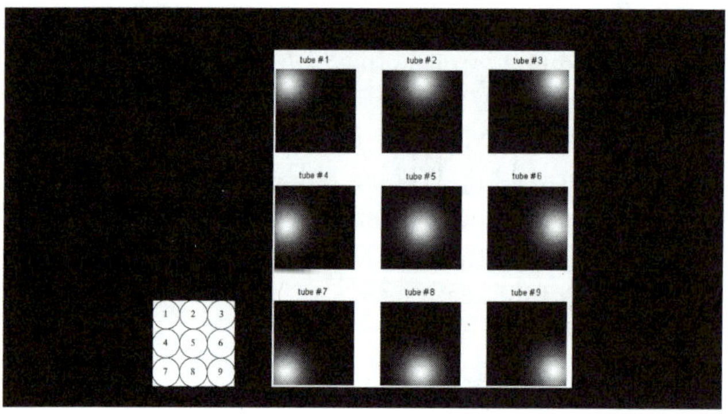

Figure 12.2. The tube arrangement of a scintillation camera and the mean response of all nine PMTs as a function of collimated source location.

4. Interpolation of the *H* matrix

The span of the calibration grid points in the ***H*** matrix acquisition defines the FOV, while the spacing between the calibration grid points defines the voxel size. This span and spacing act as the ultimate limits on system FOV and resolution in object reconstruction. Because the whole calibration process takes about four half-lives of ^{99m}Tc, it is unrealistic to either extend the scan size or decrease the step size. Therefore, interpolation of the ***H*** matrix serves as an alternative to obtain subgrid resolution in object reconstruction. In addition, this technique can also be used to rotate an existing ***H*** matrix, and hence is useful for imaging systems that rotate the object or the imager during the imaging procedure. Two possible

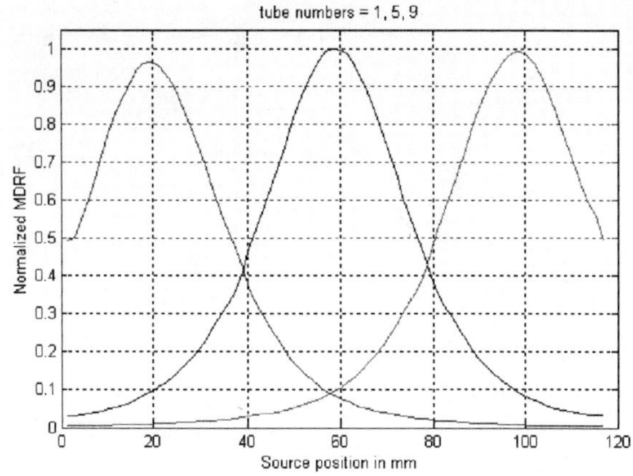

Figure 12.3. A 1D slice of the 2D MDRF of three tubes along a diagonal line across the camera face.

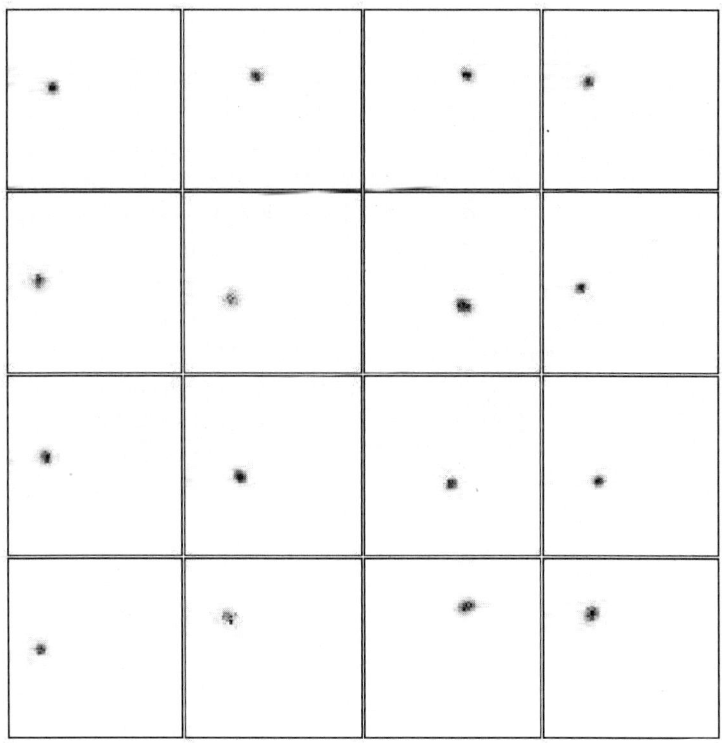

Figure 12.4. One column of $\boldsymbol{H}$, the images of the point source for all 16 projection directions.

schemes to interpolate the $\boldsymbol{H}$ matrix are discussed briefly, and preliminary results are presented.

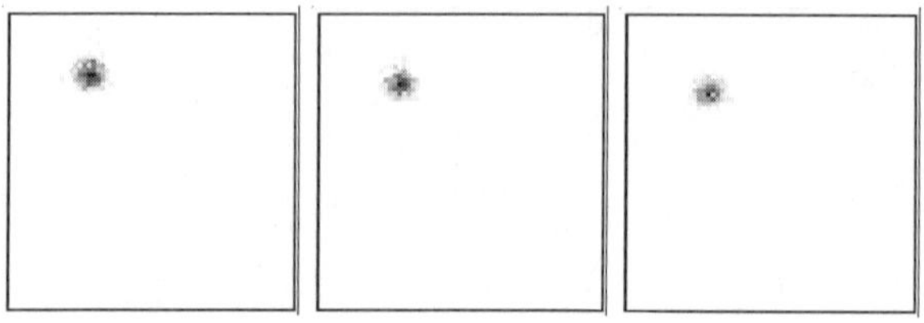

(a) (b) (c)

Figure 12.5. Sample images of $\boldsymbol{H}$, when the point source is located at three adjacent locations. (a) Projection image of the 3rd camera when source is located at (0,0,0). (b) Projection image of the 3rd camera when source is located at (0,0,1). (c) Projection image of the 3rd camera when source is located at (0,0,2).

The point response of a pinhole SPECT system is approximately shift-invariant laterally and slowly varying longitudinally with respect to the detector face. One way to interpolate the $\boldsymbol{H}$ matrix is to determine the centroid of each pinhole projection and fit a Gaussian function about the centroid. Hence, the response between adjacent point source locations can be estimated by averaging the locations of the centroids and the covariance matrices of the Gaussian fits. Another approach utilizes the fact that the point responses of adjacent source locations have approximately the same properties in their Fourier transforms and thus can be interpolated by averaging their magnitudes and phases in Fourier domain.

Figure 12.5 shows three images of adjacent point response when the source is located at (0,0,0), (0,0,1), and (0,0,2) in the object space. The Gaussian and Fourier-interpolated responses of Figures 12.5(a) and (c) are displayed in Figure 12.6. Comparison between Figure 12.5 and Figure 12.6 shows a close correspondence between the acquired and the interpolated data. The actual interpolation of the entire $\boldsymbol{H}$ matrix will be more complex, because interpolation will be between multiple points rather than two, but this study gives an encouraging demonstration that the interpolation methods will allow us to achieve better resolution in object reconstruction.

5. Summary and conclusions

The system matrix (referred to as $\boldsymbol{H}$) specific to pinhole SPECT imaging was described in a probabilistic viewpoint and decomposed into the system-specific and object-related components. Calibration methods to provide the system-specific component of $\boldsymbol{H}$ for scintillation cameras and pinhole SPECT systems were described. Two interpolation schemes of $\boldsymbol{H}$ were introduced, including centroid interpolation with Gaussian fitting and Fourier-interpolation methods.

The use of a measured MDRF and $\boldsymbol{H}$ matrix avoids the assumption of an idealized model for the cameras and imaging systems. As a measured $\boldsymbol{H}$ matrix incorporates the imperfections or misalignment of the imaging system, as well as

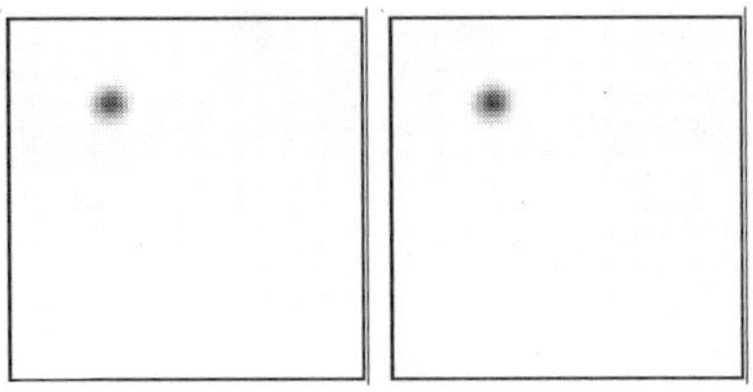

(a) (b)

Figure 12.6. Interpolated response of $\boldsymbol{H}$ using different interpolation methods. (a) Interpolated image of Figures 12.5(a) and (c) using the Gaussian-interpolation scheme. (b) Interpolated image of Figures 12.5(a) and (c) using the Fourier-interpolation scheme.

the non-uniformity in the camera response, this calibration procedure should be applicable to various imaging systems. As implemented here, however, it does not account for the scatter component $\boldsymbol{H}^{(\mathrm{sc})}$.

Acknowledgments

This project was supported by the Center for Gamma-Ray Imaging (NIH/NIBIB Grant P41 EB002035-05) and the Southwest Animal Imaging Resource (NCI Grant R24 CA83148).

Notes

1. Composition of Cerrobend is 50% bismuth, 26.7% lead, 13.3% tin, and 10% cadmium. Melting point is 158° F.

References

[Barrett and Myers, 2004] H. H. Barrett, and K. J. Myers, 2004, *Foundations of Image Science*, Wiley-Interscience, New York, pp. 1200-1206, 2004.

[Milster, 1990] T. D. Milster, J. N. Aarsvold, H. H. Barrett, A. L. Landesman, L. S. Mar, D. D. Patton, T. J. Roney, R. K. Rowe, R. H. Seacat III, "A full-field modular gamma camera", *J. Nucl. Med.*, vol. 31(5), pp. 632, 1990.

[Sain, 2001] J. D. Sain, *Optical Modeling, Design Optimization, and Performance Analysis of a Gamma Camera for Detection of Breast Cancer*, Ph.D. Dissertation, University of Arizona, Tucson, Arizona, pp. 75-90, 2001.

Chapter 13

Imaging Dopamine Transporters in a Mouse Brain with Single-Pinhole SPECT

Jan Booij, Gerda Andringa, Kora de Bruin, Jan Habraken, and Benjamin Drukarch*

1. Introduction

Parkinsonism is a feature of a number of neurodegenerative diseases, including Parkinson's disease (PD). The results of post-mortem studies point to dysfunction of dopaminergic neurotransmission in parkinsonism, with degeneration of dopaminergic neurons in PD. Dopamine neurons reside primarily in the mesencephalon, which is a part of the brain stem, and project predominantly to the striatum (presynaptic nigrostriatal projection). The high affinity dopamine transporter (DAT), or reuptake site, is presumably a unique constituent of the membrane of dopaminergic nerve terminals. The integrity of the nigrostriatal projection can now be studied *in vivo* with radiotracers whose striatal uptake reflects binding to DATs.

In an effort to study in more detail the pathophysiology of dopaminergic degeneration in PD, several animal models of PD have been developed, including the 1-methyl-4-phenyl-1,2,3,6-tetrahydropyridine (MPTP) mouse model. MPTP is a neurotoxin that leads to neurochemical and histopathological alterations that replicate very closely the well-known alterations in PD and render currently the most favored animal model of PD, which is of interest to study, among others, therapeutic intervention strategies. Until recently, all studies on these models needed to rely on a cross-sectional study design, because, for clear reasons, it is not possible to perform repeated *ex vivo* studies in the same group of animals. In comparison with *ex vivo* measurements (a cross-sectional study design), a serial study design, however, may have the advantage of detecting statistically significant changes between groups with a lower number of animals per group under study. Such an *in vivo* approach could be used to study progression of dopaminergic degeneration in, e.g., MPTP-treated mice, or to study the potential neuroprotective properties of drugs to slow down degeneration.

For this purpose, we have recently developed a single-pinhole high-resolution SPECT system for studies in small animals. In this system, the collimated detector

*J. Booij, K. de Bruin, J. Habraken, University of Amsterdam, Amsterdam, The Netherlands; G. Andringa, B. Drukarch, VU University Medical Center, Amsterdam, The Netherlands

is fixed and the animal rotates. Initial phantom studies showed good uniformity and a spatial resolution of up to 1.3 mm (FWHM) using a 1-mm pinhole aperture [Habraken, 2001]. Moreover, the potential to image DATs in a rat brain has recently been reported by us [Booij, 2002].

Thus, the aim of the present study was to explore the possibility of detecting loss of striatale DATs (as a marker of nigrostriatal dopaminergic neurons) in MPTP-treated mice using our new system. Moreover, we tested the validity of the *in vivo* DATs measurements by comparing *in vivo* DAT binding with *ex vivo* DAT binding (by using immunohistochemistry).

2. Methods and materials

2.1 Control and MPTP-treated mice

Four control and 14 MPTP-treated mice participated in this study. To induce limited as well as severe dopaminergic degeneration, the MPTP-treated mice were divided into three subgroups. One subgroup received MPTP i.p. (dosage 25 mg/kg; n = 4) once, while the other two subgroups received the same dosage of MPTP for 3 (n = 5) or 5 (n = 5) consecutive days, once a day. Because MPP+ is taken up via the DAT, the ^{123}I-labeled radioligand was injected five days after the last administration of MPTP. Just before injection of the radiotracer until the end of the scanning procedure, mice were anesthetized by intraperitoneal injections of a mixture of Hypnorm/Diazepam. To prevent uptake of iodide in the thyroid, all mice were pretreated with potassium iodine. The DAT tracer [^{123}I]N-α-fluoropropyl-2β-carbomethoxy-3β-{4-iodophenyl}nor-tropane (FP-CIT; specific activity approximately 750 MBq/nmol; radiochemical purity of $>$ 97%) was injected intravenously (approximately 80 MBq), and acquisition was started 2 h p.i. At the end of the experiment, mice were killed, and *ex vivo* DAT measures were performed

2.2 Pinhole SPECT system

Our high-resolution pinhole SPECT system has been extensively described earlier [Habraken, 2001]. Shortly, a cylinder with a diameter of 25 mm (which was designed for tight fitting of the mouse) is positioned directly above the pinhole aperture. A mechanical support allows precise manual adjustment of the cylinder in two directions: the distance of the cylinder to the pinhole aperture, which equals the radius of rotation (ROR) and an adjustment along the axis of the cylinder to select the field of view. The mechanical support was designed such that the midline of the cylinder is exactly in the middle of the pinhole. Because the cylinder rotates exactly around its midline, the ROR is not affected by a rotation-induced variation. The pinhole collimator is connected to an ADAC ARC3000© scintillation camera (circular field-of-view diameter 400 mm). The pinhole collimator has a diameter of 300 mm at the base of the shielding and an opening angle of 60°. In this study, a 1 mm pinhole aperture was used (spatial resolution 1.3 mm FWHM), and 50 projections of 60 s per projection were acquired. All experiments were acquired, step and shoot, with a 20% energy window around 159 keV in a 64×64 matrix, ROR of

25 mm. Reconstruction was performed using a HERMES© application program, utilizing filtered backprojection, adapted to pinhole SPECT, according to the conversion algorithm of Feldkamp [1984]. The ramp filter was used as a reconstruction filter with a Butterworth post-reconstruction filter (4.7 cycle per cm, order 5). MR images were obtained in one mouse to provide anatomic landmarks for region of interest (ROI) definition and for positioning of ROIs on the SPECT images. MR imaging was performed with a clinical 1.5 Tesla MRI scanner (GE Signa-Lx). To maximize signal-to-noise ratio, a coil was especially developed to image the brain of small laboratory animals [Booij, 2003]. This receive-only 20-mm diameter surface coil was fixed on a Delrin¨ support directly above the mouse head. A T_1 weighted, 3D fast-spoiled gradient echo sequence was performed. Acquisition was performed in a $256 \times 256 \times 46$ matrix, with a field of view of $40 \times 40 \times 32$ mm yielding a resolution of $0.15 \times 0.15 \times 0.7$ mm.

ROIs for the striata and cerebellum were drawn on the MR images. These ROIs were saved as a template. For analysis of striatal [^{123}I]FP-CIT binding, four consecutive horizontal slices (total thickness approximately 1.6 mm) with the highest striatal binding were selected, and the template was positioned manually (without changing the size and form of the ROIs) on the SPECT images with the backing of anatomical information from the MR image. Striatal binding ratios were expressed as specific striatal binding divided by cerebellar binding.

2.3 Dopamine transporter immunohistochemistry

One day after performance of the SPECT scan, animals were deeply anesthetized with sodium pentobarbital (60 mg/kg) and transcardially perfused with 4% paraformaldehyde in phosphate-buffered saline. Brains were removed and dehydrated for 48 h in 20% sucrose. Horizontal, 12-μm sections of the striatum were cut using a cryostat. Then, sections were processed for DAT immunohistochemistry according to the avidin-biotin-peroxidase method using a rat anti-DAT monoclonal antibody (1:1000; Chemicon). The products of the antibody immunoreactions were then developed with the Vectastain elite ABC kit (Vector Laboratories, Burlingame, CA), using 3,3'-diaminobenzidine (DAB) as the chromogen. Endogenous peroxidase activity was blocked by incubation of the sections in 0.3% H_2O_2 prior to immunolabeling. Negative controls consisted of representative sections processed without the primary antibody.

Analysis of DAT immunoreactivity in the striatum was performed with the Scion Image computerized image analysis system (Scion Corporation, Frederick, MD). Images were captured using a digital camera. The left and right striatum were outlined and optical density was assessed at eight ventrodorsal levels per animal. Non-specific immunoreactivity was measured in the parietal cortex. Striatal DAT labeling was expressed as specific immunoreactivity (density striatum – density cortex) divided by non-specific (background) immunoreactivity (density parietal cortex).

3. Results

In control mice, intense symmetrical striatal [^{123}I]FP-CIT binding was observed. In addition, intense symmetric uptake in the harderian glands could be visualized. In MPTP-treated mice, striatal binding was significantly lower bilaterally, but intense symmetrical uptake in the glands could still be visualized (Fig. 1). In control rats, the specific to non-specific ratios were on the average 1.9. In MPTP-treated mice, the ratios were approximately 60%, 80%, and 75% lower for the mice that were treated for 1, 3, or 5 days, respectively.

The *ex vivo* data showed that in the control mice, the specific to non-specific binding ratios were on the average 15.2. In MPTP-treated mice, the *ex vivo* ratios were also approximately 60%, 80%, and 80% lower for the mice that were treated for 1, 3, or 5 days, respectively. The percentage loss of striatal DATs, induced by MPTP and measured *ex vivo*, is in good agreement with the *in vivo* data.

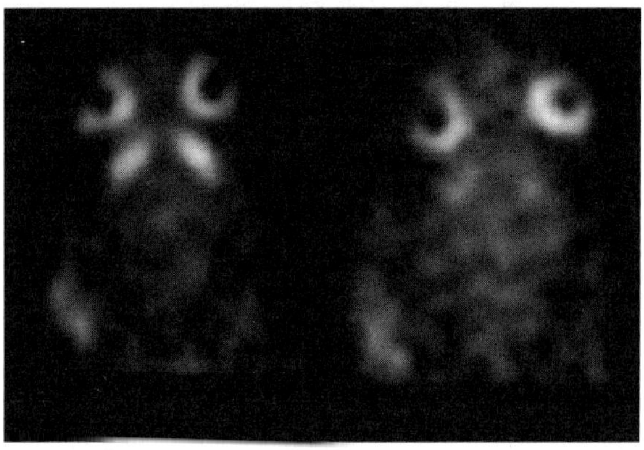

Figure 13.1. Left: control mouse, showing intense symmetrical striatal uptake. Right: MPTP-treated mouse, showing loss of striatal uptake bilaterally.

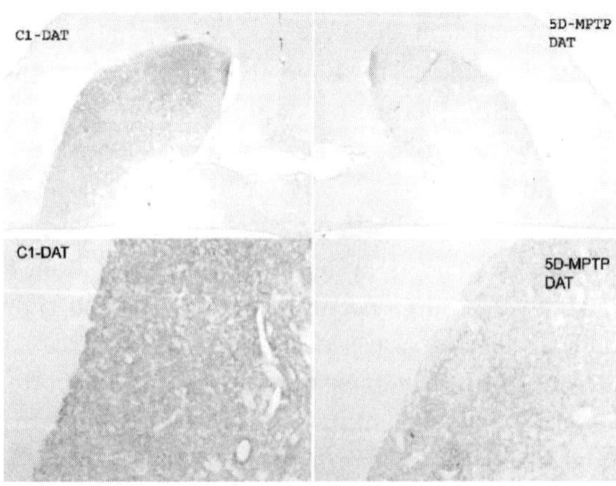

Figure 13.2. Left: control mouse showing intense striatal binding. Right side: lower binding after five days of MPTP administration.

4. Conclusion

These results indicate that assessment of loss of striatal DATs, using our recently developed SPECT system, is sensitive and feasible in living mice. Such a technique may offer the possibility of monitoring dopaminergic degeneration in experimental conditions and may provide an excellent tool for studying neuroprotective strategies *in vivo*.

References

[Booij, 2002] J. Booij, K. de Bruin, J. B. Habraken, P. Voorn, "Imaging of dopamine transporters in rats using high-resolution pinhole single-photon emission tomography," *Eur J Nucl Med Mol Imag*, vol 29, pp 1221-1224, 2002.

[Booij, 2003] J. Booij, K. de Bruin, M. M. L de Win, C. Lavini, G. J. Den Heeten, J. B. A. Babraken, "Imaging of striatal dopamine transporters in rat brain with single pinhole SPECT and co-aligned MRI is highly reproducible," *Nucl Med Biol*, vol. 30, pp. 643-649, 2003.

[Habraken, 2001] J. B.A. Habraken, K. de Bruin, M. Shehata, J. Booij, R. Bennink, B. L.F. van Eck Smit, E. B. Sokole, "Evaluation of high-resolution pinhole SPECT using a small rotating animal," *J Nucl Med*, vol. 42, pp. 1863-1869, 2001.

[Feldkamp, 1984] L. A. Feldkamp, L. C. Davis, J. W. Kress, "Practical cone-beam algorithm," *J Opt Soc Am A.*, vol. 1, pp. 612-619, 1984.

Chapter 14

A Micro-SPECT/CT System for Imaging of AA-Amyloidosis in Mice

Jens Gregor, Shaun Gleason, Stephen Kennel, Michael Paulus, Alan Solomon, Philip Hawkins, and Jonathan Wall*

1. Introduction

Amyloidosis refers to a diverse group of diseases characterized by the abnormal extracellular deposition of proteinaceous substances within the body's organs and tissues. The protein substances are known as amyloid and consist of insoluble fibrils. In general, amyloid deposits arise due to the overproduction of an amyloidogenic protein or as a result of a genetic mutation that occurs in a normally soluble, innocuous, protein that renders it amyloidogenic. Amyloid deposits have been found in virtually every organ and tissue and may be of a restricted localized form or systemic and involve multiple organ or tissue systems. More than 20 proteins have been identified as components of pathologic amyloid deposits, including the A(β) peptide in Alzheimer's disease; amylin in Type-2 diabetes; and the prion protein in the spongiform encephalopathies such as mad cow disease. Our focus is on AA- and AL-amyloidosis, which respectively are composed of apolipoprotein A synthesized during chronic inflammation and immunoglobulin light chains synthesized by abnormal plasma cells.

The understanding of amyloid, its structure and biology, has advanced with the available technology [Sipe and Cohen, 2000]. The term amyloid (meaning starch-like) was coined in 1854 when a macroscopic brain tissue abnormality was found to have staining characteristics similar to cellulose when treated with iodine. Many years later, studies revealed that amyloid-burdened organs and tissues exhibited birefringence when stained with the cotton dye Congo red; that is, when viewed microscopically through crossed polarizers, there is a striking change in color in the amyloid-bound dye from red to apple green. This test is still used to diagnose the disease. Subsequently, electron microscopic analysis showed that amyloid deposits contain rigid, non-branching fibrils (10 nm in diameter). Further chemical analysis

*J. Gregor, University of Tennessee, Department of Computer Science, Knoxville, Tennessee; S. Gleason, S. Kennel, M. Paulus, Oak Ridge National Laboratory, Engineering, Science and Technology Division, Oak Ridge, Tennessee; A. Solomon, J. Wall, University of Tennessee, Graduate School of Medicine, Knoxville, Tennessee; P. Hawkins, Royal Free and University College Medical School, National Amyloidosis Center, London, UK

revealed the presence of numerous non-fibrillar accessory proteins and carbohydrates. One such protein, called serum amyloid P-component (SAP), was found to be ubiquitously and avidly associated with amyloid deposits. In recent years, exploitation of these findings led to the advent of I-123-labeled SAP scintigraphic imaging for clinical monitoring of amyloid diseases [Hawkins, 1988].

In this paper, we give an overview of a microSPECT/CT imaging system that we are developing for the purpose of studying murine models of AA- and AL-amyloidosis *in vivo*. Preliminary experimental results are provided.

2. MicroCT instrumentation and reconstruction

We acquire CT data using a MicroCAT™ II (ImTek, Inc., TN), which is a circular orbit conebeam system is equipped with a 20-80 kVp microfocus x-ray source. The detector is a 2048×3072 CCD array, optically coupled to a minR phosphor screen. The data are downsampled on the CCD via 4×4 binning. The field of view is 57 mm transaxial by 85 mm axial. We acquire 360 projections of each animal over the course of 6 minutes. See e.g. [Paulus, 2000] for more details.

With respect to image reconstruction, we have developed a modified version of the Feldkamp algorithm [Gregor, 2003]. Modifications include focus of attention which is a data-driven preprocessing scheme that automatically precludes a large portion of the background voxels from being considered during backprojection thereby lowering the overall computational cost. We have also introduced support for multi-processor-based cluster computing. Using 12 dual-processor PCs, we can thus reconstruct a 100-μm resolution image volume in the same amount of time required to acquire the data in the first place.

Recently, we implemented a parallelized version of Fessler's mono-energetic weighted least-squares algorithm [Elbakri and Fessler, 2002]. Our conebeam system matrix is based on depth-weighted trilinear interpolation and exploits geometric symmetries to allow for pre-computation and storage to a disk for subsequent use. The iterative reconstructions are computationally intensive but of high quality.

3. MicroSPECT instrumentation and reconstruction

The microSPECT head is developed by the Detector Group at Jefferson Lab and consists of a crossed-wire, multi-anode photomultiplier tube coupled to a pixellated NaI(Tl) crystal array. See [Weisenberger, 2004] for more details. The detector has a 55×55-mm^2 active area which is discretized into a 64×64 array. The resolution is approximately 2 mm FWHM. For the experimental work presented in this paper, we configured the system with a parallel-hole collimator and acquired 60 projections over the course of 30 to 60 minutes. The microSPECT system is presently housed in a separate gantry, but will be merged with the microCT platform to yield a true dual-modality system.

We reconstruct SPECT images using a parallelized version of the EM-ML algorithm that employs a volume intersection-based system matrix. Each voxel is divided into a number of subvoxels. We compute the conic view of the image volume for each detector pixel and count the number of subvoxels seen per voxel using an inner-product computation. Due to the symmetry that results from using parallel-hole collimation, we only model the intersection pattern for a single imaginary detector column, which is then used repeatedly. As a consequence, the system matrix contains a relatively small number of non-zero elements and computes in a few seconds. A $64 \times 64 \times 64$ SPECT image volume is typically reconstructed in less than a minute.

4. Preliminary experimental results

4.1 Study 1

The Solomon group at the University of Tennessee Graduate School of Medicine has developed a transgenic mouse model of systemic AA-amyloidosis [Solomon, 1999]. The so-called H2/huIL-6 mouse expresses the human interleukin 6 (IL-6) transgene under the control of the major histocompatibility complex class 1, H2, gene promoter. Rapid induction of systemic (splenic, hepatic, renal, and pancreatic) amyloid disease in eight week old mice is achieved by injection of an amyloid-enhancing factor (AEF). See Fig. 14.1 for more detail.

In our preliminary evaluation of the microSPECT/CT system, we injected four mice intravenously with 100 μg AEF and administered control mice an equivalent amount of saline solution. After seven weeks, the mice received 600 μCi of I-125 labeled SAP, having been provided two days prior with 1% Lugol's solution in their drinking water to prevent thyroid uptake of free radioiodine. Twenty-four hourst after SAP injection, the mice were sacrificed, and image data were acquired. Figure 14.1 shows the reconstructed microSPECT and CT images co-registered for simultaneous display, with the former being a color activity map overlaying a gray scale version of the latter. To the best of our knowledge, the resulting images provide the first detailed 3D dual-modality view of systemic AA-amyloid disease in a mouse.

We computed the biodistribution of the amyloid and compared that with the equivalent I-125 SAP image counts. We obtained the former through organ biopsies and the latter by first segmenting out the relevant organs in the CT images and then summing up the activity in the corresponding regions of the SPECT images. The two data sets were in excellent agreement, clearly indicating that the SPECT images represent organ-specific amyloid deposits.

4.2 Study 2

Our second study deals with a novel mouse model of localized AL-amyloidosis. An amyloidoma composed of human AL-amyloid extract was introduced between the scapulae of Balb/c mice by administering a subcutaneous bolus of highly concentrated material (see Fig. 14.2). The Solomon group recently developed a therapeutic monoclonal antibody (mAb) designated 11-1F4, which binds to an amyloid fibril-related epitope [Hrncic, 2000]. Natural resolution of the amyloidoma in the mouse

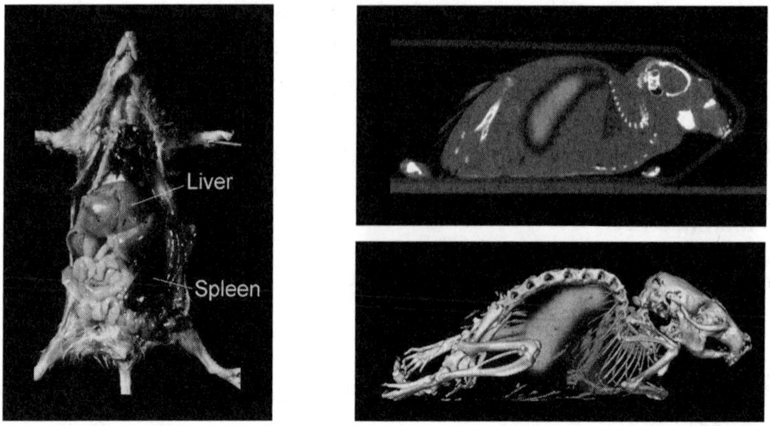

Figure 14.1. Mouse with AA-amyloidosis (left). Note the enlarged spleen and discoloration of the liver. Pseudo-colored SPECT image overlaid on top of co-registered CT image (top, right) and surface-rendered skeleton CT image (bottom, right). Bright object (high specific activity) is splenic amyloid, while cloudy object represents liver deposits.

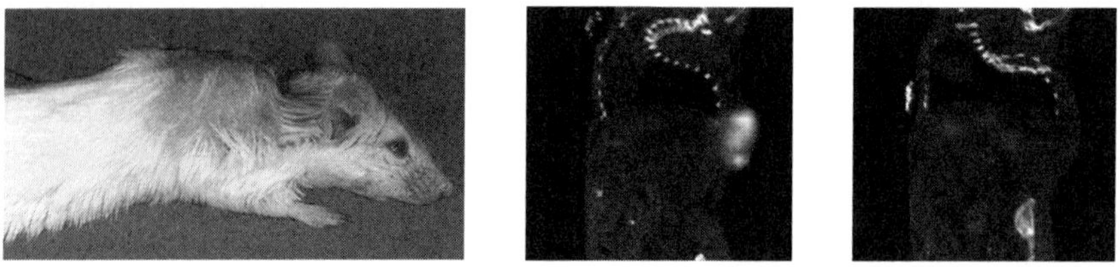

Figure 14.2. Mouse with AL-amyloidosis (left). Pseudo-colored SPECT images overlaid on top of co-registered CT images showing amyloidoma (middle) and non-specific blood pool background in the heart and liver (right).

occurs after two weeks, but can be accelerated to four days following 11-1F4 mAb treatment.

We again divided six mice into a test group of four and a control group of two. All mice received 50 mg of human-derived AL amyloid. After a week, the test mice were intravenously given I-125-labeled 11-1F4 mAb, while the control mice received an I-125 labeled isotype-matched control reagent. Following a three-day period to permit the clearance of unbound 11-1F4 mAb, the mice were sacrificed, and image data were acquired and processed as described above. The results shown in Fig. 14.2 represent the first 3D dual-modality view of localized AL-amyloidosis in a mouse model.

We again performed and compared biodistribution results with the imaging data and found the two to be correlated. In both cases, significantly higher concentrations of the 11-1F4 mAb were found in the amyloidoma compared with the heart, kidneys, and liver. The correlation indicates that radiolabeled 11-1F4 mAb is a good reagent for discerning AL amyloid deposits *in vivo*.

Our preliminary data demonstrate that the dual SPECT/CT imaging technology is capable of providing high-resolution detailed maps of amyloid deposits in mice using both SAP and amyloidophilic mAbs. Currently, a modified form of the 11-1F4 mAb is being produced in readiness for clinical trials of its efficacy as an imaging agent and therapeutic for patients with AL-amyloidosis, a devastating and invariably fatal disease.

Acknowledgments

This work was sponsored by the National Institutes of Health under grant number 1 R01 EB00789-01A2.

References

[Elbakri and Fessler, 2002] I.A. Elbakri and J.A. Fessler, "Statistical image reconstruction for polyenergetic x-ray computed tomography," *IEEE Trans. Medical Imaging*, vol. 21, pp. 89–99, 2002.

[Gregor, 2003] J. Gregor, S.S. Gleason, M.J. Paulus, and J. Cates, "Fast Feldkamp reconstruction based on focus of attention and distributed computing," *Intl. J. Imaging Systems and Technology*, vol. 12, pp. 229–234, 2003.

[Hawkins, 1988] P.N. Hawkins, M.J. Mayers, J.P. Lavender, and M.B. Pepys, "Diagnostic radionuclide imaging of amyloid: biological targeting by circulating human serum amyloid P component," *Lancet*, pp. 1413–1418, 1988.

[Hrncic, 2000] R. Hrncic, J. Wall, D. Wolfenbarger, C.L. Murphy, M. Schell, D. Weiss, and A. Solomon, "Antibody-mediated resolution of light chain-associated (AL) amyloid deposits," *Am. J. Pathol.*, vol. 157, pp. 1239–1246, 2000.

[Paulus, 2000] M.J. Paulus, S.S. Gleason, S.J. Kennel, P.R. Hunsicker, and D.K. Johnson, "High resolution x-ray computed tomography: An emerging tool for small animal cancer research," *Neoplasia*, vol. 2, pp. 62–70, 2000.

[Sipe and Cohen, 2000] J.D. Sipe and A.S. Cohen, "Review: History of the amoyloid fibril," *J. Structural Biol.*, vol. 130, pp. 88–98, 2000.

[Solomon, 1999] A. Solomon, D.T. Weiss, M. Schell, R. Hrncic, C.L. Murphy, J. Wall, M.D. McGavin, H.J. Pan, G.W. Kabalka, and M.J. Paulus, "Transgenic mouse model of AA-amyloidosis," *Am. J. Pathol.*, vol. 154, pp. 1267–1272, 1999.

[Weisenberger, 2004] A.G. Weisenberger, B. Kross, S. S. Gleason, J. Goddard S. Majewski, S.R. Meikle, M.J. Paulus, M. Pomper, V. Popov, M.F. Smith, B.L. Welch, and R. Wojcik, "Development and testing of a restraint free small animal SPECT imaging system with infrared based motion tracking," *IEEE Trans. Nuc. Sci.* To appear.

Chapter 15

Feasibility of Micro-SPECT/CT Imaging of Atherosclerotic Plaques in a Transgenic Mouse Model

Benjamin M. W. Tsui, Yuchuan Wang, Yujin Qi, Stacia Sawyer, Eric C. Frey, Stan Majewski, and Martin G. Pomper*

1. Introduction

Cardiovascular disease (CVD) is the leading cause of disability and mortality for both men and women in the United States and other developed countries. About 80% of myocardial infarctions and strokes are due to the rupture of unstable coronary and carotid plaques that are not detected by current diagnostic methods. The identification and treatment of vulnerable plaque prior to rupture will have a significant impact on health care.

The development of atherosclerotic plaque through the disruption of normal endothelial function caused by chronic inflammation has been under intense investigation in recent years [Ruberg, 2002]. In particular, the differentiation between stable and unstable (or vulnerable) plaque, and the pathophysiological mechanisms involved in the rupture of unstable plaque, remain unclear.

The current understanding of the mechanisms leading to plaque instability suggests endothelial dysfunction that leads to diffusion of low-density lipoprotein (LDL) through endothelial cell junctions into the vessel lumen [Ruberg, 2002, Virmani, 2002, Shah, 2002]. The LDL is oxidized to form ox-LDL, which attracts macrophages that become foam cells. Concurrently, induced changes occur in the surrounding endothelium, resulting in elimination of smooth muscle cells through apoptosis. Apoptosis induces degradation of the fibrous cap of the plaque, especially at the shoulder region from which plaque rupture.

Plaque destabilization involves an array of complex inflammatory cytokines. Examples are TNF-γ, 1L-1β, transforming growth factors (e.g., TGF-β), TNF-α, and lipoprotein (composed of apoliprotein B-100 and glycoprotein apo(a)). Furthermore, recent studies have demonstrated the role of sphingolipids in various

*B. M. W. Tsui, Y. Wang, Y. Qi, S. Sawyer, E. C. Frey, M. G. Pomper, Johns Hopkins University, Department of Radiology, Baltimore, Maryland; S. Majewski, Thomas Jefferson National Accelerator Facility, Newport News, Virginia

processes involved in plaque formation and destabilization [Chatterjee and Martin, 2003].

Various imaging techniques have been applied to study atherosclerotic plaque [Vallabhajosula and Fuster, 1997]. Conventional biplane angiography has been considered the "gold standard" in clinical studies to measure the degree of stenosis. Angioscopy has been used to identify thrombus. Duplex Doppler ultrasound (US) has been used to measure the degree of stenosis and plaque morphology, and intravascular US has been used to image plaque within the coronary arteries. Magnetic resonance angiography (MRA) can also delineate stenosis, although it is fraught with motion artifacts. MR imaging can characterize plaque directly.

Nuclear imaging techniques have been used to provide functional information about atherosclerotic plaque [Vallabhajosula and Fuster, 1997]. Positron emission tomography (PET) with ^{18}F-fluorodeoxyglucose (FDG) has been used to study metabolism in plaque. Planar scintigraphy and single-photon emission computed tomography (SPECT) has been used to measure specific pathophysiological aspects of plaque. For example, lipoprotein, platelets, and various immunoglobulins have been labeled with ^{125}I, ^{131}I, and ^{111}In. Unfortunately, images of these radiolabeled agents give poor target-to-blood ratios, resulting in poor image quality. Technetium-99m-labeled peptides and monoclonal antibody fragments tend to clear from the blood rapidly and can be used to bind various components of the plaque [Dinkelborg, 1998, Narula, 1997].

Because apoptosis of macrophages and smooth muscle cells are involved in the formation and destabilization of plaque, imaging apoptosis allows the detection and characterization of such lesions. During apoptosis, translocase enzyme permits phosphatidylserine (PS) to migrate from inside of the cell membrane to the outer surface, marking the apoptotic cells for elimination by phagocytes. Annexin V is a human protein that binds to PS with high affinity. Hynic-Annexin-V is a commercial kit that enables linking of ^{99m}Tc to Annexin-V. Upon intravenous injection, the ^{99m}Tc-Hynic-Annexin V binds to apoptotic cells. High uptake of ^{99m}Tc-Hynic-annexin V in atherosclerotic plaque has been demonstrated in rabbits and mice [Blankenberg, 1998, Tait, 2000, Blankenberg and Strauss, 2001]. However, planar and SPECT images from those studies were obtained using standard clinical equipment or earlier generations of microSPECT systems with relatively poor spatial resolution.

In this study, we investigated the feasibility of applying a new generation of microSPECT systems for imaging plaque in a unique transgenic mouse model that produces plaque with thin and thick fibrous caps, which are purported to be consistent with stable and unstable plaques. The microSPECT systems used have spatial resolution on the order of 1 mm.

2. Methods

2.1 Transgenic mouse model

A newly genetically engineered transgenic mouse model developed at the University of North Carolina at Chapel Hill (UNC-CH) was used in our investigation. The Gulo-/-Apoe-/- mouse model [Nakata and Maeda, 2002] is a cross between the Apoe-/- genotype that spontaneously develops atherosclerotic plaques and the Gulo-/- genotype that is unable to synthesize ascorbic acid (Vitamin C) [Maeda, 2000]. The Gulo-/-Apoe-/- mice were fed diets that were either high or low in ascorbic acid to produce plaques with thick and thin caps, respectively.

2.2 MicroSPECT and MicroCT imaging systems

Three microSPECT systems with similar imaging characteristics were used in the study. As shown in Fig. 15.1, they include a prototype system developed in our laboratory at the Johns Hopkins University (JHU) with assistance from the Detector Group at the Thomas Jefferson National Accelerator Facility (TJNAF) (see Chapter 21), a prototype system developed by the TJNAF Detector Group and an earlier commercial A-SPECT system from Gamma Medica, Inc. with a new pixellated detector. The JHU and TJNAF systems are based on a mini-camera consisting of a 5" Hamamatsu R3292 position-sensitive photomultiplier tube (PSPMT) and a Saint-Gobain pixellated NaI(Tl) crystal array (JHU system: 11 cm $\times$ 11 cm array size, 1.2 mm $\times$ 1.2 mm $\times$ 6.0-mm pixels, 0.2-mm gaps and 73 $\times$ 73 pixel array, TJNAF system: $\sim$ 10-cm diameter, 1.0 mm $\times$ 1.0 mm $\times$ 5.0-mm pixels, 0.25-mm gaps and 77 $\times$ 77 pixel array). The A-SPECT system (from Gamma Medica Inc. consists of a 12.5 $\times$ 12.5 cm^2 pixellated NaI(Tl) crystal with 1.3 $\times$ 1.3 mm^2 pixels, 0.2 mm gaps and an 82 $\times$ 82 pixel array coupled to an array of 5 $\times$ 5 R8520-00-12 PSPMTs.

All three systems were fitted with pinhole collimators with interchangeable tungsten pinhole apertures of different diameters. The aperture-to-crystal distances for the pinhole collimator of the JHU, TJNAF, and A-SPECT systems were 10 cm, 11 cm, and 9.1 cm, respectively. A pinhole aperture with 1-mm diameter was used in all three systems. The spatial resolution at 3 cm from the pinhole aperture was $\sim 1.1 - 1.2$ mm for all three microSPECT systems. The mini-cameras in all of the microSPECT systems are stationary, and projection data were acquired by rotating the animal in front of the pinhole collimator. Additionally, images were acquired in a planar mode on a Gamma Medica system using a parallel-hole collimator.

The microCT system used in the study was developed in our laboratory. It consists of an Oxford Apogee X-ray tube and a Medoptics 1024 $\times$ 1024 2" CCD detector. The small animal was vertically rotated inbetween the x-ray tube and the CCD detector in CT data acquisition.

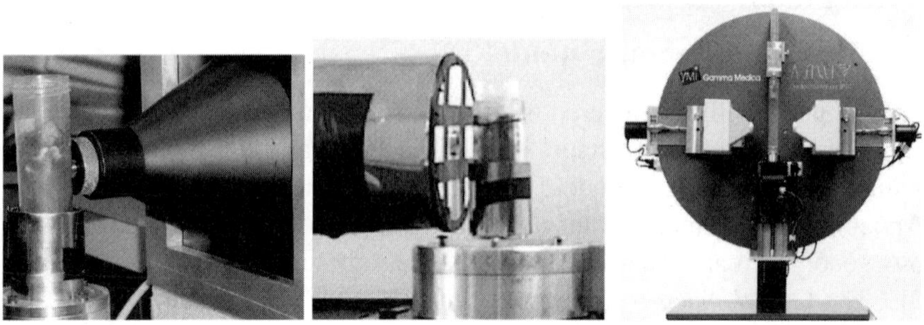

(a) (b) (c)

Figure 15.1. The three microSPECT systems used in the study. The (a) JHU and (b) TJNAF systems are based on a Saint Gobain pixellated NaI(Tl) crystal array and a 5" Hamamatsu R3292 PSPMT. (c) A commercial A-SPECT system from Gamma Medica, Inc. with one new 12.5 cm x 12.5 cm detector with 82×82 pixellated NaI(Tl) crystal array and an array of 1" flat-panel PSPMT. Only single-detector head was used for the mouse plaque imaging. All three systems were fitted with a pinhole collimator with an interchangeable aperture. The small animal was rotated in front of the pinhole aperture in SPECT data acquisition.

2.3 Data acquisition

The Gulo-/-Apoe-/- mice received $\sim$3-5 mCi of ^{99m}Tc-labeled Annexin-V (Theseus Imaging Corp. of North American Scientific, Inc.) in 0.2 mL of saline vehicle via tail vein injection. One hour after administration of ^{99m}Tc-Hynic-Annexin V, mice were anesthetized by intraperitoneal injection with 20 μL of 1:1.5:3 acepromazine:ketamine:saline. Anesthetized mice were placed inside a holder that consisted of a 1"-diameter plastic tube marked with two fiducials which were short capillary tubes filled with $^{99m}TcO_4$. The fiducials were visible on both SPECT and CT images and were used to co-register images obtained from those modalities.

The mouse holder was fitted into a rotational stage that rotated in front of the pinhole aperture with a radius-of-rotation (ROR) of $\sim$3 cm. Ninety emission projections over 360° were acquired with $\sim$40 sec/view for a total acquisition time of $\sim$1 hour.

After SPECT data acquisition, the holder containing the transgenic mouse was transferred to the microCT system. A total of 180 CT projections in 256×256 matrices and 0.17-mm bins over 186° (180° plus cone-angle) were acquired.

In a couple of animals, additional ultrasound scans and pathological studies were performed to verify the existence of plaques.

2.4 Image reconstruction and co-registration

The emission projections were reconstructed using an iterative 3D pixel-driven pinhole OS-EM algorithm. The reconstructed image size was $80 \times 80 \times 80$ for the JHU and the TJNAF systems and $82 \times 82 \times 82$ for the A-SPECT system with

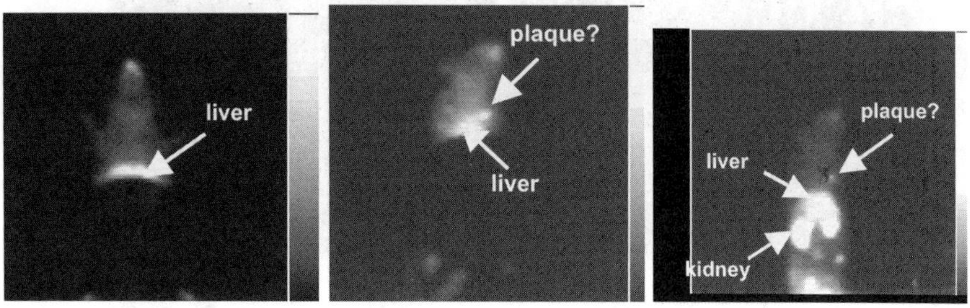

Figure 15.2. Planar images obtained from (a) a normal control mouse at 2 hours after injection of ~4 mCi of ^{99m}Tc-Hynic-Annexin V and a Gulo-/- Apoe-/- transgenic mouse (#3973) at (b) 1 hour and (c) 5 hours after injection of ~4 mCi of ^{99m}Tc-Hynic-Annexin V using the Gamma Medica A-SPECT system fitted with a parallel-hole collimator. In (a) and (b), emissions from organs in the abdomen with a high level of radioactivity uptake were blocked using a lead shield. The focal areas of high radiopharmaceutical uptake in the transgenic mouse indicate possible plaque (arrows).

an 0.35-mm pixel size. The OS-EM reconstructed images were postfiltered with a Butterworth smoothing filter. The microCT data were reconstructed using a 3D Feldkamp cone-beam image reconstruction method in 256 × 256 × 256 matrices with an 0.17-mm pixel size.

The 3D microCT image was first collapsed into a 128 × 128 × 128 matrix and cropped to 82 × 82 × 82 that contained the image of the animal. The cropped microCT image was then co-registered with the microSPECT image using the ends of the ^{99m}Tc solution in the two capillary tubes of the fiducial markers. The co-registration involved rigid transformation, including scaling and 3D rotation, of the microCT and microSPECT images.

3. Results

Figure 15.2 shows planar images from a normal control mouse and from a Gulo-/- Apoe-/- transgenic mouse (#3973) at different times after injection of ~4 mCi of ^{99m}Tc-Hynic-Annexin V. The images show focal areas of the high activity uptake in the transgenic mouse but not in the normal control animal indicating possible plaque uptakes.

Figure 15.3 shows sample coronal pinhole microSPECT image slices of the same Gulo-/- Apoe-/- transgenic mouse (#3973) obtained using the Gamma Medica A-SPECT system fitted with a pinhole collimator with 1-mm diameter aperture. The microSPECT data acquisition was initiated ~1 hour after injection of ~4 mCi of ^{99m}Tc-Hynic-Annexin V. Unfortunately, the animal expired at the beginning of the data acquisition. Nevertheless, the microSPECT images depicted in Figure 15.3 have the advantage of omitting cardiac and respiratory motion, producing high-quality images. Several focal areas of high radiopharmaceutical uptake were found

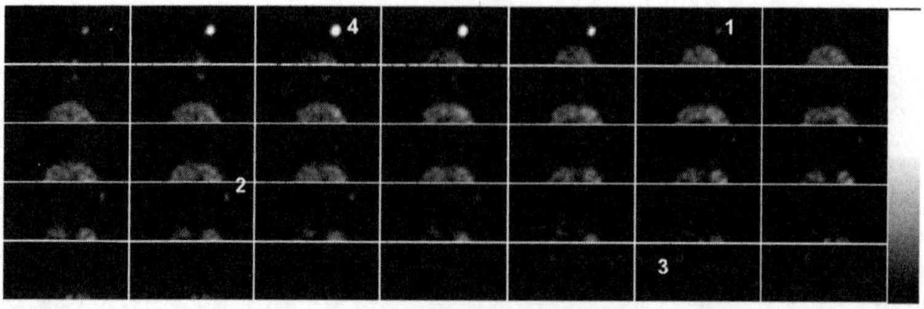

Figure 15.3. Sample coronal pinhole microSPECT images of a Gulo-/- Apoe-/- transgenic mouse (#3973) obtained using the Gamma Medica A-SPECT system fitted with a pinhole collimator with a 1-mm diameter aperture. The image pixel size is 0.35 mm. Data acquisition was initiated ~1 hour after injection of ~4 mCi of ^{99m}Tc-Hynic-Annexin V. The animal expired at the beginning of the data acquisition. Several focal areas of high-activity concentration were found in the images.

Table 15.1. Contrast and signal-to-noise ratios of the areas of focal radiopharmaceutical uptake noted in Fig. 15.3.

Focal Uptake Area	Contrast Ratio	Signal-to-Noise Ratio
#1	7.3	13.3
#2	7.8	14.3
#3	5.8	10.1
#4	16.9	133.7

in the images. Table 15.1 shows the contrast and signal-to-noise ratios of the four identified focal areas with the highest radiopharmaceutical uptake.

Figure 15.4 shows fused microSPECT/CT images of the same transgenic animal. The microCT images provide exquisite anatomical detail for correlation with the focal areas of high radiopharmaceutical uptake identified on the microSPECT images. The co-registered images indicate that focal uptake area #1 is located just above the heart, suggesting plaque in the aorta. Comparing the images of Fig. 15.4 with an atlas of mouse anatomy [Iwaki, 2001], focal uptake areas #2, #3, and #4 indicate possible plaque within the thoracic vessels.

To further verify the presence of plaque in these animals, one of the mice were imaged using US and histopathological analysis. Figure 15.5 (a) and (b) show a B-mode US image of the long axis view of the left ventricle and a pulsed wave Doppler spectrum recording. When compared to similar images from normal mice, they indicate the existence of plaque in the aorta. Histopathological analysis of a specimen through the aorta of the animal, shown in Fig. 15.6, confirmed plaque near the aorta valve.

4. Conclusions

We demonstrated the feasibility of microSPECT/CT imaging of atherosclerotic plaques labeled with ^{99m}Tc-Hynic-Annexin V in a Gulo-/- Apoe-/- transgenic

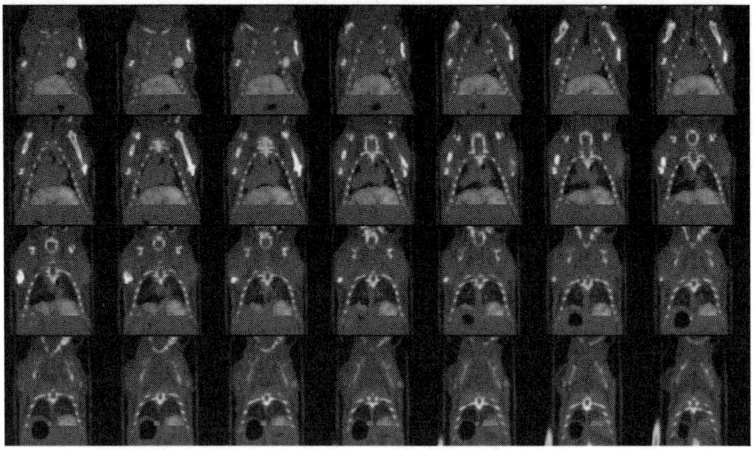

Figure 15.4. Sample fused microSPECT/CT coronal images of the same transgenic mouse shown in Fig. 15.3. The image pixel size is ~0.35 mm. The microCT images provide anatomical correlation of the focal areas of high radiopharmaceutical uptake, indicating possible presence of plaque in the thoracic vessels.

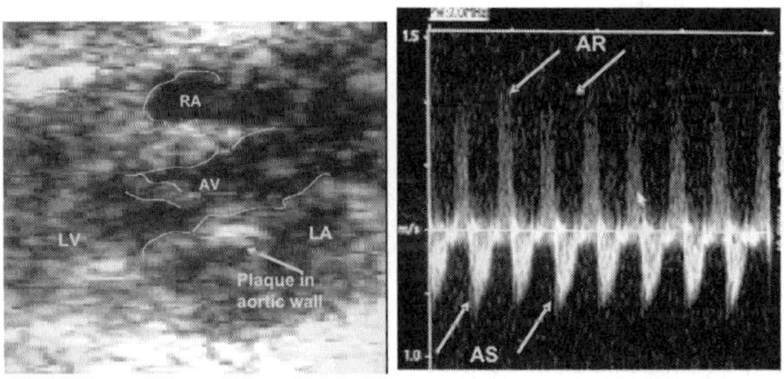

(a) (b)

Figure 15.5. (a) B-mode US image of a 2D long axis view of the left ventricle (LV) showing a thickened aortic valve with echogenic deposits on the aortic posterior wall consistent with the pathology shown in Figure 15.6. RA: right atrium; LA: left atrium and AV: aortic valve. (b) Pulsed wave Doppler spectrum recorded from the LV outflow tract (aorta). Flow disturbance indicating significant aortic regurgitation (AR) and aortic stenosis (AS) are also shown (arrows).

mouse model. Focal areas with high-radioactivity contrast and signal-to-noise ratios were found on the microSPECT images of the transgenic mice, but not in normal control animals, indicating likely uptake of ^{99m}Tc-Hynic-Annexin V in atherosclerotic plaque in the transgenic mouse. Further US studies and histopathological analysis of specimens through the aorta of the transgenic mouse confirmed the presence of plaque near the aortic valve.

Further validation of the uptake of ^{99m}Tc-Hynic-Annexin V in the plaque of these transgenic animal requires whole-body autoradiography, which will obviate cardiac and respiratory motion, with their attendant image quality degradation (see Chapter

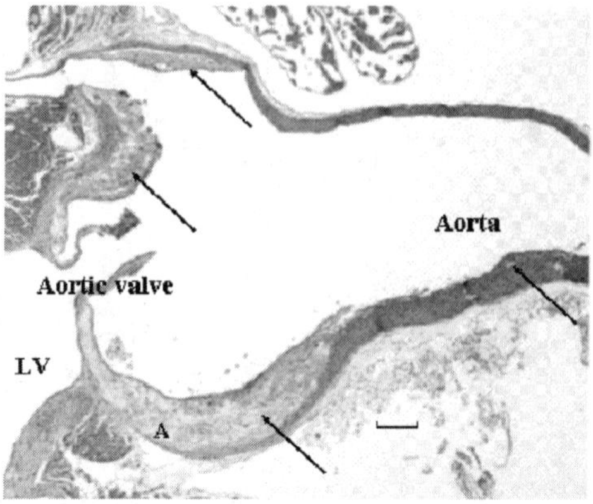

Figure 15.6. Pathological analysis of a specimen through the aorta indicating plaque near the aortic valve (arrows).

16), inherent to the imaging procedures described herein. However, that degradation can be reduced with cardiac and respiration gating techniques now increasingly used for *in vivo* small-animal imaging studies. Despite the encouraging results of this preliminary study, characterization of plaque in transgenic animals needs further improvement in the spatial resolution and quantitation of microSPECT imaging.

Acknowledgments

This work is partially supported by the Public Health Service Grant CA92871. The authors are grateful to Theseus Imaging Corp. of North American Scientific Inc. for providing the Hynic Annexin-V kits, N. Maeda, Ph.D. of the University of North Carolina at Chapel Hill for providing the Gulo-/- Apoe-/- transgenic mice and H. William Strauss, M.D. of the Memorial Sloan Kettering Cancer Center for valuable advice on plaque imaging using Annexin-V.

We also thank several collaborators at Johns Hopkins University including Kathleen Gabrielson, D.V.M., Ph.D., for expert US and histological analysis, Catherine Foss, Ph.D., for labeling ^{99m}Tc with the Hynic-Annexin-V, and Ruth Hageman for animal handling.

References

[Blankenberg, 1998] F.G. Blankenberg, P.D. Katsikis, J.F. Tait, R.E. Davis, L. Naumovski, K. Ohtsuki, S. Kopiwoda, M.J. Abrams, M. Darkes, R.C. Robbins, H.T. Maecker, and H.W. Strauss, "*In vivo* detection and imaging of phosphatidylserine expression during programmed cell death," *Proc. Natl. Acad. Sci.*, vol. 95, pp. 6349-6354, 1998.

[Blankenberg and Strauss, 2001] F.G. Blankenberg and H.W. Strauss, "Noninvasive strategies to image cardiovascular apoptosis," *Cardiovascular Disease*, vol. 19, pp. 165-172, 2001.

[Chatterjee and Martin, 2003] S. Chatterjee and S.F. Martin, "Sphingolipid metabolism and signaling in atherosclerosis," *Advances in cell aging and gerontology*, vol. 12, pp.71-96, 2003.

[Dinkelborg, 1998] L.M. Dinkelborg, S.H. Duda, H. Hanke, G. Tepe, C.S. Hilger and W. Semmler, "Molecular imaging of atherosclerosis using a Technetium-99m-labeled endothelin derivative," *J. of Nucl. Med.*, vol. 39, pp. 1819-1822, 1998.

[Iwaki, 2001] T. Iwaki, H. Yamashita and T. Hayakawa, "A Color Atlas of Sectional Anatomy of the Mouse," *Braintree Scientific Inc.*, 2001.

[Maeda, 2000] N. Maeda, H. Hagihara, Y. Nakata, S. Hiller, J. Wilder, and R. Reddick, "Aortic wall damage in mice unable to synthesize ascorbic acid," *Proceedings of the National Academy of Sciences of the United States of America*, vol. 97, pp. 841-846, 2000.

[Nakata and Maeda, 2002] Y. Nakata and N. Maeda, "Vulnerable atherosclerotic plaque morphology in apolipoprotein E-deficient mice unable to make ascorbic acid," *Circulation*, vol. 105, pp. 1485-1490, 2002.

[Narula, 1997] J. Narula, A. Petrov, K.-Y. Pak, C. Ditlow, F. Chen and B.-A. Khaw, "Noninvasive detection of atherosclerotic lesions by 99mTc-based immunoscintigraphic targeting of proliferating smooth muscle cells," *Chest*, vol. 111, pp.1684-1690, 1997.

[Ruberg, 2002] F.L. Ruberg, J.A. Leopold and J. Loscalzo, "Atherothrombosis: Plaque instability and thrombogenesis," *Progress in Cardiovascular Diseases*, vol. 44, pp. 381-394, 2002.

[Shah, 2002] P.K. Shah, "Pathophysiology of coronary thrombosis: Role of plaque rupture and plaque erosion," *Progress in Cardiovascular Diseases*, vol. 44, pp. 357-368, 2002.

[Tait, 2000] J.F. Tait, D.S. Brown, D.F. Gibson, F.G. Blankenberg, and H.W. Strauss, "Development and characterization of annexin V mutants with endogenous chelation sites for 99mTc," *Bioconjugate Chemistry*, vol. 11, pp. 918-925, 2000.

[Vallabhajosula and Fuster, 1997] S. Vallabhajosula and V. Fuster, "Atherosclerosis: Imaging techniques and the evolving role of nuclear medicine," *J. of Nucl. Med.*, vol. 38, pp. 1788-1796, 1997.

[Virmani, 2002] R. Virmani, A.P. Burke, A. Farb and F.D. Kolodgie, "Pathology of the unstable plaque," *Progress in Cardiovascular Diseases*, vol. 44, pp. 349-356, 2002.

Chapter 16

Effect of Respiratory Motion on Plaque Imaging in the Mouse Using Tc-99m Labeled Annexin-V

William P. Segars, Yuchuan Wang, and Benjamin M. W. Tsui*

1. Introduction

The main cause of death in coronary artery disease (CAD) is the rupture of unstable or "vulnerable" atherosclerotic plaque which leads to a sudden occlusion. The structure and composition of an atherosclerotic plaque is an important determinant in its stability. Vulnerable plaque tend to have a thin fibrous cap and a large lipid core and are softer and more likely to rupture than more stable plaque with thicker caps. Currently, a great deal of research is ongoing to investigate different imaging techniques to differentiate stable and vulnerable plaque. The technique could significantly enhance the screening and management of patients with CAD. It would have great potential in identifying patients who are at a high risk for acute events.

Transgenic mouse models bred to develop atherosclerotic plaque are currently being used to investigate imaging techniques to differentiate stable and vulnerable plaque. A group at the University of North Carolina (UNC) headed by Dr. Nobuyo Maeda, Ph.D., recently developed a unique Gulo-/-Apoe-/- mouse model [Nakata and Maeda, 2002] that is a cross between Gulo-/- mice that are unable to synthesize ascorbic acid or vitamin C [Maeda, 2000] and Apoe-/- mice that spontaneously develop advanced atherosclerotic plaque. By feeding these mice diets that differ in levels of ascorbic acid (vitamin C), they found that mice with a diet low in ascorbic acid tend to develop plaque that have a thinner wall that is consistent to those of vulnerable plaque.

Technetium-99m labeled Hynic-Annexin-V has been investigated as a hot spot agent for imaging apoptotic cell death [Tait, et al., 2000, Blankenberg and Strauss, 2001, Blankenberg, 1998]. High uptake of Hynic-Annexin-V in plaque in Apoe-/- mice was found to be as high as 18:1 with respect to the background.

Movement of the heart due to respiratory motion is a major factor that can cause blurring and artifacts in plaque imaging. The total movement of the heart with the diaphragm during respiration may greatly exceed the coronary wall thickness,

*Johns Hopkins University, Department of Radiology, Division of Medical Imaging Physics, Baltimore, Maryland

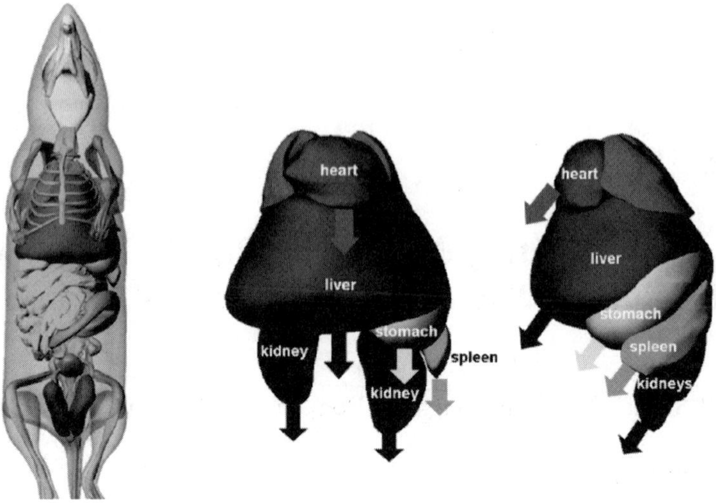

Figure 16.1. (Left) Anterior view of the digital mouse phantom. (Right) Inspiratory motions simulated in the phantom. The heart can be seen to move downward and forward as the diaphragm contracts during inspiration.

significantly decreasing the visibility of plaque due to motion blur. Our goal in this study is to investigate the effects of respiratory motion on microSPECT imaging of atherosclerotic plaque in the mouse using Hynic-Annexin-V. To do this, we use the new, realistic 4D digital mouse phantom developed in our laboratory.

The 4D digital mouse phantom (Fig. 16.1) [Segars, 2003] was developed to provide a realistic and flexible model of the mouse anatomy and cardiac and respiratory motions for use in molecular imaging research. The organ shapes were modeled with non-uniform rational b-spline (NURBS) surfaces using high-resolution 3D magnetic resonance microscopy (MRM) data obtained from the Duke Center for *in vivo* Microscopy as the basis for the formation of the surfaces. With its basis upon actual imaging data and the inherent flexibility of the NURBS primitives, the phantom model's organ shapes realistically while maintaining the flexibility to model anatomical variations and involuntary motions such as the cardiac and respiratory motions. These motions were modeled using a gated black-blood magnetic resonance imaging (bb-MRI) data set of a normal mouse as the basis for the cardiac model and respiratory-gated MRI and known respiratory mechanics as the basis for the respiratory model, using images obtained from the University of Virginia. The 4D mouse phantom provides an excellent tool with which to study the effects of anatomy and motion on molecular imaging data.

2. Methods

For our study, we modeled atherosclerotic plaque of three different sizes inside the aortic arch of the mouse heart phantom using 3D NURBS surfaces (Fig. 16.2).

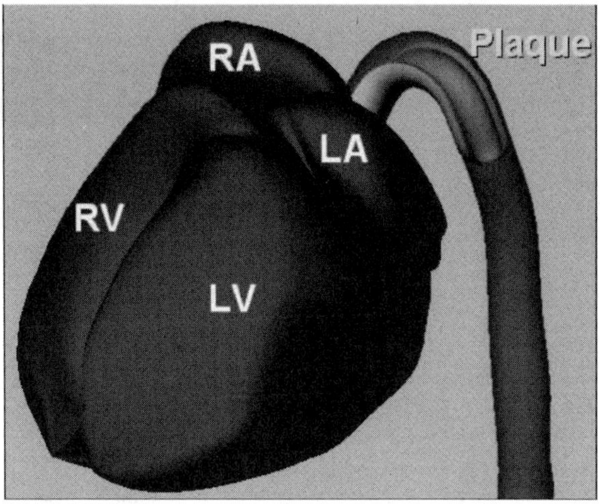

Figure 16.2. Mouse heart phantom with plaque placed in the aortic arch.

The different plaque sizes were $1.0 \times 1.0 \times 0.5$ mm^3, $2.0 \times 2.0 \times 1.0$ mm^3, and $3.0 \times 3.0 \times 1.5$ mm^3 corresponding to blockages of 25%, 50%, and 75%, respectively.

Using the mouse phantom software application, we generated pairs of 3D voxelized phantoms that represented the average distributions of attenuation coefficients and the average radioactivity concentrations in the different organs. Each phantom was generated into a $160 \times 160 \times 160$ array with a pixel width and slice thickness of 0.15 mm. The radioactivity concentrations were set to model a typical Tc-99m labeled Hynic-Annexin-V study. Three different activity uptake ratios (relative to the background) were simulated: 9 to 1, 18 to 1, and 36 to 1. Phantoms were generated without any respiratory motion and with respiratory motion consisting of the diaphragm and heart moving downward a maximum of 0.5 mm, 1.0 mm, and 2.0 mm during inspiration.

Emission projection data were generated from the voxelized phantoms using a realistic pinhole SPECT projection model. The projection data matrices were collapsed to 80×80 to simulate sampling. Noise-free projections were generated in addition to projections with Poisson noise added roughly equivalent to that of a typical Tc-99m-labeled Hynic-Annexin-V mouse SPECT study. The emission projection data were then reconstructed using the iterative OS-EM reconstruction method. The images were reconstructed into $80 \times 80 \times 80$ arrays with a pixel width and slice thickness of 0.3 mm.

Regions of interest (ROIs) were defined for the plaque (ROIp) and background (ROIbg) in the reconstructed images. For each reconstruction, the mean intensity and standard deviation for the two ROIs were calculated. To assess the visibility of the plaque in the resulting images, the signal-to-noise ratio (SNR) for the plaque was calculated as shown in Eq. (16.1), and the plaque contrast ratio was calculated

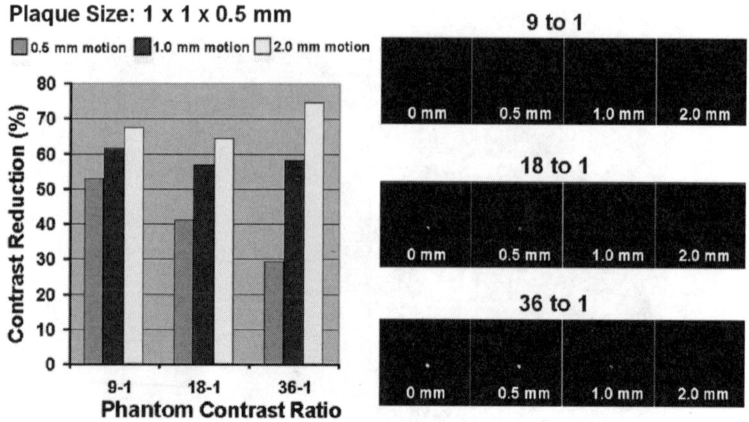

Figure 16.3. Effect of respiratory motion on the contrast of the smallest plaque as measured from noise-free reconstructions.

as shown in Eq. (16.2).

$$\text{SNR} = \frac{\text{mean}(\text{ROI}_p) - \text{mean}(\text{ROI}_{bg})}{\text{stdev}(\text{ROI}_{bg})} \tag{16.1}$$

$$\text{CR} = \frac{\text{mean}(\text{ROI}_p)}{\text{mean}(\text{ROI}_{bg})}. \tag{16.2}$$

3. Results

Fig. 16.3 shows the effect of respiratory motion on the contrast of the smallest plaque ($1 \times 1 \times 0.5$ mm^3) as measured on noise-free reconstructions. For each contrast ratio simulated, the contrast of the plaque to the background is further reduced with increasing respiratory motion. The decrease in contrast can be seen in the reconstructed transaxial slices shown in the figure for each case. The plaque is less and less visible with increasing amounts of respiratory motion. The medium ($2 \times 2 \times 1.0$ mm^3) and large plaque ($3 \times 3 \times 1.5$ mm^3) also show a similar result (figures not shown). The amount of reduction is less and less severe as the plaque size increases.

Fig. 16.4 illustrates the effect of respiratory motion on the SNR of the smallest plaque as measured on noise-added reconstructions. For each phantom contrast ratio simulated, the SNR decreases with an increase in the amount of respiratory motion. In the reconstructed images, the plaque becomes less and less visible with increasing amounts of respiratory motion. The plaque with the highest initial contrast ratio (36 to 1) is the most visible. However, even it disappears with a respiratory motion of 1.0 mm or higher. The medium and large plaque show a similar result (figures not shown). With the increased size, the plaque is more visible at the different contrasts and levels of respiratory motion. For the largest size, the plaque becomes even slightly visible with a respiratory motion of 2 mm and an uptake contrast ratio of 36 to 1.

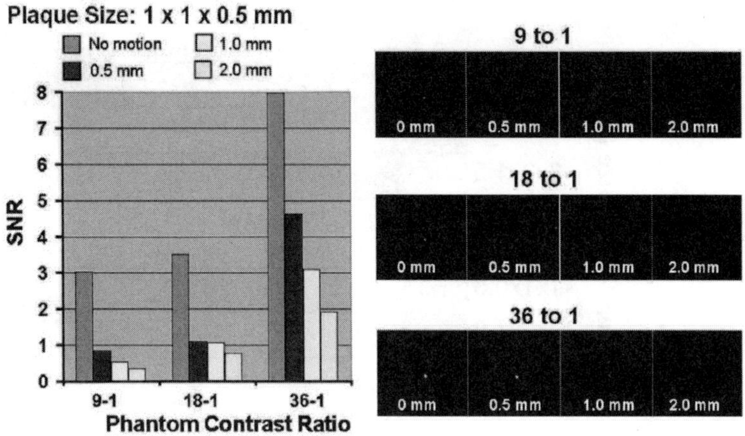

Figure 16.4. Effect of respiratory motion on the SNR of the smallest plaque as measured from noise-added reconstructions.

Fig. 16.5 summarizes the effect of respiratory motion on measured contrast ratio and SNR of the plaque. A signal-to-noise ratio of $\sim$4 and above typically means that an object is visible to the naked eye. Fig. 16.5 is color-coded according to the calculated SNR values for each case. Considering the different plaque sizes and the different levels of respiratory motion, the plaque was visible in the most cases with the activity uptake ratio of the plaque set to 36 to 1 in the phantom. When the activity uptake ratio was 18 to 1, the plaque is visible only when it is greater than $1 \times 1 \times 0.5$ mm^3 in size and with no respiratory motion. If the activity uptake ratio is 9 to 1, the plaque is only slightly visible when there is no respiratory motion.

The numbers given in Fig. 16.5 are the measured contrast ratios for the plaque relative to the background as measured from the noise-added reconstructed images. These numbers reflect the contrast reduction due to respiratory motion and noise. From the figure, one can get an idea of how much contrast ratio is needed in order for the plaque to be visible (SNR $\geq$ 4) in the images. The plaque was found to be visible when the measured uptake ratio was greater than 7.5. The measured contrast ratio for plaque using Hynic-Annexin-V has been shown to be as high as 18 to 1, which would make it a good agent for plaque imaging under various conditions. These results demonstrate the utility of the mouse phantom to assess the effects of respiratory motion on and investigate optimal parameters for plaque imaging in small animals.

4. Conclusions

We conclude that respiratory motion contributes significantly to blurring and artifacts in microSPECT plaque imaging in small animals. For each contrast ratio and plaque size simulated, the contrast and signal-to-noise ratio of the plaque was further reduced with increasing respiratory motion. The contrast reduction was as high as 60% for a plaque size of $2 \times 2 \times 1.0$ mm^3 and a respiratory motion of 2 mm.

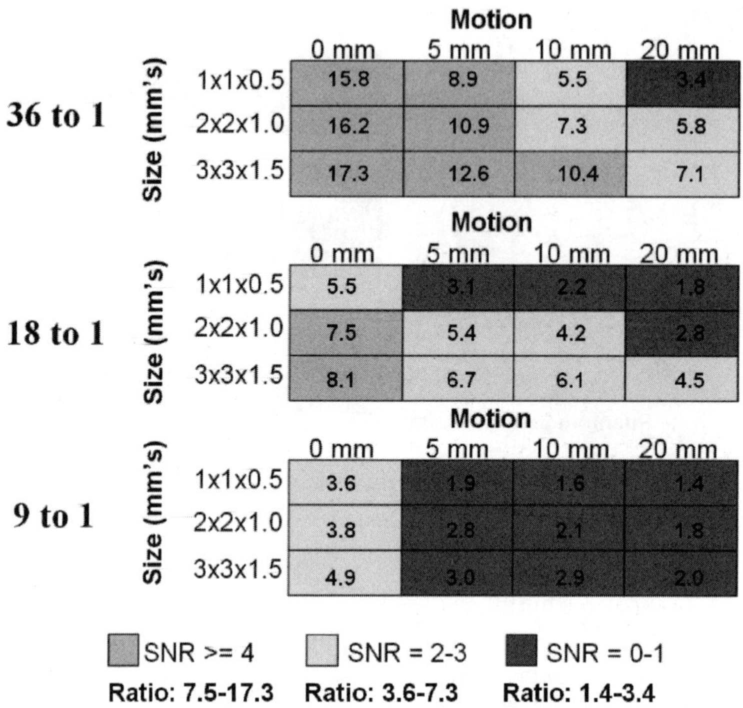

Figure 16.5. Summary of the effect of respiratory motion on the measured contrast ratio and signal-to-noise ratio of simulated plaque. SNR is color-coded, while the numbers are the measured contrast ratios for each case.

Therefore, accurate respiratory motion compensation is critical for atherosclerotic plaque imaging. The 4D digital mouse phantom is a useful tool for assessing the effects of respiratory motion, for investigating optimal imaging parameters, and for designing respiratory compensation methods for improved microSPECT imaging of plaque.

References

[Blankenberg, 1998] F.G. Blankenberg, P.D. Katsikis, J.F. Tait, R.E. Davis, L. Naumovski, K. Ohtsuki, S. Kopiwoda, M.J. Abrams, M. Darkes, R.C. Robbins, H.T. Maecker, and H.W. Strauss, "*In vivo* detection and imaging of phosphatidylserine expression during programmed cell death," *Proc. Natl. Acad. Sci.*, vol. 95, pp. 6349-6354, 1998.

[Blankenberg and Strauss, 2001] F.G. Blankenberg and H.W. Strauss, "Noninvasive strategies to image cardiovascular apoptosis," *Cardiovascular Disease*, vol. 19, pp. 165-172, 2001.

[Maeda, 2000] N. Maeda, H. Hagihara, Y. Nakata, S. Hiller, J. Wilder, and R. Reddick, "Aortic wall damage in mice unable to synthesize ascorbic acid," *Pro-*

ceedings of the National Academy of Sciences of the United States of America, vol. 97, pp. 841-846, 2000.

[Nakata and Maeda, 2002] Y. Nakata and N. Maeda, "Vulnerable atherosclerotic plaque morphology in apolipoprotein E-deficient mice unable to make ascorbic acid," *Circulation*, vol. 105, pp. 1485-1490, 2002.

[Segars, 2003] W.P. Segars, B.W.M. Tsui, E.C. Frey, and G.A. Johnson, "Development of a 4D digital mouse phantom for molecular imaging research," *Molecular Imaging and Biology*, vol. 5, no. 3 pp. 126-127, 2003.

[Tait, et al., 2000] J.F. Tait, D.S. Brown, D.F. Gibson, F.G. Blankenberg, and H.W. Strauss, "Development and characterization of annexin V mutants with endogenous chelation sites for 99mTc," *Bioconjugate Chemistry*, vol. 11, pp. 918-925, 2000.

Chapter 17

Calibration and Performance of the Fully Engineered YAP-(S)PET Scanner for Small Rodents

Alberto Del Guerra, Nicola Belcari, Deborah Herbert, Alfonso Motta, Angela Vaiano, Giovanni Di Domenico, Elena Moretti, Nicola Sabba, Guido Zavattini, Marco Lazzorotti, Luca Sensi, and Aldo Pinchera*

1. Introduction

Functional imaging of small animals, such as mice and rats, using high-performance positron emission tomography (PET) and single-photon emission tomography (SPECT), is becoming a valuable tool for studying animal models of human disease. The possibility to use either PET or SPECT allows the scientist to exploit the advantages of both techniques, e.g., the wide range of easily accessible single-photon radiotracers for SPECT and the exquisite performance of PET. The combination of PET and SPECT techniques for small-animal studies could offer the unique possibility of developing new and interesting protocols for the investigation of many biological phenomena more effectively than with PET or SPECT modality alone.

In this paper, we present the characteristics and the performance of the fully engineered version of the YAP-(S)PET scanner. The scanner was originally developed [Del Guerra, et al., 1998, 2000] at the Department of Physics at the University of Ferrara, Italy, and is now commercially available [WebRef]. The YAP-(S)PET scanner allows one to perform both PET or SPECT as well as simultaneous PET/SPECT acquisitions [Del Guerra, et al., 2002].

2. YAP-(S)PET scanner design

At the Department of Physics at the University of Pisa, a new and fully engineered version of the YAP-(S)PET small-animal scanner has been recently installed.

The scanner is made up of four detector heads: each one is composed of a 4 $\times$ 4 cm^2 $YAlO_3$:Ce (or YAP:Ce) matrix of 20 $\times$ 20 elements, 2 $\times$ 2 $\times$ 25 mm^3 each. The matrix is directly coupled to a PS-PMT (Hamamatsu R2486). The four modules are positioned on a rotating gantry; the opposite detectors are in

*A. Del Guerra, N. Belcari, D. Herbert, A. Motta, A. Vaiano, A. Pinchera, University of Pisa, Pisa, Italy; G. Di Domenico, E. Moretti, N. Sabba, G. Zavattini, University of Ferrara and INFN, Ferrara, Italy; M. Lazzorotti, L. Sensi, I.S.E Ingegneria dei Sistemi Elettronici s.r.l., Pisa, Italy

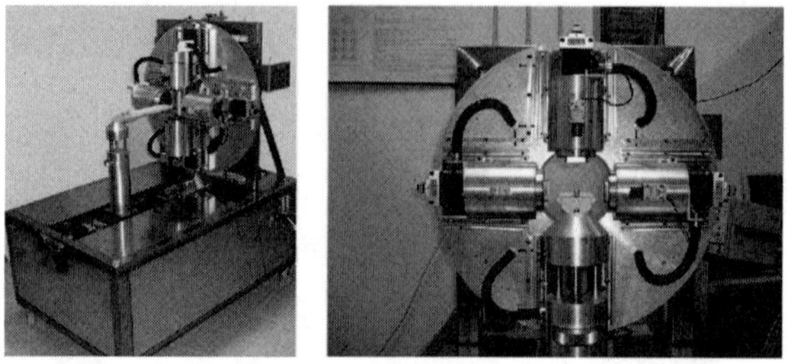

Figure 17.1. Photograph of the YAP-(S)PET scanner (left) and the four rotating heads (right).

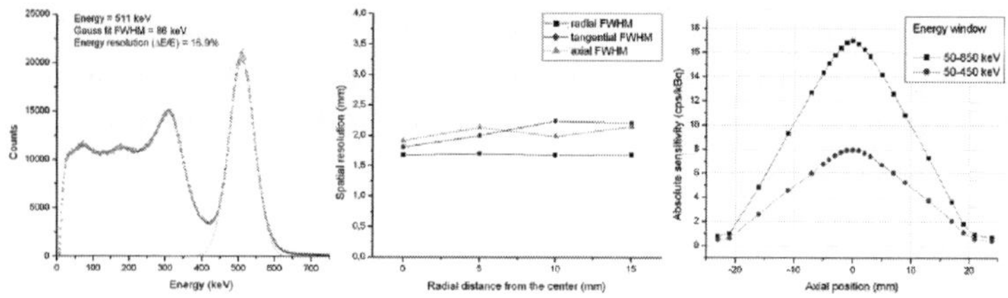

Figure 17.2. Graphs of the energy spectrum at 511 keV (left) and the spatial resolution (center) and absolute sensitivity (right) measured in PET mode.

time coincidence when used in PET mode. The rotation is controlled via PC thus permitting the acquisition of the tomographic views. The scanner is equipped with a laser system and motorized bed for the animal positioning and motion within the FoV. Dedicated, compact electronic boards are used for the signal amplification and digitization. The system is managed by an on site PC performing the data acquisition and the motion control and can be controlled by a remote PC connected to a local network. The system operates in 3-D data acquisition mode and both FBP (Filtered Back Projection) and EM (Expectation Maximization) algorithms can be used for image reconstruction [Motta, et al., 2002].

The switching to the SPECT modality can be easily made by replacing the tungsten septum (used in PET for shielding the scintillators from the background outside the FoV) with a high-resolution parallel-hole, lead collimator (0.6 mm $\emptyset$, 0.15 mm septum) in front of each crystal.

For both PET and SPECT modalities, the scanner has an axial field of view of 4 cm, and the diameter of the transaxial FoV is 4 cm.

3. YAP-(S)PET scanner performance

3.1 Energy resolution

Figure 17.2 (left) shows the energy spectrum obtained with a complete detector head at 511 keV. The measured energy resolution for the four heads of the YAP-(S)PET ranges between 17% and 20%, with an average value of 19% at 511keV and 25% at 122 keV.

3.2 Intrinsic axial spatial resolution (PET)

A ^{22}Na source has been moved across the two pairs of detector heads along the rotational axis with a step size of 0.5 mm. The source is a small cylinder (nominal size 1 mm ∅, 1 mm thick). A tomographic acquisition has been performed for each source position. The number of coincidences recorded in each plane, defined by a single row of pixels in each matrix, is plotted against the known source location. The FWHM of the count distribution for each plane was measured as an estimation of the intrinsic axial resolution. Using the 50-850 keV energy window, the mean measured FWHM is 2.6 mm, without correction for the source dimensions, while using the 50-350 keV window, the FWHM is reduced down to 2.1 mm. This improvement is due to the fact that by selecting the Compton fraction of the spectrum, single interactions are preferentially selected with respect to multiple interactions that mainly contribute to the photopeak [Del Guerra, et al., 1998].

3.3 Image spatial resolution

In PET mode, a ^{22}Na point source (nominal size 1 mm ∅, 1 mm thick) was positioned at the center of the FoV and moved radially with a 5-mm step size. For each position, the radial, transaxial, and axial FWHM are plotted in Fig. 17.2 (center). The volume resolution is below 8 mm^3 and is nearly constant over the whole FoV. The highest spatial resolution is measured at the center of the FOV and is 1.7 × 1.8 × 1.9 mm^3 (R × T × A) FWHM. No source dimension subtraction was made.

In SPECT mode, a capillary (1.0-mm internal diameter) filled with ^{99m}Tc was positioned parallel to the scanner axis 1 cm away. The image was reconstructed with EM obtaining a FWHM of 2.9 mm × 2.9 mm (R × T) FWHM. No source dimension subtraction was made.

3.4 System sensitivity

In PET mode, a ^{22}Na point source (5.4 μCi) was moved along the scanner axial axis. In Fig. 17.2 (right), the results are plotted against the actual position of the source. Two different curves are produced for different energy windows: 50-850 keV (high sensitivity) and 50-450 keV (high resolution); the maximum absolute sensitivity, measured at the center of the FOV, is 1.7% (17 cps/kBq) and 0.8% (8 cps/kBq), respectively.

In SPECT mode, the sensitivity, measured with the YAP-(S)PET prototype, is 30 cps/MBq [Di Domenico, et al., 2003], constant over the whole FOV.

3.5 Phantom images

A mini-Derenzo phantom was scanned in both PET and SPECT mode. In PET mode, the rods of the Derenzo phantom were filled with 100μCi of an ^{18}F-FDG solution and scanned for 75 minute, while for SPECT, 3 mCi of ^{99m}Tc were used and scanned for 2.5 hours. The sizes of the rods were 3.0, 2.5, 2.0, and 1.5 mm

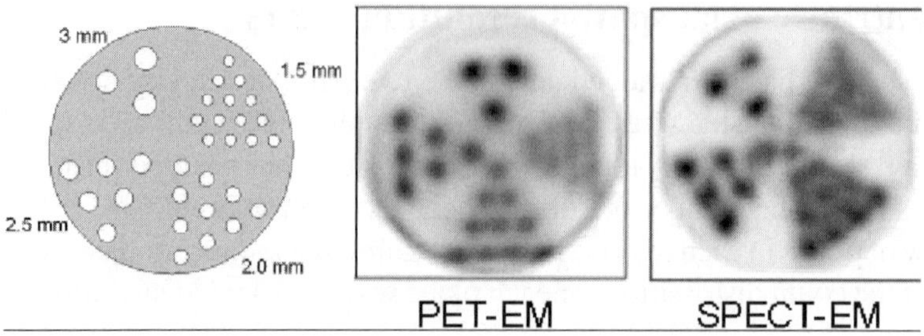

Figure 17.3. Drawing and reconstructed images of the mini Derenzo phantom.

∅. The center-to-center distance between adjacent rods is twice the rod diameter. The time required for the EM reconstruction is 8 minutes using a PC Pentium 4 (2.8 GHz). Figure 17.3 shows the images for both modalities. In PET mode, the 2.0-mm rods and in SPECT mode the 2.5-mm rods can be clearly distinguished.

4. Conclusions

The YAP-(S)PET small-animal scanner is able to perform both PET and SPECT investigation on small rodents. The switching from PET to SPECT modality can be easily made by simply installing the lead collimators and selecting the new modality on the user interface.

In PET mode, the scanner shows a volume resolution ≤ 8 mm^3 over the whole FOV and an absolute sensitivity of 1.7% at the center of the FOV. In SPECT, the scanner shows a spatial resolution ≤ 3.1 mm FWHM and an absolute sensitivity of 30 cps/MBq over the whole FOV.

References

[Del Guerra, 1998] A. Del Guerra, Di Domenico, M. Scandola, G. Zavattini, "High spatial resolution small animal YAPPET," *Nucl. Instr. and Meth. Phys. Res.*, vol. A409, pp. 537-541, 1998.

[Del Guerra, 2000] A. Del Guerra, C. Damiani, G. Di Domenico, A. Motta, L. Sartori, G. Zavattini, "An integrated PET-SPECT small animal imager: preliminary results," *IEEE Trans Nucl Sci,* vol. 47, pp. 1537-1540, 2000.

[Del Guerra, 2002] A. Del Guerra, G. Di Domenico, M. Gambaccini, E. Moretti, N. Sabba, G. Zavattini, "Simultaneous PET/SPECT imaging with the small animal YAP-(S)PET scanner," presented at the *2002 annual conference of the Academy of Molecular Imaging*, October 23-27, 2002, San Diego, CA, (USA) (abstract)

[Di Domenico, 2003] G. Di Domenico, G. Zavattini, Moretti, A. Piffanelli, M. Giganti et al., "YAP-(S)PET small animal scanner: quantitative results," *IEEE Trans Nucl Sci,* vol. 50, pp. 1351-1356, 2003.

[Motta, 2002] A. Motta, C. Damiani, A. Del Guerra, G. Di Domenico, G. Zavattini, "Use of a fast deconvolution EM algorithm for 3-D imaging reconstruction with the YAP-PET tomograph," *Comp. Med. Im. and Graph,* vol. 26, pp. 293-302, 2002.

[WebRef] I.S.E. Ingegneria dei Sistemi Elettronici s.r.l., Vecchiano, Pisa, Italy http://www.ise-srl.com.

Chapter 18

A Small-Animal SPECT Imaging System Utilizing Position Tracking of Unanesthetized Mice

Andrew G. Weisenberger, Brian Kross, Stan Majewski, Vladimir Popov, Mark F. Smith, Benjamin Welch, Randolph Wojcik, James S. Goddard, Shaun S. Gleason, Michael J. Paulus, Steven R. Meikle, and Martin Pomper*

1. Introduction

Recent advances in nuclear-medicine based small-animal imaging technology have enabled researchers to acquire *in vivo* images of the biodistribution of radio-labeled molecules in small-animal models such as mice. The standard imaging method requires the use of anesthetic and/or physical restraint to immobilize the mouse during image acquisition of the radioisotope tracer biodistribution. This has the potential to interfere with neurological or other processes that are being studied. With this in mind, Oak Ridge National Laboratory (ORNL) and Thomas Jefferson National Accelerator Facility (Jefferson Lab), in collaboration with Royal Prince Alfred Hospital (RPAH) in Sydney, Australia and Johns Hopkins University, designed and constructed a high-resolution single-photon emission tomography (SPECT) system to study unrestrained, unanesthetized mice. Others have reported development of scintillator based PET isotope probes and systems to study the brain of unanesthetized rodents [Woody, 2001, Zimmer, 2002, Vaska, 2001].

2. Imaging methodology

We have built a SPECT gantry with an infrared (IR) tracking system and a 3-cm diameter cylindrical mouse burrow at the center of rotation (Fig. 18.1). The imaging methodology we have designed digitally records the mouse position and pose during a SPECT scan. The gamma-ray projection data are reconstructed into a fixed small-animal reference frame (SARF) based on the time-varying animal orientation data. The goal of this project is to develop an apparatus to acquire high-resolution volumetric SPECT images of the head region of an unrestrained,

*A. G. Weisenberger, B. Kross, S. Majewski, V. Popov, M. F. Smith, B. Welch, R. Wojcik, Thomas Jefferson National Accelerator Facility, Newport News, Virginia; J. S. Goddard, S. S. Gleason, M. J. Paulus, Oak Ridge National Accelerator Laboratory, Oak Ridge, Tennessee; S. R. Meikle, Royal Prince Alfred Hospital, Sydney, Australia; M. Pomper, Johns Hopkins University, Baltimore, Maryland

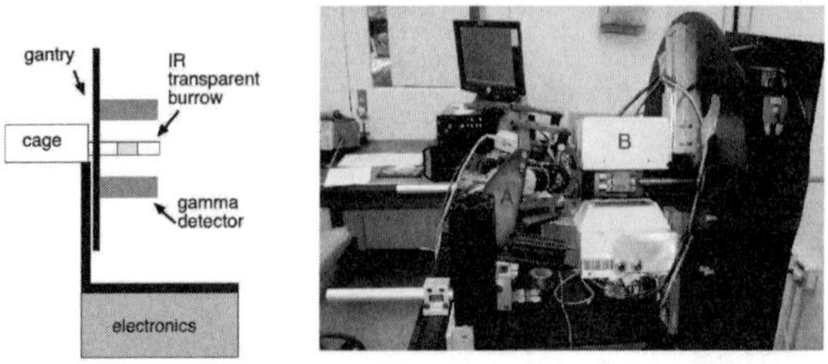

Figure 18.1. Diagram (left) and photograph (right) of the gantry. The IR tracking system (A) and the SPECT cameras (B) are shown in the photograph. The top camera labeled B is shown equipped with a parallel-hole collimator, while the lower camera has a single pinhole collimator.

unanesthetized mouse and to register these image volumes with previously acquired microCT data sets of the same mouse. The animal will be anesthetized during the microCT scan. The microCT images serve as a reference frame for the SPECT data.

An IR-based tracking system developed at ORNL provides the position and pose of the mouse's head during the imaging session. The infrared tracking system is composed of two high-speed CMOS cameras mounted horizontally on a platform facing an IR transparent tubular "burrow" in which the animal is unrestrained during scanning.

The SPECT imaging system is equipped with two 10 cm × 20 cm detector heads based on an array of position-sensitive photomultiplier tubes (PSPMT). A NaI(Tl) scintillator crystal array is optically coupled to the array of PSPMTs. The system is optimized for iodine-125 imaging, but also is capable of technetium-99m imaging. The use of parallel-hole and multi-pinhole collimation for improved sensitivity with high resolution is being investigated.

Prototype gamma cameras with an active area of 5 cm × 5 cm, which we have described elsewhere [Weisenberger, 2003], were based on the 3" Hamamatsu R2487 PSPMT coupled to 5 cm × 5 cm NaI(Tl) scintillator crystal arrays with individual crystal elements 1 mm × 1 mm × 5 mm in size with a pitch of 1.25 mm. These cameras were installed in a SPECT gantry at ORNL to perform initial SPECT studies. Time-correlated list-mode data containing the tracking coordinates and the gamma-imaging data acquired from the gamma cameras equipped with a parallel-hole collimator have been obtained of a moving radioactive phantom.

3. Apparatus description

The present apparatus is composed of three subsystems: 1) IR animal tracking system, 2) gamma camera data acquisition system, and 3) gantry control system. Each subsystem is controlled by a separate CPU (Dell desktop PCs). A central clock is read by all three CPUs to generate time-stamped list-mode data so that the projection angle, animal pose, and gamma camera projection data can be used to reconstruct image data in the SARF.

The IR position tracking system was built by ORNL and has been tested with live mice [Goddard, 2002, WebRef]. The IR tracking apparatus is attached to the rotating SPECT gantry. Jefferson Lab has built and installed two 10 cm × 20 cm compact high-resolution, high-sensitivity gamma-ray imaging detectors for the small-animal SPECT imaging system.

3.1 Infrared animal tracking system

We are developing two different IR tracking methods. The first makes use of extrinsic IR refectors attached to the head of a mouse. The second method uses intrinsic features on the mouse acquired through laser profile tracking. The infrared tracking systems have been described in detail elsewhere [Goddard, 2002, WebRef]. It is composed of two high-speed CMOS IR cameras mounted horizontally on a platform facing a tubular "burrow" in which the animal is unrestrained while being imaged. For the first method, infrared LED arrays and beam splitters are mounted in front of the cameras to coaxially illuminate hemispherical retro-reflective markers placed on the mouse's head. The tracking apparatus is designed to measure the spatial position of the mouse's head at a rate of 10-15 frames per second with submillimeter accuracy.

The tracking system has been tested with live mice such that the position coordinates of mouse's head were successfully tracked. The second method using laser profile tracking (also known as profilimetry [WebRef]) has been tested only with phantoms and is in the initial stages of development.

3.2 SPECT system

Two SPECT gamma camera detector heads are based on a 4 × 8 array of the Hamamatsu R8520-C12 (1" × 1"; 6X × 6Y anodes) PSPMTs. Optically coupled to the array of PSPMTs for each detector head is a NaI(Tl) scintillator crystal array, which has individual crystal elements 2 mm × 2 mm × 15 mm in size with a pitch of 2.5 mm. The detectors extend axially so that the entire animal in the burrow can be imaged on the 10 cm wide × 20 cm long NaI(Tl) scintillator crystal array. The detector heads can be equipped with either parallel-hole or pinhole collimators. We are investigating improving system sensitivity by employing multi-pinhole collimation with image overlap [Smith, 2003, Meikle, 2003]. The detector heads are calibrated and are being tested with SPECT phantoms. Initial phantom studies and modeling studies with multi-pinhole masks have been underway.

The gamma camera data-acquisition system is composed of two 16-channel ADC cards (Datel, Inc., Mansfield, MA), a discriminator circuit, a millisecond clock to time stamp the gamma-ray data, and a 10-millisecond clock used to synchronize the gamma-ray event data with the mouse IR tracking data. A more in-depth description of our data-acquisition system can be found elsewhere [Welch, 2003].

4. Discussion

The overall system concept has been tested with the prototype system in which we have obtained gamma-ray images of a moving phantom source by making use of time-correlated list-mode position tracking data and gamma-ray event data. Preparations for an iodine-125 study are underway to obtain time-correlated list-mode data of a mouse's head position and the gamma-ray event data of an unrestrained, unanesthetized mouse. From the time-correlated tracking and gamma-ray data sets, the iodine-125 uptake in the moving animal's head will be imaged.

Acknowledgments

This work is supported by the U.S. Department of Energy Office of Biological and Environmental Research in the Office of Science through the DOE Medical Imaging Program and by the DOE Office of Nuclear Physics. The Southeastern Universities Research Association (SURA) operates the Thomas Jefferson National Accelerator Facility (Jefferson Lab) for the U.S. Department of Energy under contract DE-AC05-84ER40150.

References

[Goddard, 2002] J. S. Goddard, S. S. Gleason, M. J. Paulus, A. Weisenberger, M. Smith, B. Welch, and R. Wojcik, "Real-time landmark-based unrestrained animal tracking system for motion-corrected PET/SPECT imaging," *2002 IEEE Medical Imaging Conference Record*, October 2002.

[Meikle, 2003] S. R. Meikle, P. Kench, R. Wojcik, M. F. Smith, A. G. Weisenberger, S. Majewski, M. L. F. Lerch, and A. B. Rozenfeld, "Performance evaluation of a multipinhole small animal SPECT system," *2003 IEEE Medical Imaging Conference Record*, October 2003.

[Smith, 2003] M. F. Smith, S. R. Meikle, S. Majewski, A. G. Weisenberger, "Design of multipinhole collimators for small animal SPECT," *2003 IEEE Medical Imaging Conference Record*, October 2003.

[Vaska, 2001] P. Vaska, D. J. Schlyer, C. L. Woody, S. P. Stoll, V. Radeka, and N. Volkow, "Imaging the unanesthetized rat brain with PET: a feasibility study," *2001 IEEE Medical Imaging Conference Record*, October 2001.

[WebRef] http://www.ivp.se/documentation/technology/LaserTriangulation.pdf

[Weisenberger, 2003] A. G. Weisenberger, B. Kross, S. S. Gleason, J. Goddard, S. Majewski, S. R. Meikle, M. J. Paulus, M. Pomper, V. Popov, M. F. Smith, B. L. Welch and R. Wojcik, "Development and testing of a restraint free small animal SPECT imaging system with infrared based motion tracking," *2003 IEEE Medical Imaging Conference Record*, October 2003.

[Welch, 2003] B. L. Welch, S. Majewski, V. Popov, A. G. Weisenberger, R. Wojcik, J. S. Goddard, S. S. Gleason and M. J. Paulus, "Acquisition and control for a combined SPECT/infrared tracking system for restraint-free small animal imaging," *2003 IEEE Medical Imaging Conference Record*, October 2003.

[Woody, 2001] C. L. Woody, S. P. Stoll, D. J. Schlyer, M. Gerasimov, P. Vaska, S.Shokouhi, N. Volkow, J. S. Fowler, and S. L. Dewey, "A study of scintillation beta microprobes," *2001 IEEE Medical Imaging Conference Record*, October 2001.

[Zimmer, 2002] L. Zimmer, W. Hassoun, F. Pain, F. Bonnefoi, P. Laniece, R. Mastrippolito, L. Pinot, J. F. Pujol, and V. Leviel, "SIC, an intracerebral beta(+)-range-sensitive probe for radiopharmacology investigations in small laboratory animals: binding studies with (11)C-raclopride," *Journal of Nuclear Medicine*, vol. 43(2), pp. 227-233, 2002.

Chapter 19

A Multidetector High-Resolution SPECT/CT Scanner with Continuous Scanning Capability

Tobias Funk, Mingshan Sun, Andrew B. Hwang, James Carver, Steve Thompson, Kevin B. Parnham, R. Luu, Bradley E. Patt, J. Li, and Bruce H. Hasegawa*

1. Introduction

Small animal imaging has become an important tool in research of human biology and disease. These techniques include high-resolution ultrasound, computed tomography (CT), positron emission tomography (PET), and single-photon emission computed tomography (SPECT), all of which have a role in answering biological questions in animal models. However, techniques such as MRI and CT primarily reveal information about the organism's structure or anatomy. In comparison, radionuclide imaging methods such as PET and SPECT provide functional and physiological information. For this reason, several laboratories are developing methods to combine SPECT and CT (or PET and CT) in an integrated imaging device as a means of correlating structure and function to obtain a more complete assessment of the animals studied. Furthermore, the CT data inherently provide a map of attenuation coefficients that can be used to correct the correlated emission data for photon attenuation errors, with the goal of improving both the visual quality and the quantitative accuracy of the radionuclide image.

Radionuclide imaging with SPECT is developing an important role in the functional imaging of small animals. Small-animal SPECT can be performed with a wide spectrum of radiopharmaceuticals, including those labeled with ^{125}I, ^{99m}Tc, and ^{111}In. ^{125}I is inexpensive and is widely available for *in vitro* studies. Furthermore, ^{125}I emits low-energy photons (e.g., 27-32 keV) at high yield that are suitable for *in vivo* small-animal imaging. ^{111}In is well suited for radioimmunoscintigraphy because it binds easily to proteins and has a long half-life that matches the uptake and washout characteristics of most radiolabeled antibodies [Koziol, et al. 1995]. However, its rather high γ-ray energies are less favorable for imaging. ^{99m}T is

*T. Funk, M. Sun, A. B. Hwang, B. H. Hasegawa, University of California, San Francisco, California; M. Sun, A. B. Hwang, B. H. Hasegawsa, University of California, Berkeley, California; J. Carver, S. Thompson, Jamco Engineering, Cottage Grove, Oregon; K. B. Parnham, R. Luu, B. E. Patt, J. Li, GammaMedica, Inc., Northridge, California

very cost effective and readily available, and it remains the most commonly used radiolabel for clinical and small-animal SPECT.

Over the past few years, several corporate and academic investigators have developed SPECT and SPECT/CT scanners for small-animal imaging, including those capable of imaging ^{125}I. For example, Beekman et al. constructed a micropinhole camera (with a bore diameter as small as 0.1 mm) that produced a spatial resolution of 0.19 mm [Beekman, et al. 2002]. Slightly lower spatial resolution has been achieved by Peterson et al. using a silicon strip detector operated with a collimator having 21 pinholes [Peterson, et al. 2003]. Unfortunately, radionuclide detectors that rely on absorptive collimation typically achieve improved spatial resolution by sacrificing geometric efficiency. Gamma Medica, Inc. (Northridge CA) developed and now markets a combined SPECT/CT imager ("X-SPECT") that enables dual-modality imaging of small animals. X-SPECT can be equipped with up to two 12.8×12.8 cm^2 gamma cameras having a pixelated NaI(Tl) scintillator and an array of position-sensitive photomultiplier tubes.

In general, both higher detection efficiency and improved spatial resolution are two important factors that drive the development of new SPECT systems. Higher efficiency reduces the scan time and allows studies to be performed with a smaller amount of injected radioactivity to reduce the radiation burden delivered to the animal, which can be high for mouse SPECT imaging [Funk, et al. 2004]. Higher spatial resolution is especially important for small animal imaging, particularly in molecular imaging with agents that have high functional specificity.

SPECT also offers dual-isotope imaging for simultaneous monitoring of more than one physiological parameter with multiple radiotracers. However, this requires excellent energy resolution to resolve the different photon energies encountered in dual-isotope studies.

For these reasons, we are developing a next generation SPECT/CT scanner that will offer both high efficiency and excellent spatial resolution, and that will be suitable for imaging a range of single-photon labels with energies from ^{125}I (i.e., 27.5 keV) to ^{111}In (i.e., 245 keV), in both single and multiple isotope imaging applications. The system also will offer high-resolution CT for anatomical imaging and to obtain an object-specific attenuation map to achieve the best possible image quality and quantitative accuracy of the correlated radionuclide data. Finally, the gantry is designed to be highly flexible so that new detector technologies and imaging configurations can be implemented and tested.

2. Design of the SPECT/CT system

The primary components of the SPECT/CT system include the x-ray source and detector, four radionuclide detectors and pinhole collimators, and a gantry to support and rotate the imaging components around a common rotational axis. The CT system will produce 70 μm spatial resolution, with submillimeter resolution achieved the by SPECT system. This implies that the gantry must be moved with high stability and precision that is maintained in spite of the heavy weight of the

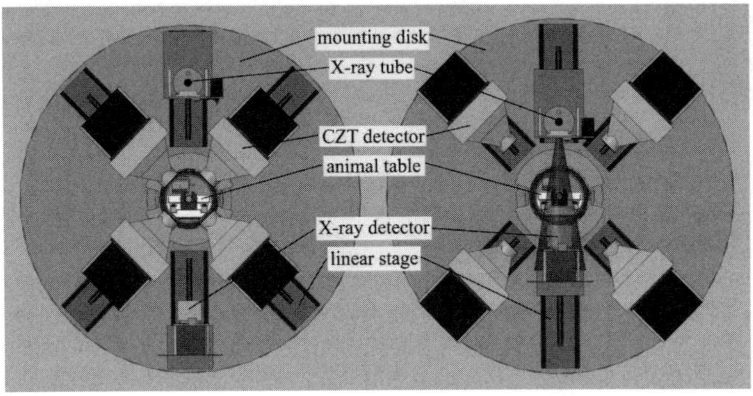

Figure 19.1. Front view of the SPECT/CT scanner. Left side of the picture shows the SPECT system with the CZT detectors. The right side of the picture shows the CZT detectors retracted and the CT components positioned for CT scanning.

components. Finally, the gantry will offer an open configuration, making components easily accessible and interchangeable if needed.

2.1 Gantry

The rotating platform of the gantry (Figure 19.1) will be supported on high-precision bearings and rotated in a stationary frame, with a slip ring for the electrical and data connections to allow continuous and helical acquisitions. One side of the rotating platform will support the SPECT detectors and the CT components, with the power supplies, data-acquisition electronics, and control electronics mounted on the opposite side. The x-ray source, x-ray detector, and radionuclide detectors will be positioned at the appropriate radial distance from the rotational axis during imaging with linear translation stages. That gantry will include a horizontal animal table can be translated under computer control to position the animal in the reconstruction volume of the rotating SPECT and CT subsystems.

We designed the gantry to acquire tomographic images in either a "stop-and-shoot" or a "non-stop" mode. In the stop-and-shoot mode, the gantry positions the imaging components at angular increments for image acquisition. In the non-stop mode, the system acquires data continuously while the imaging components are rotated continuously. An angular encoder will provide the exact angular position of the gantry and read by the host computer.

We performed a finite element analysis to determine if the proposed design offers sufficient stability and precision for both SPECT and CT. These calculations show that the slight mechanical errors are caused both by gravitational and active drive forces, causing displacement of the rotating imaging components from their ideal position. These deflections force the X-ray tube and detector into a slightly distorted orbit with a maximum deviation of 10 μm and a minimum deviation of 6 μm from the ideal circular orbit. Furthermore, the angular positioning accuracy is approximately 6 arcsec.

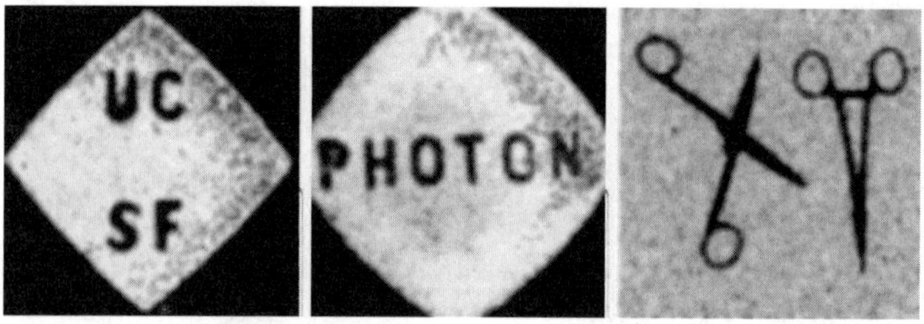

Figure 19.2. Dual isotope imaging of a phantom containing ^{201}Tl and ^{99m}Tc. Left panel: Image is obtained with energy resolution to select photons from the ^{99m}Tc source. Middle panel: Image obtained from the same phantom from the ^{201}Tl source. Right panel: Transmission images taken with an external ^{125}I source placed 1 m away from the detector.

2.2 SPECT subsystem

The SPECT subsystem includes four cadmium zinc telluride (CZT) detectors, each 20×20 cm^2 configured as an 80×80 pixel array with a pixel pitch of 2.5 mm. The detectors incorporate the room-temperature solid-state semiconductor CZT which offers direct charge conversion and good stopping power for radionuclides used for small-animal SPECT. In addition, CZT has intrinsically good energy resolution, making it a material of choice for dual-isotope imaging. The operating temperature of the detector is stabilized to optimize low energy photon detection, and the detector has been designed to minimize absorption losses for photons entering the active detector material. We have designed lead buckets enclosing the back and sides of the detectors to prevent background radiation from entering the detectors. Furthermore, a specially designed pinhole or parallel-hole collimator is attached to the detector. We made the buckets from a lead-antimony alloy offering almost the same stopping power as lead but having better structural properties. Lead bucket and collimator add considerable weight to the detectors.

We estimate that a fully shielded camera weighs about 55 kg. We bench-tested the CZT detector, and our preliminary results show the integral uniformity to be better than 5% and the energy resolution better than 9% for ^{99m}Tc [Funk, et al. 2003]. Dual-isotope imaging is possible with the current setup. Figure 19.2 shows images of a phantom consisting of two layers of stacked containers containing different isotope sources. The bottom container contained a 1.2 mCi solution of ^{201}Tl with the plastic letters "PHOTON", while the top container contained a 1.3 mCi solution of ^{99m}Tc with the letters "UCSF". Thus, the letters of the phantom were cold while the surrounding solution was hot.

We have taken a transmission image using an ^{125}I sealed source to demonstrate that our detector is also well suited for low-energy imaging. These data were acquired with an ^{125}I source (90 μCi) placed 1 m away from the detector on which we placed two metal objects as absorbers. The transmission image (Figure 19.2) was acquired for 900 s and uniformity corrected using a uniform image acquired for 9000 s with an energy window placed around the K_α line of ^{125}I (27.5 keV).

The CZT detectors embedded in the lead buckets are designed to image radionuclides with photon energies ranging from 27.5 keV (^{125}I) to 245 keV (^{111}In). We expect that our system will have very high counting efficiency due to large detector area and the use of a direct conversion semiconductor. Furthermore, energy resolution will be excellent and will provide the ability to perform dual-isotope imaging with various isotopes.

2.3 CT subsystem

The CT subsystem will be implemented using a microfocus x-ray source (Oxford Instruments Series 6000) and a CCD camera coupled to a gadolinium oxysulfide phosphor (Dalsa AC70) with a pixel size of 70 μm. The fan angle of the tube is about 20° and the distance of detector to tube will be about 20 cm.

We performed simulations to determine if the gantry stability is sufficient to achieve the proposed spatial resolution and focused the simulations on the CT subsystem which must operate at a higher spatial resolution than the SPECT subsystem. We developed a one-dimensional projector that simulates the component movement determined by the finite element analysis to evaluate the impact of angular deviations in the source and detector positions during the stop-and-shoot scanning mode. The simulated projected data are recontructed using a filtered backprojection algorithm. Comparative calculations have been performed for the ideal system and for an extreme case, where we assumed 10-fold bigger deflections and angular uncertainties than predicted by our finite element analysis. The impact on the image quality is not significant even for the 10-fold limit. Furthermore, we simulated the impact of non-stop imaging on the image quality. Assuming the covered angle is about 0.12°, which is 1/3 of the angular increment with 1024 projections, we do not see a significant degradation of the image quality. These results predict that our open and flexible design will be sufficiently rigid to perform high spatial resolution CT and SPECT imaging.

3. Conclusion

We are building a new SPECT/CT small-animal scanner with continuous scanning capability. The gantry is configured with an open architecture that will allow flexibility in configuring the imaging components. The SPECT/CT system will incorporate four large area CZT cameras with shielding designed for ^{111}In imaging. One of the radionuclide detectors has undergone bench-testing and has demonstrated good characteristics for dual-isotope and ^{125}I imaging. We also performed finite element analysis and other mechanical simulation testing to show that the rigidity of our scanner will be sufficient for CT scanning at 70 μm spatial resolution. The gantry is now in the final stage of design and is expected to be operational in summer 2004.

Acknowledgments

This work is supported by a Bioengineering Research Partnership award from the National Institute of Biomedical Imaging and Bioengineering (NIBIB), NIH Grant 8 R01 EB00348.

References

[Beekman, 2002] F. J. Beekman, D. P. McElroy, et al. "Towards *in vivo* nuclear microscopy: iodine-125 imaging in mice using micro-pinholes," *Eur J Nucl Med Mol Imaging,* vol. 29(7), pp. 933-938, 2002.

[Funk, 2003] T. K. Funk, K. B. Parnham, et al. "A new CdZnTe-based gamma camera for high resolution pinhole SPECT," *IEEE NSS Conference Record*, 2003.

[Funk, 2004] T. Funk, M. Sun, et al. "Radiation dose estimate in small animal SPECT and PET," to be published.

[Koziol, 1995] J. A. Koziol, P. P. Lee, et al. "Pharmacokinetics of ^{111}In-labelled monoclonal antibody ZCE-025 and fragments in tumour-bearing mice," *Nucl Med Commun*, vol. 16(4), pp. 299-305, 1995.

[Peterson, 2003] T. E. Peterson, D. W. Wilson, et al. "Ultrahigh-resolution small-animal Imaging using a silicon detector," *IEEE NSS Conference Record*, 2003.

Chapter 20

High-Resolution Multi-Pinhole Imaging Using Silicon Detectors

Todd E. Peterson, Donald W. Wilson, and Harrison H. Barrett*

1. Introduction

The use of pinhole collimation for small-animal SPECT imaging has been recognized as a powerful tool for about a decade now [Jaszczak, 1994, Weber, 1994]. A common approach has been to fit clinical gamma cameras with pinhole apertures for this purpose. Large magnification factors can be used with this method, making it possible to attain good image resolution despite the modest spatial resolution of the gamma camera. A chief drawback to pinhole SPECT is the poor sensitivity overall due to the rapid falloff with increasing distance from the pinhole and with increasing distance away from the pinhole axis. Several researchers have recently begun using multiple pinhole collimation to improve the overall sensitivity [Schramm, 2002, Meikle, 2002]. Multi-pinhole collimation schemes can result in multiplexing of the image projections on the detector, which can be thought of as a reduction in the information content of each detected photon owing to the uncertainty in which pinhole it passed through.

Our approach is to utilize a detector with a spatial resolution more than an order of magnitude better than a conventional gamma camera. Use of a high-resolution detector means that, for a given image resolution, lower magnification can be used than would be required for a gamma camera. Lower magnification means that the projection data cover a smaller area on the detector. This in turn means that a multiple-pinhole scheme would have less multiplexing. We are using silicon double-sided strip detectors for this purpose. Detectors of this sort can be obtained with strip pitches down to 20 μm and in thicknesses from 0.3 mm to 2 mm. While silicon is not suitable for detecting 140 keV photons, its detection efficiency is reasonable for the photon energies observed in ^{125}I decay.

*T. E. Peterson, Vanderbilt University, Nashville, Tennessee; D. W. Wilson, H. H. Barrett, Department of Radiology, The University of Arizona, Tucson, Arizona

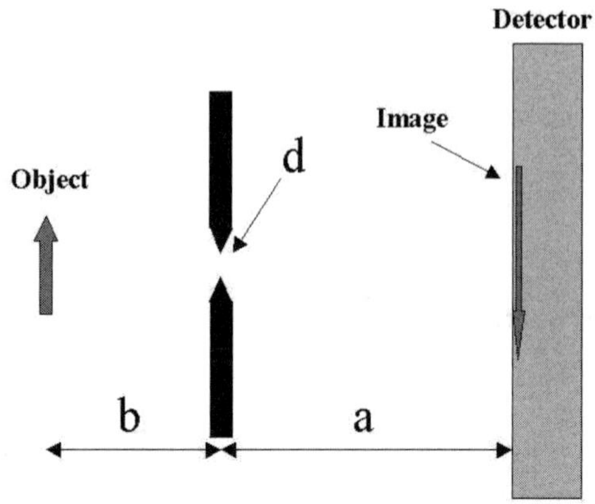

Figure 20.1. A schematic showing the basic pinhole-imaging configuration.

2. Impact of detector resolution on pinhole imaging

It is possible to get an idea of the potential impact of high-resolution detectors on SPECT imaging via the well-known, basic equations for planar pinhole imaging [Anger, 1967]. From the basic pinhole imaging scheme depicted in Fig. 20.1, and ignoring pinhole penetration (a reasonable assumption at low energies), the planar spatial resolution is:

$$R_g = d\frac{(a+b)}{a}, \tag{20.1}$$

where d is the diameter of the pinhole, a is the aperture-detector distance, and b is the object-aperture distance. Figure 20.1 shows the basic layout of the pinhole imaging configuration. The final spatial resolution, however, depends on the detector resolution as well as the geometric resolution due to the pinhole. The total resolution is:

$$R_{total} \approx \sqrt{(R_i/M)^2 + R_g^2} \tag{20.2}$$

where $M = \frac{a}{b}$ is the image magnification. Based on this equation, we can easily test the impact that detector spatial resolution can have on the performance of an imaging system. Figure 20.2 shows the planar image resolution as a function of pinhole magnification for the four combinations that can be formed using a 0.25-mm pinhole or a 0.5-mm pinhole with a detector of 0.05-mm or 1-mm intrinsic resolution. While the detector resolution has only a minor impact on the image resolution for larger magnifications, the higher-resolution detector has a dramatic impact at smaller values of the magnification. This difference is important if detectors of a limited size are used or if multiple pinholes are to be used with a single detector.

As an example of how the use of a high-resolution detector can impact what can be done in pinhole SPECT, consider doing rotational SPECT at a 3-cm radius of rotation using a detector of 10.5 cm × 10.5 cm active area. For a detector with

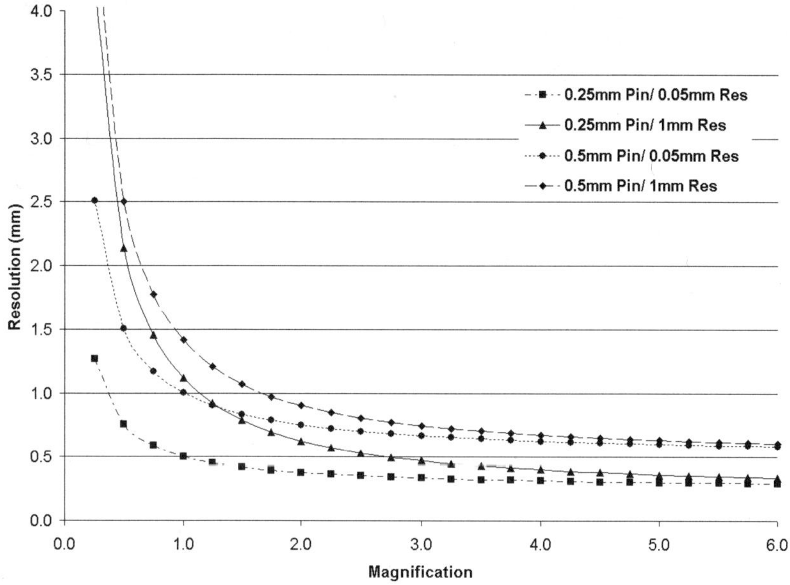

Figure 20.2. The planar image resolution as a function of pinhole magnification is plotted for the combinations of 0.25-mm or 0.5-mm diameter pinhole with a detector of 0.05-mm or 1-mm intrinsic resolution. The object-to-pinhole distance was fixed at 2 cm.

1-mm spatial resolution, a reasonable approach would be to use a single pinhole with 500-μm diameter and 45° opening angle, with the detector positioned 5 cm away from the aperture in order to obtain the best resolution over the full field of view. If one instead had a detector of the same size with 50-μm spatial resolution, it would be possible to use an aperture with 81 pinholes of 250-μm diameter and 30° opening angle equally spaced in a 9×9 array. By positioning the detector 1 cm behind this aperture, the 81 pinhole projections would not overlap on the detector (i.e., no multiplexing). Figure 20.3 shows that the 81-pinhole configuration would actually have superior planar resolution out to a distance equal to the radius of rotation (based on equation 20.2).

The sensitivity of a pinhole, the fraction of gamma-rays emitted that pass through the pinhole, as a function of position is:

$$g = \frac{d \cos^3 \theta}{16 b^2}, \tag{20.3}$$

where θ is the angle between a gamma-ray path passing through the pinhole and the normal to the surface of the detector. This simple equation reveals that, while the single pinhole with larger diameter would have higher sensitivity along the pinhole axis out to a distance just beyond one centimeter from the pinhole, overall the multi-pinhole aperture would yield a higher, more uniform sensitivity over a larger field of view. As an example of this, Fig. 20.4 shows the difference in sensitivity between the two approaches along the axis of rotation for a single projection view. The

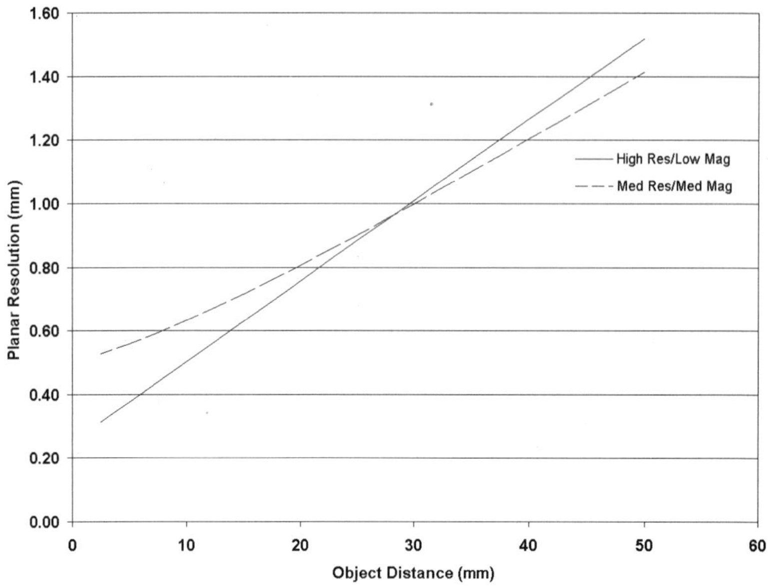

Figure 20.3. The planar image resolution is plotted as a function of the object distance from the pinhole aperture for a high-resolution detector (0.05 mm) with low magnification (1-cm aperture to detector distance) and for a medium-resolution detector (1 mm) with medium magnification (5-cm aperture to detector distance).

multi-pinhole approach offers additional advantages in increased angular sampling of the object space. Clearly, one would want to employ a more sophisticated multi-pinhole aperture design in a practical system, but this example does illustrate the potential of detectors with superior spatial resolution to impact imager design.

3. Silicon imager prototype

We have obtained a silicon double-sided strip detector with which to develop a prototype imaging system. This detector has a strip pitch of 50 μm and is 300-μm thick. It possesses over 700,000 resolvable detector elements across a 28 mm $\times$ 63 mm active area. The electronic readout is based around the VaTaGP2.2 ASIC, manufactured by IDEAS ASA, Hovik, Norway. This 128-channel ASIC provides an individual preamplifier, shaper amp, comparator, and sample-and-hold for each channel. It is an event-driven system with a sparse readout consisting of the address of the strip that triggered the event, the pulse height of that channel, and the pulse heights of its nearest neighbors.

The first imaging aperture developed for the prototype has 21 pinholes formed in a 500-μm-thick piece of molybdenum. Molybdenum has a K-edge at 20 keV, resulting in high attenuation for photons from ^{125}I decay. The pinholes are each 100 μm in diameter with a half-angle of 45° and were fashioned using electron-discharge machining.

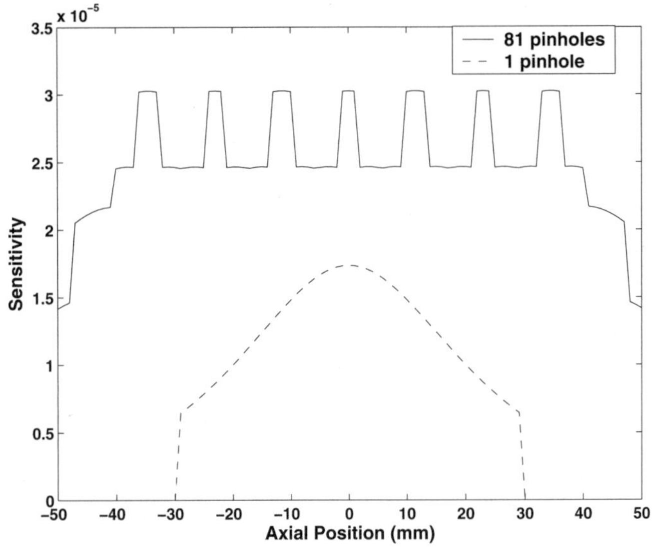

Figure 20.4. The sensitivity profile along the axis of rotation is shown for both the 81-pinhole aperture and the single pinhole.

A planar projection image of two ^{125}I-filled capillary tubes has been obtained using this 21-pinhole aperture. The tubes had inner diameters of 200 μm and were filled at a concentration of 11 μCi/mm. These line sources were placed 1 cm above the aperture in a parallel configuration with 660 μm center to center spacing. The detector was located approximately 5 mm below the aperture (magnification $\sim$0.5) for the two-hour acquisition. Figure 20.5 shows the count profile along a one-strip-wide segment of the detector. The pair of line sources is clearly resolved in each of the three projections subtended by this detector segment.

4. The synthetic collimator

The spatial resolution attainable with silicon DSSDs allows for schemes in which multi-pinhole imaging can be performed with little or no multiplexing. However, multiplexing is not necessarily a bad thing when combined with maximum-likelihood-based iterative reconstruction schemes for SPECT imaging. In particular, simulation studies have shown that tomographic reconstructions are possible even without any rotation when the synthetic-collimator approach is used [Wilson, 2000]. The basic idea of the synthetic collimator is to use a high-resolution detector together with a multiple-pinhole aperture to collect projection data at different magnfications and then use a maximum-likelihood expectation-maximization algorithm for reconstruction.

While the modest stopping power of silicon is generally thought of as an impediment to its use in gamma-ray imaging, this liability can be turned into an asset by stacking more than one detector behind the imaging aperture. This detector stacking increases the total detection efficiency while also allowing data to be acquired at

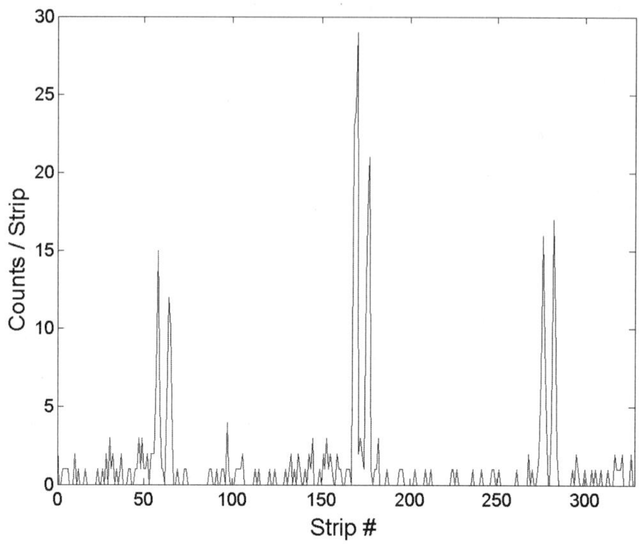

Figure 20.5. A one-strip wide count profile shows three projections in which a pair of 200 μm line sources with center-to-center spacing of 660 μm are clearly resolved.

the different magnifications required for the synthetic-collimator approach simultaneously. Double-sided strip detectors are particularly well suited to this approach because the electrical connections for readout are near the edges. Consequently, DSSDs can be stacked with a minimum of inactive volume.

One potential concern with a stacked detector approach is that there might be a degradation in image quality arising from events where photons underwent a scattering in one detector before stopping in another. Given that a 27 keV photon loses a maximum of 2.6 keV in a Compton scatter, energy windowing would be of little use in reducing the contribution of these scattered photons. To study the influence of these scattering events within the imaging system, a simulation was done using the EGSnrc Monte Carlo software [Kawrakow, 2000]. A point source emitting 27 keV photons located 2 cm directly above a 500-μm pinhole was simulated. The detector stack simulated consisted of two detectors each with thickness 1 mm and a transverse area of 10.5×10.5 cm^2. One detector was located 1 cm below the pinhole ($0.5\times$ magnification), and the other 2 cm below ($1\times$ magnification). The first detector stopped 32% of the incident photons, while 21% were detected in the second layer. Of the photons detected in the second layer, 6.1% of them underwent a Compton and/or Rayleigh scattering in the first detector before detection in the second. However, the full-width-at-half-maximum (FWHM) in the back detector was unchanged whether or not a detector was placed between it and the pinhole. Figure 20.6 shows a line profile through the center of the back detector, indicating the distribution of all detected events and of those that first underwent a scattering in the first detector.

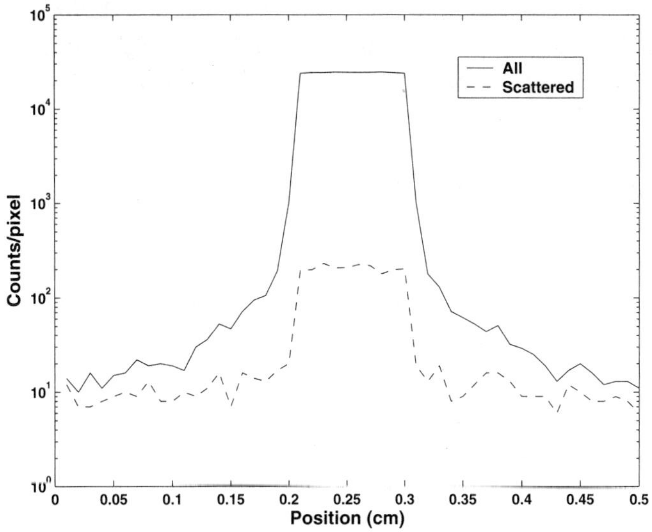

Figure 20.6. The count profile for a one-pixel wide slice through the center of the second detector is shown for all detected events and for only those events where a photon underwent either a Compton or Rayleigh scattering in the first detector before being detected in the second.

5. Summary

The ability to obtain high-resolution images at low magnification makes detectors with high spatial resolution particularly appealing for multi-pinhole SPECT imaging. We are developing an imager prototype using a silicon double-sided strip detector to explore the potential of this approach. While the superior planar imaging capability has already been demonstrated, we plan to employ the synthetic-collimator technique to obtain tomographic images.

Acknowledgments

The authors gratefully acknowledge the support of NIH/NIBIB under grant numbers EB000776 and EB002035. This research of Todd E. Peterson, Ph.D., is supported in part by a Career Award at the Scientific Interface from the Burroughs Wellcome Fund.

References

[Anger, 1967] H. Anger, "Radioisotope Cameras," *Instrumentation in Nuclear Medicine*, vol. 1, ed. G.J. Hine (New York:Academic), pp. 516-517, 1967.

[Jaszczak, 1994] R.J. Jaszczak, J. Li, H. Wang, M.R. Zalutsky, R.E. Coleman, "Pinhole collimation for ultra-high-raesolution, small-field-of-view SPECT," *Phys. Med. Biol.*, vol. 39, pp. 425-437, 1994.

[Kawrakow, 2000] I. Kawrakow, D.W.O. Rogers, The EGSnrc code system, NRC Report PIRS-701, NRC, Ottawa, 2000.

[Meikle, 2002] S.R. Meikle, P. Kench, A.G. Weisenberger, R. Wojcik, M.F. Smith, S. Majewski, S. Eberl, R.R. Fulton, A.B. Rosenfeld, M.J. Fulham, "A prototype coded aperture detector for small animal SPECT," *IEEE Trans. Nucl. Sci.*, vol. 49, no. 5, pp. 2167-2171, 2002.

[Schramm, 2002] N.U. Schramm, G. Ebel, U. Engeland, T. Schurrat, M. Béhé, T.M. Behr, "High-Resolution SPECT using multi-pinhole collimation," *IEEE Trans. Nucl. Sci.*, vol. 50, no. 3, pp. 315-320, 2003.

[Weber, 1994] D.A. Weber, M. Ivanovic, D. Franceschi, S.E. Strand, K. Erlandsson, M. Franceschi, H.L. Atkins, J.A. Coderre, H. Susskind, T. Button, K. Ljunggren, "Pinhole SPECT–An approach to in-vivo high-resolution SPECT imaging in small laboratory animals," *J. Nucl. Med.*, vol. 35, pp. 342-348, 1994.

[Wilson, 2000] D.W. Wilson, E.W. Clarkson, H.H. Barrett, "Reconstruction of two- and three-dimensional images from synthetic collimator data," *IEEE Trans. Med. Im.*, vol. 19, no. 5, pp. 412-422, 2000.

Chapter 21

Development and Characterization of a High-Resolution MicroSPECT System for Small-Animal Imaging

Yujin Qi, Benjamin M.W. Tsui, Yuchuan Wang, Bryan Yoder, Randolph Wojcik, Stan Majewski, and Andrew G. Weisenberger*

1. Introduction

The rapid growth in molecular genetics and the development of mouse models of human diseases have led to significant interest in *in vivo* small animal-imaging. Several instrumentation approaches [Weber, 1994, Tsui, 2001, McElroy, 2002, Peterson, 2002] have been utilized to develop high-resolution animal SPECT for functional small-animal imaging. Compact modular cameras based on pixelated crystal and position sensitive photomultiplier tube (PSPMT) are a low-cost alternative to conventional gamma cameras for use in pinhole SPECT systems with high detection efficiency and resolution [Qi, 2003]. We have developed a compact, high-resolution microSPECT system in our laboratory for small-animal imaging. Our approach was to use a dedicated mini camera with pinhole collimator. The modular camera was based on a pixelated NaI(Tl) crystal array and a single 5" Hamamatsu PSPMT. The system performance was characterized using small point source. The system spatial resolution and sensitivity were measured. High-resolution phantom and *in vivo* mouse imaging were performed to demonstrate the system capability.

2. Imaging system and method

Figure 21.1 shows the microSPECT system developed in our lab. The system was designed to have a simple motion control scheme where the camera was placed in horizontal stationary position while the imaging object was rotated vertically in front of the collimator. The rotary stage was mounted on an (x, y, z) linear translation stage from Velmex, Inc. for accurate three-dimensional positioning of the object.

*Y. Qi, B. M. W. Tsui, Y. Wang, B. Yoder, Johns Hopkins University, Department of Radiology, Baltimore, Maryland; R. Wojcik, S. Majewski, A. Weisenberger, Thomas Jefferson National Accelerator Facility, Detector Group, Newport News, Virginia

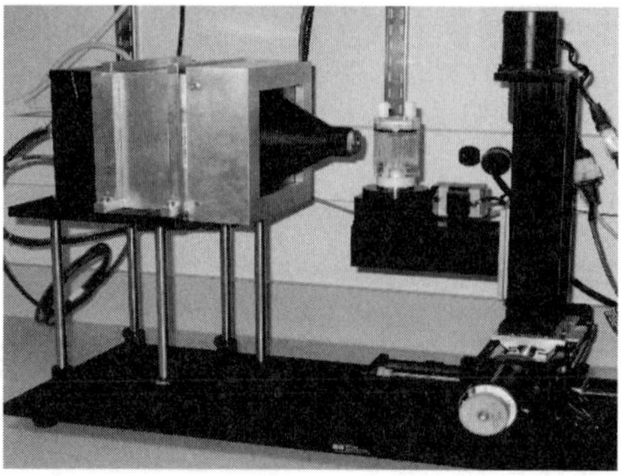

Figure 21.1. A photograph of the microSPECT system based on a compact gamma camera using a pixelated Na(Tl) crystal array and a 5" Hamamatsu R3292 PSPMT. The camera was placed in a stationary position and the object was rotated vertically in front of the collimator.

2.1 Compact gamma camera

The compact gamma camera is based on a pixellatted NaI(Tl) scintillation crystal array from Saint Gobain Crystals and Detectors, Inc. attached to a 5" diameter Hamamatsu R3292 position-sensitive PMT (PSPMT). The 11.2 cm $\times$ 11.2 cm pixelated crystal array consists of 1.2 $\times$ 1.2 $\times$ 6 mm^3 pixel elements separated by 0.2-mm gaps that are filled with optically opaque and reflective materials. The light output from the scintillator is detected by the optically coupled PSPMT using a subtractive resistive readout [Wojcik, 2001] to lead out four signal outputs (X^+, X^-, Y^+ and Y^-). The signals were digitized by a 12-bit PCI-6110E ADC card from National Instruments. The data-acquisition system was based on a Macintosh G3 workstation using the Kmax software package from Sparrow, Inc. A truncated centroid algorithm [Wojcik, 1998] was used to calculate the position and energy of the detected gamma photons. The effective field-of-view (FOV) of the camera was $\sim$10.2 cm in diameter within a useful pixel array of 73 $\times$ 73. The camera was optimized for ^{99m}Tc imaging. The measured energy resolution was $\sim$ 16% FWHM for 140-KeV photons. The energy window was set at 130-155 KeV for ^{99m}Tc imaging.

The camera can be fitted with interchangeable pinhole and parallel-hole collimators. The parallel-hole collimator was designed for imaging the whole body of small animals, and the pinhole collimator was used in imaging regional activity uptakes in the animals. The pinhole collimator has a focal length of $\sim$10 cm and an acceptance angle of 62°. The pinhole apertures were interchangeable and were made of tungsten alloy with diameters of 1.0, 1.5, and 2.0 mm. The pinhole apertures had keel-edge design to minimize the photon penetration. Two general-purpose parallel-hole collimators were designed for the camera: one for high-resolution and the other for high-sensitivity imaging. The design parameters of the two parallel-hole collimators are listed in Table 21.1. The design of all the collimators was optimized for 140-KeV photons.

Table 21.1. Design parameters of the two parallel-hole collimators.

Type	Material	Technique	Hole Length (mm)	Hole Size (mm)	Septa (mm)
HRES	Lead	Cast	40	1.4	0.16
HSEN	Lead	Foil	23	1.5	0.20

The system was carefully calibrated for the system misalignments using a novel calibration method developed in our group [Wang, 2004]. The measured distance from the pinhole aperture to the image plane of the detector was 10.8 cm.

2.2 Experimental method

The performance of the microSPECT system was carefully characterized by its point source response function (PSRF) at different source positions. The full-width-at-half-maximum (FWHM) of the PSRF was used to determine the system spatial resolution, while the volume under the PSRF was used to determine the system sensitivity.

The point sources used in the PSRF measurements were made with $\sim$ 300-μm resin beads that absorbed high $^{99\text{m}}$Tc concentrations up to 0.1- 0.2 mCi. We scanned the point source along the central axis and transaxially across the FOV of the pinhole collimator. For each source position, a 10-minute planar image of the point source was acquired. From the measured PSRF, the system spatial resolution and sensitivity were determined as a function of source-to-collimator distance, source position offset from the central axis, and the pinhole diameter.

The system performance in pinhole SPECT imaging was evaluated using a microSPECT phantom from Data Spectrum, Inc. This cylindrical phantom has two types of inserts of 4.5 cm in diameter. The first insert is made with six sets of small plastic rods, while the second insert has the same sets of hole channels. The rod and hole diameters are 1.2, 1.6, 2.4, 3.2, 4.0, and 4.8 mm, respectively. The phantoms with either cold-rods or hot-channels were imaged using the 1.0-mm pinhole aperture. The microSPECT phantoms were filled with $\sim$5 mCi of $^{99\text{m}}$Tc-pertechnetate in water solution. To avoid truncation in the projection data, the phantoms was placed at a distance of $\sim$ 5 cm from the pinhole aperture, resulting in a magnification factor of $\sim$ 2.

The projection data were acquired using 120 angular views equally spaced over 360°, and the acquisition time was 40 seconds per view. The radius-of-rotation (ROR) was $\sim$ 5 cm, resulting in a magnification of $\sim$ 2. The projection data were reconstructed using a 3D pinhole OS-EM algorithm with 10 iterations and 10 subsets. Reconstruction matrix size was $80 \times 80 \times 80$ with a voxel size of 0.35 mm. A 3D Butterworth filter with a cutoff frequency of 0.25 cycles/voxel was used for the post-reconstruction.

A mouse bone scan with $^{99\text{m}}$Tc-MDP injection was also performed using a 1.0-mm pinhole aperture to evaluate the pinhole microSPECT image quality. The mouse was IV-injected with 10 mCi $^{99\text{m}}$Tc-MDP through the tail vein. The mouse was

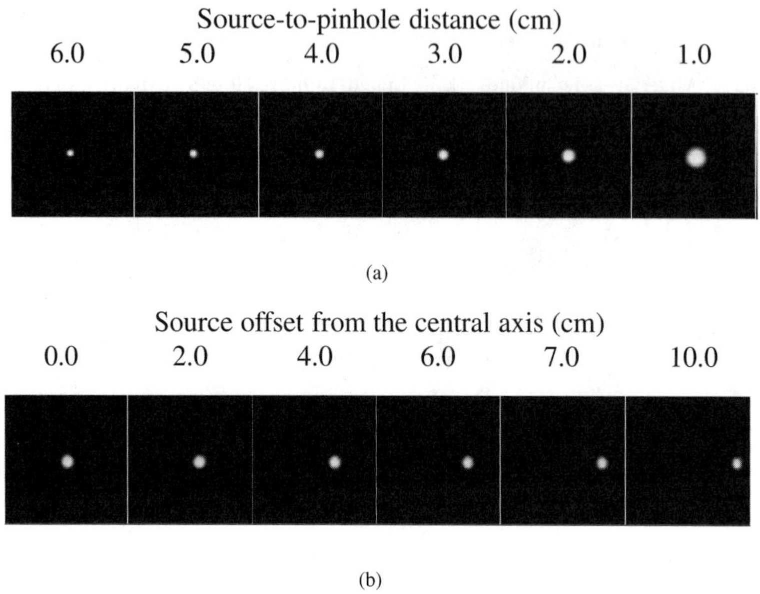

Figure 21.2. Sample of point source response function results obtained using a 300-μm diameter resin bead soaked with 0.15 mCi ^{99m}Tc and 2.0-mm pinhole aperture with keel-edge design: (a) along the axis direction, and (b) along the transaxial direction at the source-to-pinhole distance of 2.5 cm.

sacrificed and scanned after 2.5 hours of post-injection. A total of 120 projections with angular views equally spaced over 360° were acquired from the animal. The scan interval was 40 seconds per view. The ROR was $\sim$ 2.6 cm, resulting in a magnification of $\sim$ 4. The projection data were reconstructed using a 3D pinhole OS-EM algorithm with six iterations and 10 subsets and with correction of system geometric misalignments. Reconstruction matrix size was $80 \times 80 \times 80$ with a voxel size of 0.35 mm. A 3D Butterworth filter with a cutoff frequency of 0.3 cycle/voxel was used for the post-reconstruction.

3. Results

The measured point source response functions for the keel-edge pinhole aperture using ^{99m}Tc point source are shown in Fig. 21.2. In the central axis direction, the image of the point source grows larger as the point source moves closer to the pinhole due to the magnification nature of the pinhole collimation. However, in the transaxial direction across the FOV of the pinhole collimator, the PSRF becomes increasingly asymmetric as the point source moves further off the central axis of the pinhole collimator. The shape of the PSRF is narrower in the radial than in the tangential direction.

Figure 21.3 gives the axial spatial resolution and sensitivity as a function of source-to-collimator distance for the three pinhole apertures and two parallel-hole collimators. All three pinhole apertures provide much improved spatial resolution

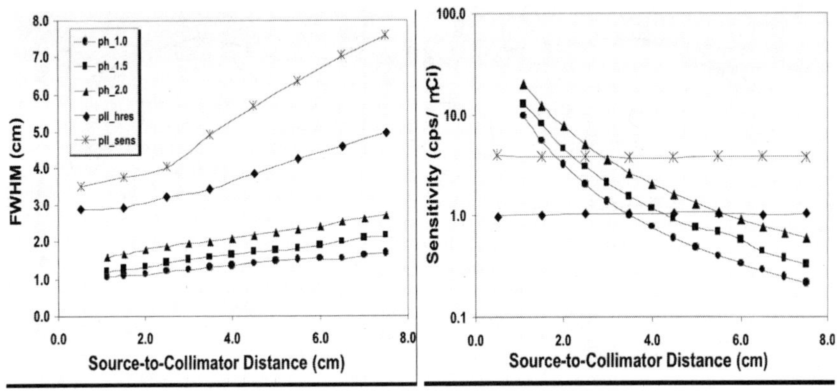

(a) (b)

Figure 21.3. Measured axial (a) spatial resolution and (b) sensitivity of the microSPECT system as a function of source-to-collimator distance.

as compared to the parallel-hole collimators. In contrast with the parallel-hole collimators, the pinhole collimator exhibits a rapid increase in detection efficiency as the source-to-collimator distance decreases. However, the useful field-of-view is reduced as the distance is decreased. When imaging a mouse with a diameter of 2.5 cm, we can place the center of the mouse as close as $\sim$ 2.6 cm from the pinhole aperture. Our system can achieve a spatial resolution and sensitivity of $\sim$ 1.2 mm and $\sim$ 2 cps/μCi using the 1-mm pinhole aperture.

The transaxial spatial resolution and sensitivity for the three pinhole apertures are shown in Fig. 21.4. The measurements were made at a source-to-pinhole distance of 2.5 cm using a 300-μm diameter point source with 0.15 mCi ^{99m}Tc. The detection efficiencies for the three pinhole apertures show a significant falloff from the central axis to the edge of the FOV of the pinhole collimator. The PSRF shows increased asymmetry as the point source moves off the central axis to the edge of FOV of pinhole collimator with smaller FWHM values in the radial than in the tangential direction.

Figure 21.5 shows the reconstructed transaxial images of the microSPECT phantoms with cold-rods and hot-channels. With the $\sim$ 5 cm ROR and $\sim$ 2 magnification, the microSPECT system with 1-mm pinhole aperture can clearly resolve both cold-rods and hot-channels from 4.8 mm down to 1.6 mm, but not the 1.2-mm rods and hot-channels.

Figure 21.6 gives the reconstructed coronal images through the chest of a normal mouse. Individual ribs of the mouse are clearly resolved in the high-resolution reconstructed images. The results demonstrate that our microSPECT system based on a compact camera is capable of high-quality small-animal imaging.

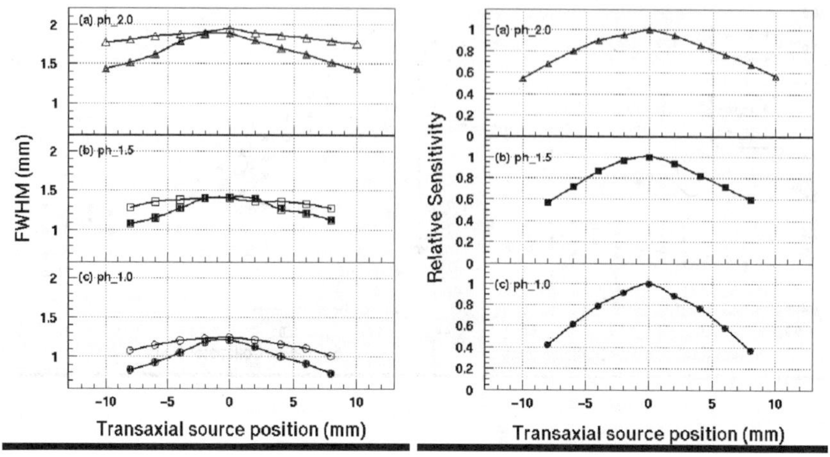

(a) (b)

Figure 21.4. Measured (a) spatial resolution and (b) sensitivity of the microSPECT system in the transaxial direction for three pinhole apertures at source-to-pinhole distance of 2.5 cm. In (a), the solid symbols denote the FWHM values in the radial direction, while the open symbols represent the FWHM values in the tangential direction in the image plane.

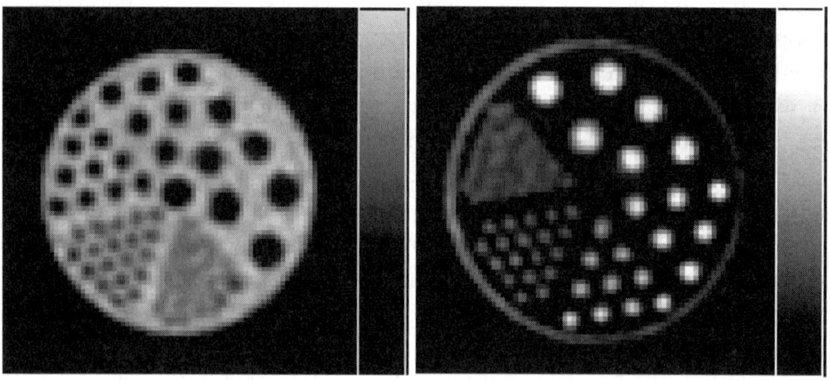

(a) (b)

Figure 21.5. Reconstructed transaxial images of the micro SPECT phantoms with (a) cold-rods and (b) hot-channels obtained from the microSPECT system using the 1.0-mm pinhole aperture. The radius-of-rotation was $\sim$ 5 cm in both cases. The phantom was filled with $\sim$ 5 mCi ^{99m}Tc-pertechnetate in a water solution. The rod and hole diameters in the six sectors are 1.2, 1.6, 2.4, 3.2, 4.0, and 4.8 mm.

4. Discussion

We characterized the performance of a high-resolution microSPECT system based on a compact gamma camera with a pixelated crystal array and a 5" Hama-

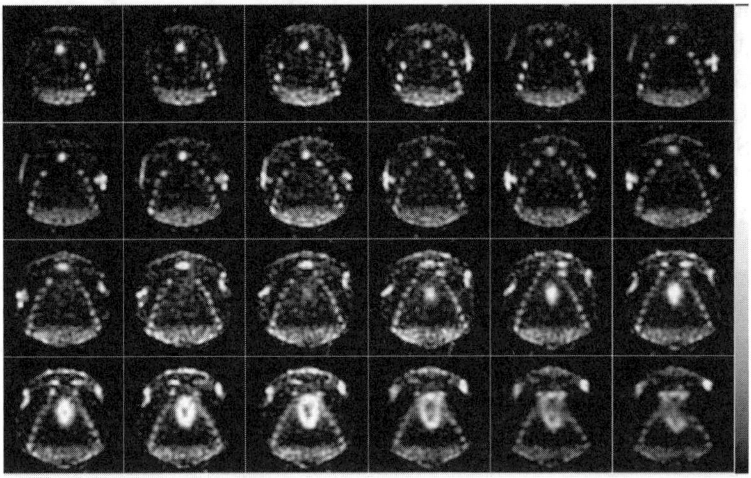

Figure 21.6. Pinhole SPECT bone scan of a normal mouse: coronal image slices through the chest of the mouse.

matsu PSPMT. As shown in the micro SPECT phantom images using ^{99m}Tc, our microSPECT system with pinhole collimator can clearly resolve the 1.6-mm cold-rods and hot-channels with an ROR of ~5 cm. When imaging a smaller object such as a mouse using a smaller ROR and larger magnification factor, improved resolution in order of 1-1.5 mm can be achieved. The measured point source sensitivities at 2.5 cm from the pinhole are approximately 2, 3 and 5.2 counts/sec/μCi for the 1.0, 1.5, and 2.0 mm pinhole apertures, respectively.

The PSRF of a pinhole collimator with keel-edge pinhole apertures becomes increasingly asymmetric toward the edge of the field-of-view of the collimator with concurrent decrease in sensitivity. The variations in PSRF and sensitivity are dependent on the aperture design parameters, including hole diameter and keel thickness, and position of the activity source relative to the pinhole aperture. These factors are important considerations in the specifications and design of a pinhole collimator for high-resolution SPECT imaging.

5. Conclusions

The modular camera based on a pixelated crystal array and a single 5" Hamamatsu PSPMT is an effective approach to a high-resolution microSPECT system for small-animal imaging. However, to achieve high-resolution SPECT images, careful collimator design, system calibration, and iterative image reconstruction methods with accurate correction of system geometric misalignments are required.

Acknowledgments

This investigation was supported by a startup fund from the Department of Radiology of the Johns Hopkins Medical Institutions. The authors thank Mrs. Ruth

Hagemann for her assistance in the small-animal experiments. Ray Visions, Inc. provided the electronic circuitry for the resistive readout on the PSPMT. R. Wojcik, S. Majewski, and A.G. Weisenberger would like to acknowledge the partial support from the Office of Biological and Environmental Research of the Office of Science of the U.S. Department of Energy.

References

[McElroy, 2002] D. P. McElroy, L. R. MacDonald, F. J. Beekman, Y. Wang, B. E. Patt, J. S. Iwanczyk, B. M. W. Tsui, and E. J. Hoffman, "Performance evaluation of A-SPECT: A high-resolution desktop pinhole SPECT system for imaging small animals," *IEEE Trans. Nucl. Sci.*, vol. 49, pp. 2139-2147, 2002.

[Peterson, 2002] T. E. Peterson, H. Kim, M. J. Crawford, B. M. Cershman, W. C. J. Hunter, H. B. Barber, L. R. Furenlid, D. W. Wilson, J. M. Woolfenden, and H. H. Barratt, "SemiSPECT: A small-animal imaging system based on eight CdZnTe pixel detectors," *2002 IEEE NSS-MIC Conference Record*, Norfolk, Nov.10-16, 2002.

[Qi, 2003] Y. J. Qi, B. M. W. Tsui, Y. Wang, B. Yoder, R. Wojcik and S. Majewski, "Performance characteristics of a new modular camera based on pixelated crystal for high-resolution pinhole SPECT with comparison to a standard camera with continuous crystal," *Conference Record: M7-60, IEEE Nuclear Science Symposium* ,2003.

[Tsui, 2001] B. M. W. Tsui, Y. Wang, E. C. Frey, and D. E. Wessell, "Application of ultra high-resolution pinhole SPECT system based on a conventional camera for small animal imaging," *J. Nucl. Med.*, vol. 42, pp. 54P-55P, 2001.

[Wang, 2004] Y. Wang, B. M. W. Tsui, and E. C. Frey. "Theoretical analysis of conditions for unique solutions in geometric calibrations for cone-beam and pinhole tomography," submitted to *Phys. Med. Bio.*, 2004

[Weber, 1994] D. A. Weber, M. Ivanovic, D. Franceschi, S-E. Strand, K. Erlandsson, M. Franceschi, H. L. Atkins, J. A. Coderre, H. Susskind, T. Button and K. Ljunggren, "Pinhole SPECT: An approach to *in vivo* high resolution SPECT imaging in small laboratory animals," *J. Nucl. Med.*, vol. 35, pp. 342-348, 1994.

[Wojcik, 2001] R. Wojcik, S. Majewski, B. Kross, V. Popov, and A. G. Weisenberger, "Optimized readout of small gamma cameras for high resolution single gamma and positron emission imaging," *2001 IEEE NSS-MIC Conference Record, San Diego*, Nov.4-10, 2001.

[Wojcik, 1998] R.Wojcik, S. Majewski, D. Steinbach and A. G. Weisenberger, "High spatial resolution gamma imaging detector based on 5" diameter R3292 Hamamatsu PSPMT," *IEEE Trans. Nucl. Sci.*, vol. 45, pp.487-491, 1998.

Chapter 22

High-Resolution Radionuclide Imaging Using Focusing Gamma-Ray Optics

Michael Pivovaroff, William Barber, Tobias Funk, Bruce Hasegawa, Carmen Taylor, William Craig, and Klaus Ziock*

1. Introduction

Animal models, especially transgenic and knock-out mice, now affect research in every area of biomedical science and are available for a diverse range of human conditions [Bernstein and Breitman, 1989]. The emergence of transgenic animal technology as a key component along the entire research path, ranging from fundamental investigations to pharmacological development, requires high-resolution techniques suitable for noninvasive imaging of small animals. While magnetic resonance imaging (MRI), magnetic resonance spectroscopy, and CT provide spatial resolution in the range 25-50 μm, these techniques are best-suited for anatomical or metabolite concentration studies. Noninvasive metabolic and functional assessments are best performed using positron emission tomography (PET) and single-photon computed tomography (SPECT).

Although dedicated small-animal PET systems are being developed with spatial resolution of 1-2 mm, it will be impossible to significantly improve the resolution beyond this due to the uncertainty in the position of the positron annihilation. (The mean positron range in water is 0.6 mm for ^{18}F and is much larger for other PET isotopes like ^{11}C, ^{13}N, and ^{124}I [Bailey, 2003].) On the other hand, radionuclide imaging techniques using single-photon agents such as ^{125}I and ^{99m}Tc do not have a fundamental physics limit to their resolution.

2. Radionuclide imaging: Traditional approach

Current imaging methods for single-photon radionuclide studies rely on absorptive collimation, with either a converging parallel-hole collimator or a pinhole collimator serving as the optical element. Figure 22.1 sketches the basic geometry of a pinhole collimator, which will serve to illustrate the basic properties of both

*M. Pivovaroff, University of California, Berkeley, California; W. Barber, T. Funk, B. Hasegawa, C. Taylor, University of California, San Francisco, California; K. Ziock, Lawrence Livermore National Laboratory, Livermore, California

types of systems. To first order, the resolution R of a pinhole imager scales with aperture diameter, while the efficiency η scales as the square of the aperture. Along with R and η, the third important parameter that determines the types of imaging studies that can be performed is the field-of-view (FOV). Accounting for all relevant effects, the complete on-axis system characteristics are defined by:

$$R = \sqrt{\left(d\left[\frac{b+l}{l}\right]\right)^2 + \left(\frac{p}{M}\right)^2} \tag{22.1}$$

$$\eta = \frac{d^2}{16b^2} \tag{22.2}$$

$$\mathrm{FOV} = 2b\tan\alpha, \tag{22.3}$$

where d is the pinhole diameter (assuming no septal penetration at the edges of the pinhole), l is the separation between the pinhole and the detector, p is the pixel size of the detector, b is the separation between the source and the pinhole, α is the half-angle of the collimator, and M is the magnification, $M \equiv l/b$.

In order to achieve sub-mm spatial resolution, either FOV or η must be reduced. This is easiest to see by rearranging Eqns. 22.1-22.3, eliminating d, and solving for R as a function of FOV:

$$R = \sqrt{\frac{\eta \times \mathrm{FOV}^2\,(1+1/M)^2}{\tan^2\alpha} + \frac{p^2}{M^2}} \tag{22.4}$$

Figure 22.2 plots a family of curves for detector pixel sizes of 1 and 3 mm (representing current technology) and magnification $M = 20$. For efficiencies, we choose two values: $\eta = 1 \times 10^{-5}$ (or 0.4 cps/μCi), representing the lowest possible sensitivity allowed for practical measurements and $\eta = 1 \times 10^{-4}$ (or 4 cps/μCi). To understand the best possible resolution that can be achieved, we plot R vs FOV as $p \rightarrow 0$ (i.e., detector with infinitely good resolution) and $M \rightarrow \infty$. Finally, for context, Fig. 22.2 shows R and FOV for three small-animal SPECT systems; #1-[Choong, 2004], parallel-hole collimator; #2-[Wu, 2002], #3-[Beekman, 2002], pinhole collimators.

Restricting attention to FOVs of at least 5 mm, the best spatial resolution possible with a pinhole collimator using modern detectors ($p \approx 2$ mm) and requiring a useful efficiency ($\eta > 10^{-5}$) is $\sim$100 μm. Even with an ideal detector or very high M, the theoretically best resolution only improves to 55 μm for a 5-mm FOV or 220 μm for a 20-mm FOV. Given this limit to absorptive collimation techniques, another approach is needed to perform radionuclide imaging at a spatial resolution of 100 μm or better.

3. Radionuclide imaging: Focusing γ-ray optics

Reflective X-ray or γ-ray optics are one choice for high-spatial resolution radionuclide imaging. It is beyond the scope of this paper to discuss the underlying

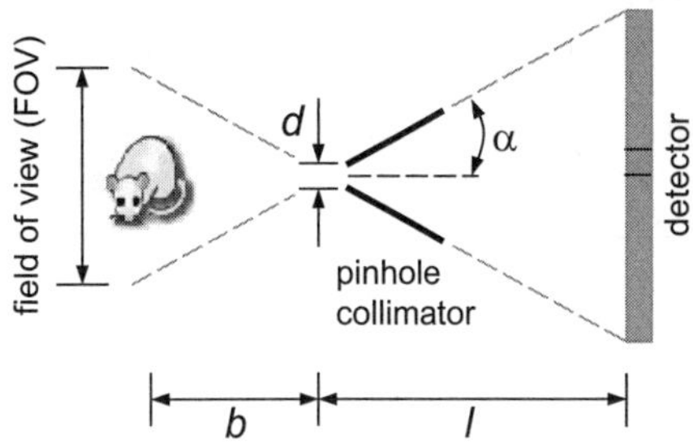

Figure 22.1. Schematic view of a pinhole collimator, indicating the relevant parameters that determine the system resolution, efficiency, and the FOV.

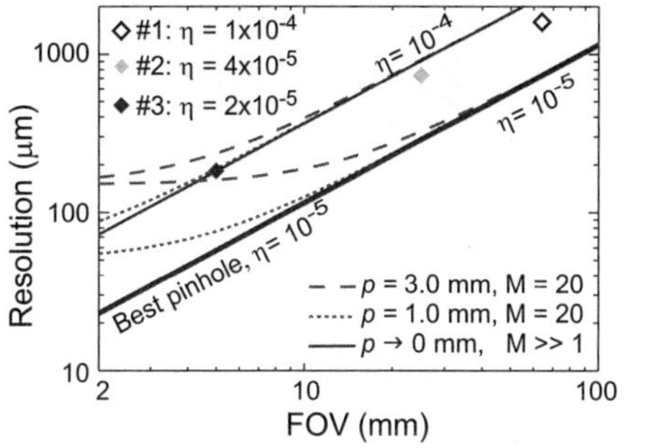

Figure 22.2. Resolution vs. FOV assuming different values of p and η. The diamonds indicate the performance of actual SPECT systems. Refer to the text for references.

physics of these systems and the important design drivers for biomedical applications. Instead, we briefly summarize the salient points and refer the interested reader to [Pivovaroff, 2003] for a detailed discussion.

Figure 22.3 sketches the basic geometry of the γ-ray lens. In order to maximize sensitivity, the reflective surfaces are coated with multilayers. For systems designed to focus 17-20 keV photons (the low-energy lines emitted by ^{95m}Tc, ^{96}Tc, or ^{99m}Tc) or 27.5 keV photons (the primary energy emitted by I^{125}), the efficiency is $\eta \approx (1-5)\times 10^{-5}$, and to first order, is determined solely by the multilayer reflectivity. The other design parameters have little or no influence on η. R and FOV are given approximately by:

$$R = \sqrt{\frac{8(b+l)^2}{(1+M)^2}\tan^2\alpha + \frac{p^2}{M^2}} \tag{22.5}$$

$$\text{FOV} = 2b\tan\theta, \tag{22.6}$$

where α is the angular quality of the mirror surface, θ is the graze angle which the photons reflect off the mirror, and the other parameters l, b, M, and p are the same as above.

It is also possible to re-arrange the system equations to solve for R as a function of FOV:

$$R = \sqrt{2\times \text{FOV}^2\left[\frac{\tan\alpha}{\tan\theta}\right]^2 + \frac{p^2}{M^2}}. \tag{22.7}$$

Figure shows the resultant curves for a range of magnifications, $M = \{1,4,12\}$, pixel size $p = 25$ μm, and mirror performance $\alpha = \{40,10,1\}$ arc seconds. These values of α represent the quality of mirrors currently produced by a thermal-forming process (40":[Craig, 2000]), a replication process (10":[Ramsey, 2002]), and a high-precision replication process under investigation (1":[Nederbragt, 2003]). Optical designs are limited such that $b+l < 4.57$ m to minimize the amount of space needed for imaging experiments. The two diamonds indicate a prototype lens already tested (#1:[Pivovaroff, 2003]) and one under construction (#2). Figure 22.4 also plots the

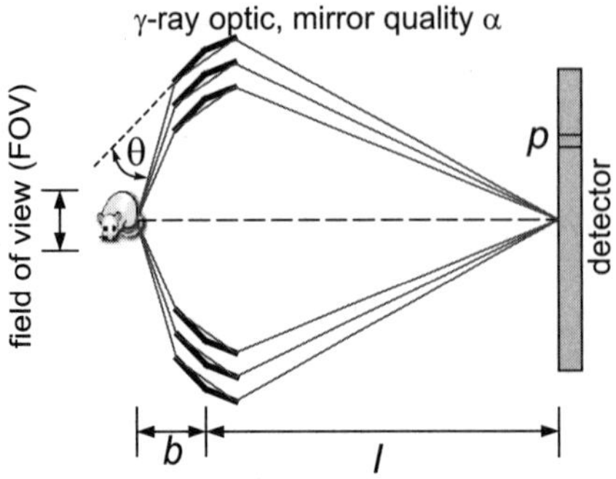

Figure 22.3. Schematic view of a γ-ray lens with three nested mirrors, indicating the relevant parameters that determine the system resolution and FOV.

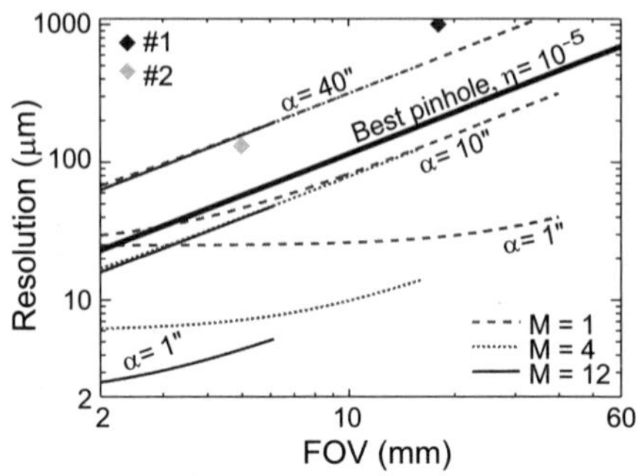

Figure 22.4. Resolution vs. FOV assuming different values of p and η. The diamonds indicate the performance of two prototype γ-ray lenses. Refer to the text for details.

theoretical best R-FOV curve for a pinhole collimator with $\eta = 10^{-5}$, an efficiency comparable to what a γ-ray lens can achieve.

As seen in Fig. 22.4, the use of X-ray focusing optics opens a large part of high-spatial resolution parameter space unobtainable with traditional pinhole collimation techniques. For example, with modest 10" mirrors, it is possible to achieve 40-μm resolution over a 16-mm FOV, using an optical design with $M = 4$ and a detector with pixels no larger than 80 μm. As mirror fabrication improves in the future [Nederbragt, 2003], it will be possible to build a radionuclide imaging system with better than 10-μm resolution over a 5-mm FOV, using an optical design with $M = 12$ and a detector with 25-μm pixels.

Of course, the use of reflective γ-ray optics also has disadvantages, when compared to absorptive collimation techniques. First, the only way to improve the sensitivity of the system beyond a few times 10^{-5} ($\sim$1 cps/μCi) is to increase the number of lenses. The atomic physics sets up an upper limit on how well multilayer coatings can reflect high-energy photons. This is analogous to the hard spatial resolution limit which PET suffers from due to the uncertainty in the location of the position annihilation. Second, a single lens will consist of several tens of nested mirror pairs, at a fabrication cost significantly more expensive than a single collimator element [Pivovaroff, 2003]. Finally, a complete focusing system will require more laboratory space than an absorptive collimation system, with separation distances between the small animal and detector equal to a few meters.

Acknowledgments

This work was supported in part by grant KP1401030, issued by the U.S. Department of Energy (DoE), and by Contract No. W-7405-ENG-48, issued by the U.S. DoE, Office of Biological and Environmental Research, by the University of California, Lawrence Livermore National Laboratory. The project received generous support from the University of California, Office of the President, under the auspices of the Campus-Laboratory Collaboration (CLC) program. The project has used resources supported in part by NIH grant 5 R01 EB00348-02, "Imaging Structure and Function in Small Animals."

References

[Bailey, 2003] D. L. Bailey, J. S. Karp, and S. Surti, *Physics and Instrumentation in PET*, in *Positron Emission Tomography: Basic Science and Clinical Practice*, pages 41-67. Springer-Verlag, Philadelphia, 2003.

[Beekman, 2002] F. J. Beekman, D. P McElroy, F. Berger, S. S. Gambhir, E. J. Hoffman, "Toward *in vivo* nuclear microscopy: iodine-125 imaging in mice using micro-pinholes," *Eur J of Nucl Med*, vol. 29, pp. 933-938, 2002.

[Bernstein and Breitman, 1989] A. Bernstein, M. Breitman, "Genetic ablation in transgenic mice," *Molecular Biol Med*, vol. 6, pp. 523-530, 1989.

[Choong, 2004] W. S. Choong, W. W. Moses, C. S. Tindall, P. N. Lunk, "Design for a high-resolution small-animal SPECT system using pixellated Si(Li) detector for *in vivo* ^{125}I imaging," *IEEE Trans Nucl Sci, submitted.*

[Craig, 2000] W. W. Craig, et al., "Development of thermally formed glass optics for astronomical hard x-ray telescopes," *Optics Exp*, vol, 7, pp. 178-185, 2000.

[Nederbragt, 2003] W. Nederbragt, "Fabrication of a precision mandrel for replicating wolter x-ray optics," *Proceedings of the 18th Annual Meeting of the ASPE*,
High-Resolution Radionuclide Imaging Using Focusing Gamma-Ray Opticshttp://www.llnl.gov/tid/lof/documents/pdf/243999.pdf, 2003.

[Pivovaroff, 2003] M. J. Pivovaroff, et al., "Small animal radionuclide imaging system with focusing gamma-ray optics," *Proc SPIE*, vol. 5199, pp.147-161, 2003.

[Ramsey, 2002] B. D. Ramsey, et al., "First image from HERO, a hard x-ray focusing telescope," *Astrophys J*, vol. 568, pp. 432-435, 2002.

[Wu, 2002] M. C. Wu, B. H. Hasegawa, M. W. Dae, "Peformance evaluation of a pinhole SPECT system for myocardial perfusion imaging of mice," *Med Phys*, vol. 9, pp. 2830-2839, 2002.

Chapter 23

SPECT/Micro-CT Imaging of Bronchial Angiogenesis in a Rat

Anne V. Clough, Christian Wietholt, Robert C. Molthen, John C. Gordon, and David L. Roerig*

1. Introduction

The bronchial circulation provides the lung with an oxygenated blood supply, derived from the aorta, whose primary purpose under normal conditions is thought to be nourishment of the airway walls [Guyton, 1996]. However, the study of the bronchial circulation and its development is particularly important with regard to lung tumors whose blood supply is via the bronchial circulation rather than the pulmonary circulation [Hirsch, 2001, Ohta, 2002]. Thus, we have developed a rat model of bronchial circulation angiogenesis, induced by complete occlusion of the left pulmonary artery. We have been observing the resulting perfusion changes in the left lung using dual-modality SPECT/micro-CT imaging. The initial objective of this study is to develop the necessary imaging system, protocol, and analysis methods for determining the time course of this angiogenesis, with the subsequent goal of using this approach to study the particular angiogenic mechanisms that might be involved.

Complete occlusion of one pulmonary artery results in very extensive development of the bronchial circulation to the occluded lung [Mitzner and Lee 2000]. Hence, we have developed a rat model that involves complete surgical occlusion of the left pulmonary artery followed by a recovery period during which recovery flow to the left lung via the bronchial circulation is observed. This observation is performed using SPECT detection of radiolabeled macroaggregated albumin (MAA) that deposits in the microvasculature in proportion to local flow. Because the recovery flow to the left lung originates from the aorta rather than the occluded left pulmonary artery, the MAA injection is made into the aorta via the carotid artery, and accumulation of MAA in the lung is used as an index of flow. Finally, we use micro-CT to obtain anatomical thorax images so that the lung field can be identified

*A. V. Clough, C. Wietholt, Marquette University, Milwaukee, Wisconsin; R. C. Molthen, J. C. Gordon, D. L. Roerig, Medical College of Wisconsin, Milwaukee, Wisconsin; A. V. Clough, R. C. Molthen, F. C. Gordon, D. L. Roerig, Zablocki VA Medical Center, Milwaukee, Wisconsin

within the SPECT images, because the entire systemic vasculature is radiolabeled. Registration of the micro-CT and SPECT volumes then enables segmentation of the SPECT images of the left lung for subsequent flow quantification.

2. Methods

The left pulmonary artery (LPA) of anesthetized rats (70 mg/kg ketamine, 0.5 mg/kg medetomidine hydrochloride IP) was surgically occluded followed by IP administration of 0.3 mg/kg of atipamezole hydrocholoride to facilitate recovery. The rats were allowed to recover prior to subsequent imaging at $\sim$10, 20, or 34 days post-surgery, with three animals studied at each time point for this preliminary study. In addition, three rats without surgical occlusion were studied as controls. For SPECT imaging, the rats were anesthetized (82 mg/kg ketamine, 1.8 mg/kg acepromazine IM), and a retrograde left carotid artery injection of 2.0 mCi of Tc99m labeled MAA (1 ml) was made. The rat was suspended vertically in a plastic tube on a rotary stage and imaged with a gamma camera (Picker DYNATM MO) equipped with a pinhole collimator (5-mm diameter) using 128 angular views with an acquisition time of 20 sec/view. Subsequently, without relocation, the rat was imaged using micro-CT (Feinfocus FXE/FXT 0.20 microfocal x-ray source and Thomson TH9438 image intensifier coupled to a Silicon Mountain Design 1M-15 CCD camera) with 360 angular views with an acquisition time of 0.3 sec/view as described previously [Karau, 2001, Wietholt, 2003].

SPECT reconstruction was performed using an ordered subset Ð expectation maximization algorithm [Hudson 1994] with seven iterations. Micro-CT reconstruction using a Feldkamp-type algorithm [Feldkamp, 1984] was performed as described previously [Karau, 2001]. The resulting 128^3 reconstructed SPECT image volume was scaled and registered to the 512^3 reconstructed micro-CT image volume using the geometric imaging parameters. The lung field was segmented out of the micro-CT volume using seeded region growing followed by morphological closing, the corresponding lung field was identified in the SPECT volume, and the total number of counts within each lung was determined. All rats were imaged again 2 - 5 days later using the same SPECT and micro-CT protocol as described above, except with an intravenous injection into the left femoral vein, resulting in MAA accumulation in the right (non-occluded) lung via the pulmonary circulation. Because more than 99% of the radioactivity accumulated within the right lung field in the LPA occluded rats, right lung MAA accumulation was used as an index of total cardiac output. Left lung MAA accumulation from the arterial injection was compared with right lung MAA accumulation from the intravenous injection to determine the flow to the bronchial circulation as a fraction of cardiac output.

3. Results

Figure 23.1 shows examples of co-registered SPECT and micro-CT lung images following injection of MAA in a control rat (no LPA occlusion). Here, the SPECT images were superimposed upon the corresponding micro-CT images with

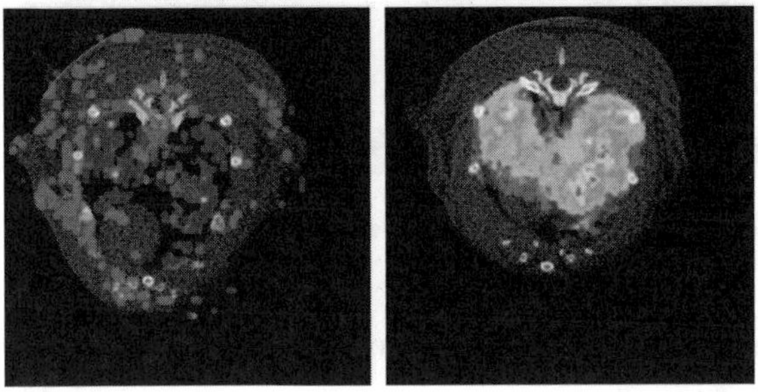

Figure 23.1. **CONTROL**: SPECT images of MAA accumulation in the lungs of a control rat are co-registered with micro-CT images and superimposed for this display. Left: Arterial injection results in accumulation in the lungs via the bronchial circulation. Right: Intravenous injection in the same rat results in accumulation via the pulmonary circulation. SPECT image scale for bronchial and pulmonary circulation is different to visualize relatively very low activity level in bronchial circulation.

the intensity scale of the SPECT bronchial circulation images (left) and pulmonary circulation images (right) different for visualization purposes only. The left image of Fig. 23.1 shows MAA accumulation in the right and left lung fields via the bronchial circulation, following an arterial injection. The right image shows significantly more MAA accumulation in both lungs via the pulmonary circulation, following an intravenous injection. In this control rat, the counts in the bronchial circulation were 1.2% of the counts in the pulmonary circulation.

Images obtained from a rat 40 days following LPA occlusion are shown in Fig. 23.2. A substantial increase in activity within the left lung due to development of the bronchial circulation (as compared to Fig. 23.1, left) can be observed in the image on the left. The right image was obtained following an intravenous injection and shows MAA accumulation in the right lung only via the pulmonary circulation, because the LPA has been occluded. In this rat, the counts in the left lung bronchial circulation (left) were 14.0% of the counts in the right lung pulmonary circulation (right).

Comparison of left lung MAA accumulation from the arterial injection with right lung MAA accumulation from the intravenous injection results in a measure of bronchial circulation blood flow as a fraction of total cardiac output. Preliminary results obtained from three animals at each time point suggest that flow in the bronchial circulation increases from an average of 1% of cardiac output in control rats to 4%, 10%, and 16% at 10, 20 and 34 days, respectively, following LPA occlusion.

4. Discussion

The results of this study suggest that occlusion of one pulmonary artery provides a useful model for studying the development of the bronchial circulation in the lung. However, additional animals will be required to more accurately determine the time course of this development. Nonetheless, this approach will be important

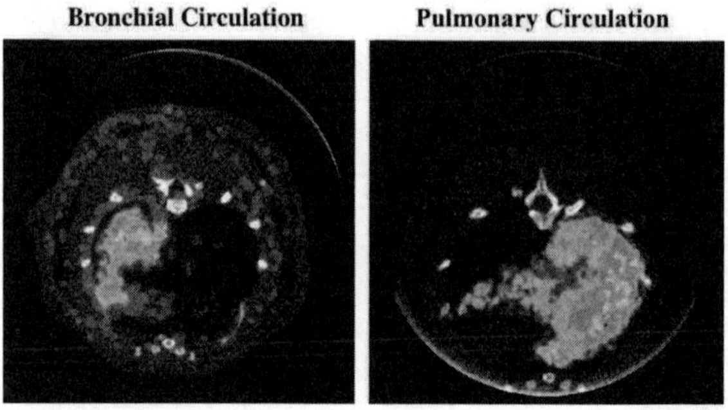

Figure 23.2. **OCCLUDED LPA**: SPECT and micro-CT images obtained from a rat forty days following occlusion of its LPA. Left: Images following an arterial injection resulting in MAA accumulation in the left lung via bronchial circulation. Right: Images from the same animal using an intravenous injection resulting in MAA accumulation in the right lung via pulmonary circulation. SPECT image scale for bronchial and pulmonary circulation is different to visualize low activity level in bronchial circulation.

in subsequent studies for observing animals subjected to treatments designed to affect angiogenic mechanisms that might be involved, as well as for monitoring the effects of antiangiogenic agents.

The imaging results illustrate that dual-modality SPECT/micro-CT imaging is an appropriate modality for small-animal lung perfusion imaging. The spatial resolution of the system described here is adequate for between-lung comparisons (i.e., right versus left) of perfusion, but improved spatial resolution obtained with up-to-date SPECT detectors will be required for quantification of the within-lung regional flow distribution.

The SPECT/micro-CT imaging protocol developed here will also be useful in other pulmonary circulation studies that are ongoing in our laboratory. One example is the study of pulmonary vascular remodeling involving partial occlusion of one pulmonary artery. In this case, the obstruction reduces the flow to that lung and increases the flow to the other lung. The objective then is to monitor pulmonary flow changes to the two lungs over a given time period to determine whether, to what degree, and how fast the pulmonary vasculature adapts to equalize the flow between the lungs in animals exposed to a variety of remodeling stimuli.

Acknowledgments

This work was supported by National Science Foundation Grant BES-9818197, National Heart, Lung, and Blood Institute Grant HL-19298, and the Department of Veterans Affairs.

References

[Feldkamp, 1984] L. A. Feldkamp, L. C. Davis, J. W. Kress, "Practical cone-beam algorithm," *J Opt Soc Amer A* vol. 1(6), pp. 612 - 619, 1984.

[Guyton, 1996] A. C. Guyton, J. E. Hall, *Textbook of Medical Physiology*, pp. 491 - 499, W.B. Saunders, 1996.

[Hirsch, 2001] F. R. Hirsch, W. A. Franklin, A. F. Gazdar, and P. A. Bunn, Jr., "Early detection of lung cancer: clinical perspectives of recent advances in biology and radiology," *Clin Cancer Res,* vol. 7, pp. 5 - 22, 2001.

[Hudson, 1994] H. M. Hudson, R. S. Larkin, "Accelerated image reconstruction using ordered subsets of projection data," *IEEE Trans Med Imag*, vol. 13, pp. 601 - 609, 1994.

[Karau, 2001] K. L. Karau, R. C. Molthen, A. Dhyani, S. T. Haworth, C. C. Hanger, D. L. Roerig, R. H. Johnson, C. A. Dawson, "Pulmonary arterial morphometry from microfocal X-ray computed tomography," *Am J Physiol Heart Circ Physiol,* vol. 281, pp. H274 7- H2756, 2001.

[Mitzner and Lee 2000] W. Mitzner W. Lee, D. Georgakopoulos, E. Wagner, "Angiogenesis in the mouse lung," *Amer J Path,* vol. 157(1), pp. 93 - 101, 2000.

[Ohta, 2002] Y. Ohta, N. Ohta, M. Tamura, J. Wu, Y. Tsunezuka, M. Oda, G. Watanabe, "Vascular endothelial growth factor expression in airways of patients with lung cancer: a possible diagnostic tool of responsive angiogenic status on the host side," *Chest*, vol. 121, pp. 1624 - 1627, 2002.

[Wietholt, 2003] C. Wietholt, S. T. Haworth, R. C. Molthen, C. A. Dawson, A. V. Clough, "SPECT imaging of pulmonary flow in a rat," *SPIE Medical Imaging 2003: Physiology and Function: Methods, Systems and Applications*, A.V. Clough and A.A. Amini, Eds, Proc. SPIE, vol. 5031, pp. 252 - 261, 2003.

Chapter 24

Projection and Pinhole-Based Data Acquisition for Small-Animal SPECT Using Storage Phosphor Technology

Matthew A. Lewis, Gary Arbique, Edmond Richer, Nikolai Slavine, M. Jennewein, Anca Constantinescu, Rolf Brekken, J. Guild, Edward N. Tsyganov, Ralph P. Mason, and Peter P. Antich*

1. Introduction

Three-dimensional Single Photon Emission Computed Tomography (SPECT) can provide high-resolution insight into biomolecular distribution and pharmacokinetics. However, instrument availability and distribution is limited at present, and imaging times can be considerable. To evaluate the large array of novel agents which are becoming available, we find that storage phosphor-based *in vivo* imaging can provide an important, rapid-throughput transition from the traditional *ex vivo* sacrifice/gamma counting and autoradiography to full-time course SPECT.

Storage phosphor (SP) technology has found widespread usage in both the radiology clinic and in the molecular biology laboratory. With a linear sensitivity latitude exceeding that of plain film, photostimulable luminescence (PSL) screens can facilitate high-throughput screening and autoradiography for a variety of small-animal models. Despite the impressive growth and improvement in small-animal nuclear imaging, the determination of appropriate time and duration of imaging for a given animal model and imaging agent is still crucial in study design and analysis. Storage phosphor technology is well-suited for addressing this issue, either by producing quantitative planar projection or low-resolution tomographic images. With γ-ray stopping cross-sections that are not radically different from film/screen systems, the phosphor image plate[1] is well-suited for low-energy gamma detection, especially for imaging studies with iodine-125 (^{125}I) where tissue scattering is minimized.

*M. A. Lewis, G. Arbique, E. Richer, N. Slavine, M. Jennewein, Johannes Gutenberg-Universität Mainz, Germany; A. Constantinescu, R. Brekken, J. Guild, E. N. Tsyganov, R. P. Mason, P. P. Antich, University of Texas Southerwestern Medical Center, Dallas, Texas

2. Background

2.1 Storage phosphor technology

Photostimulable storage phosphor (PSP[2]) screens were developed and introduced in the 1980s [Sonoda, 1983] as a replacement for film/screen x-ray detection systems. Today, SP technology is the key component in commercial filmless imaging systems grouped under the generic term Computed Radiography (CR) [Arbique, 2003]. This technology is distinct from so-called Digital Radiography (DR), where x-ray detection is digital from the moment of detection. Subsequently, SP technology was adopted by most suppliers of autoradiography equipment [Johnston, 1990]. Wile today's average molecular biologist does not have ready access to a small-animal SPECT system, he or she most likely possesses or has available an SP scanner or reader that is routinely used for gel and blot applications. Compared to the standard CR reader in a radiology clinic, these scanners typically have higher spatial resolutions (down to 50 μm) and greater digital resolution (16 vs. 12 bit). Although the current trend is toward more expensive scanners that can also read direct- or chemi-fluorescence assays, a multipurpose SP system can be obtained for a fraction of the cost of a minimal small-animal SPECT system.

A full physical description of SP technology, including image performance parameters (MTF, NPS, DQE) can be found elsewhere [von Seggern, 1999, Rowlands, 2002]. In summary, the interaction of a high-energy photon with a BaF(Br,I):Eu^{2+} phosphor grain generates electrons and holes that are trapped in the immediate fluorohalide matrix area. A latent image is formed in proportion to the density of the trapped carriers. Upon subsequent photostimulation using a red light source (typically a laser at 590-680 nm), the electron is liberated from its trap and recombines with a hole. The energy generated in this process is resonantly transfered to a doped Europium ion, which then decays with characteristic luminescence (390 nm). This luminescence is captured using a photomultiplier tube and digitized. With an appropriate reader, a typical SP image plate will have a linear dynamic range up to a thousand times greater than film, spanning 4-5 orders of magnitude, and reusable for tens of thousands of exposures. Due to thermal stimulation, the latent image does fade (decay constant approximately 9 hours), so immediate reading of PSL screens is advisable.

2.2 Low energy-integrating SPECT

The hypothesis of low energy-integrating SPECT is that reasonable images can be obtained using γ-ray detectors that integrate activity counts and have no energy discrimination for scatter rejection. Monte Carlo simulations [Tenney, 2002] have shown that, for ^{125}I in a mouse-sized cylinder of water, the scatter fraction remains below 40%, and the detective quantum efficiency (DQE) is in the reasonable range of 0.6-0.7, which can exceed the DQE of the SP screen [Rowlands, 2002]. Although dual-isotope imaging is precluded, energy-integration imaging shifts the burden of work to image reconstruction, where scatter correction represents a significant challenge, but is an active area of research for all nuclear medicine modalities.

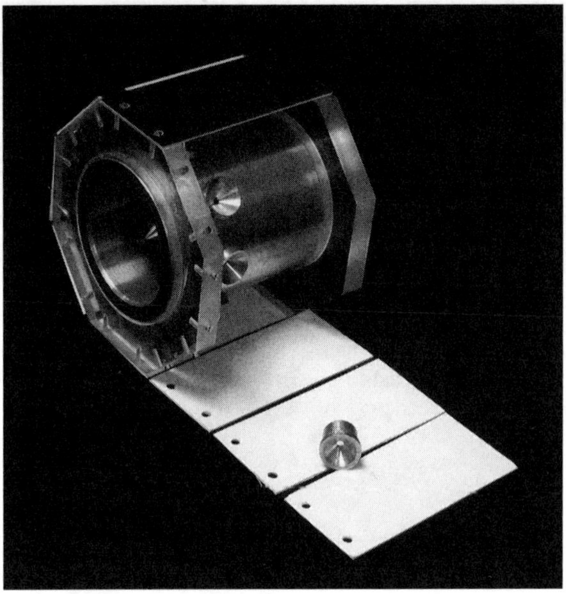

Figure 24.1. Prototype murine pinhole emission computed tomography system using energy-integrating storage phosphor technology.

A CCD-based gamma camera has been recently proposed as an efficient energy integrating detector for small-animal SPECT. Although a CCD-based camera will in general be less expensive than the traditional position-sensitive PMT, the intrinsic resolution of the CCD design will be significantly better, with characteristic resolutions below 400 μm [Antich, 2003]. At these low intrinsic resolutions, parallel-hole collimators are not well-matched. In addition, compared to a non-magnifying pinhole geometry, the packing of multiple, static projection is limited.

For lower resolution, high-throughput screening, we find that SP image plates and screens are an acceptable alternative to CCDs in an energy-integrating detector. If an infrastructure for reading SP technology is already in place, then the relative cost for detectors is further reduced, with no sacrifice in intrinsic resolution. With this savings, we believe that small-animal SPECT using SP technology may be possible for routine low-resolution, high-throughput screening.

3. Prototype

Recently, a prototype system using CR image plates for co-registered I-125 planar scintigraphy and x-ray radiography was introduced [Boone, 2003]. In this scheme, half of the image plate is used for a planar emission image. After exposure, the image plate is precisely translated so that a transmission radiography can be taken with the other half of the plate. These two images are subsequently co-registered in software, using the known displacement.

Our approach differs in that we have utilized custom-sized SP image plates as energy-integrating detectors in a low-resolution small-animal pinhole emission

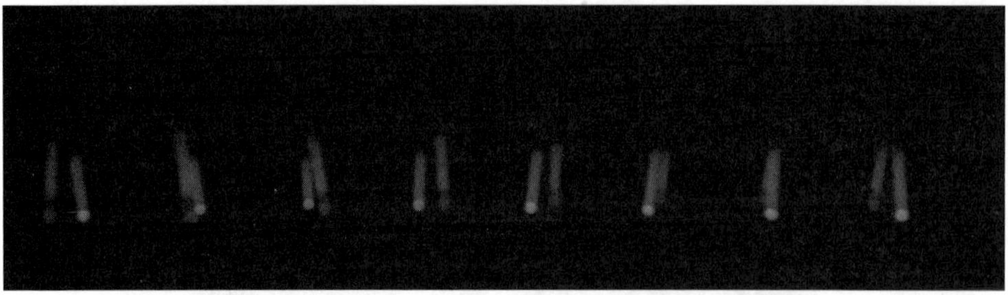

Figure 24.2. Eight pinhole projections from two 1.85 MBq ^{125}I capillaries (0.8-mm inner diameter). 15 minutes integration exposure. Signal-to-noise ratio $\approx$ 10. Heterogeneities are due to air bubbles in capillaries and infiltration of sealant.

computed tomography geometry. As shown in Fig. 24.1, a 30-mm inner diameter/5-mm thick brass cylinder serves as a support for eight 1.5-mm diameter pinholes (also in brass, with 90° cone of acceptance), spaced in 45° increments around a ring. In this geometry, the field-of-view in a plane intersecting the axis of the cylinder is equivalent to the 30-mm diameter of the cylinder. A strip of eight small SP image plates is attached to the support structure at fixed points of known distance from the pinhole centers. Each detector is placed 10 mm from the corresponding pinhole center. In this geometry, reading of the SP screen at 100-μm resolution will produce 128x128 and 256x128 projections for 60° and 90° cone-of-acceptance pinholes, respectively. For ^{125}I energies ($<$ 35.5 keV), brass is sufficient for collimation (HVL $\approx$ 80μm).

Eight 24 mm by 50 mm SP screens were cut from a 25.2×30.3 cm Fuji CR ST-VN Imaging Plate (Fuji Photo Film, Tokyo). Attachment holes of 1.6-mm diameter were milled at the end of each screen for attachment to the imaging system. The imaging plates were connected in a continuous strip using black insulating tape.

The system is placed in a light-tight enclosure with the phantom or animal placed inside the cylinder. After exposure[3], the SP detector is carefully removed and transported in a light-tight envelope to the SP reader. A SP scanner with the ability to read arbitrary size screens, such at the Molecular Dynamics Storm (Amersham Biosciences, Piscataway, NJ), is preferred, but in practice other systems may work. Special attention to the relationship between the detector coordinate system and the angular position of the detector should be maintained, because different SP readers may report data in mirror orientations.

4. Results

To evaluate the prototype system, two non-uniform 1.85 MBq ^{125}I capillaries with an inner diameter of 0.8 mm were prepared. The line sources were placed off-center in the field-of-view for the ring of pinholes and were non-parallel with an average separation of 8 mm. The sources were imaged for 15 minutes, followed by

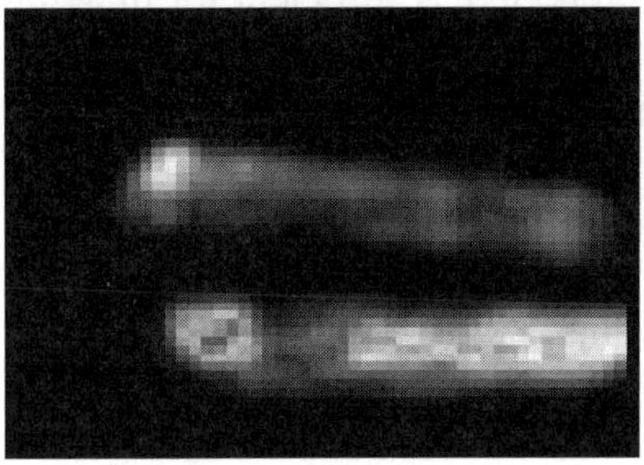

Figure 24.3. Maximum intensity projection for reconstructed, heterogenous line sources.

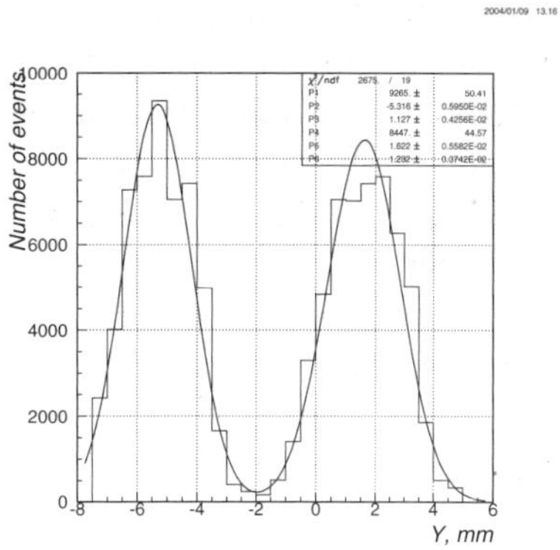

Figure 24.4. Cross-section through line sources with expected broadening due to pinhole geometry.

prompt reading of the SP image plates. Eight pinhole projections of the line source can be found in Fig. 24.2.

Using unexposed regions of the SP image plates, background noise levels were determined for windowing. Because the attachment holes appear as voids on the raw projection images, detector coordinate origins were calculated as the midpoint, and projections were corrected for rotation. A 3D image ($48 \times 48 \times 60$, 0.5-mm voxels) was reconstructed from these eight projections using the maximum-likelihood estimation maximization (MLEM) algorithm with convolution for resolution modeling [Reader, 2002, Zinchenko, 2003]. Figure 24.3 provides a maximum intensity projection (MIP) of the reconstructed volume that is consistent with the projections in Fig. 24.2. For a non-magnifying pinhole geometry, the standard pinhole collimator resolution expression

$$R_c = \frac{a+b}{a} d_e \tag{24.1}$$

(a is the pinhole-to-detector distance, b is the pinhole to object distance) indicates that the pinhole point-spread function (full-width half-maximum) at the imaging volume center is 2.5 times the pinhole diameter. Figure 24.4 demonstrates the observed and expected line broadening due to the non-magnifying geometry.

5. Conclusions and open issues

Low-resolution imaging with static pinhole geometry and energy-integrating storage phosphor detectors is a feasible, low-cost alternative for high-throughput evaluation of imaging agents and for determining optimal timing of high-resolution, small-animal SPECT studies. High resolution is not limited by the intrinsic resolution or sensitivity of the SP detector, but is due to limited angular sampling with small numbers of projections.

The current prototype possesses detector areas that allow for expansion to two rings of 90° pinholes, or three rings of 60° pinholes. The challenge for higher resolution is to increase angular sampling by increasing the number of projections in the static geometry. Sixty projections have been reported as sufficient for imaging [Palmer and Wollmer, 1990], but multiplexed multi-pinholes [Schramm, 2001], coded-apertures [Schellingerhout, 2002], and relaxed collimation [Prior, 1993] are possible solutions for efficient projection packing.

For low exposures with PS image plates, noise levels obey the expected Poisson statistics [Arbique, 2003]. However, at uniform higher exposures, it has been demonstrated that structured noise source in the image plate contributes to spatial-variant signal-to-noise ratio [Nishikawa and Yaffe, 1990]. A procedure for correcting projection images in the pre-processing stage has not been addressed.

BaF(Br,I):Eu^{2+} SP imaging plates are optimized for 80 kVp radiography. Unfortunately, a large K-edge at 40 keV reduces the sensitivity of SP detectors to ^{125}I emissions. The future commercial availability of storage phosphors more suitably matched to low-energy emissions (RbCs:Tl^{+} and CsBr:Eu^{2+}) will increase the efficiency of energy-integrated imaging with ^{125}I.

As stated above, the primary challenge remains the development of image reconstruction algorithms that provide scatter correction. Inevitably, this will probably require knowledge of the mouse topography (size and shape) for modeling scatter on a per-animal basis.

Acknowledgments

This work was supported in part by NCI P20 CA 86354.

Notes

1. The terms *screen* and *image plate* are synonymous in the context of this paper
2. The terms *storage phosphor* (SP), *photostimulable luminescence* (PSL), and *photostimulable storage phosphor* (PSP) are synonymous in the context of this paper.
3. Exposure time will depend upon collimation. Our experience is that 1 minute per 2 μCi is typically sufficient

References

[Antich, 2003] P. P Antich, M. A. Lewis, E. Richer, P. V. Kulkarni, B. J. Smith, R. P. Mason. "A novel multi-pinhole/CCD-coupled CsI(Tl) crystal gamma camera for fully 3D μSPECT/μCT small-animal imaging," *Journal of Nuclear Medicine*, vol. 44(5 (Supplement)), pp. 161P No. 523. Presented at 2003 SNM Annual Meeting, New Orleans, LA, June 2003.

[Arbique, 2003] G. Arbique, J. Guild, J. Anderson, T. Blackburn, T. Lane, J. Wang, "Clinical experience with a FUJI computed radiography quality assurance program," *Medical Physics*, vol. 30(6), pp. 1344, Presented at 2003 AAPM Annual Meeting, San Diego, California, August 2003.

[Boone, 2003] J. M. Boone, C. K. Abbey, S. R. Cherry, "A combined I-125 nuclear emission and transmission radiography system for co-registered imaging of mouse function and anatomy," *Medical Physics*, vol. 30(6), pp. 1438–1439. Presented at 2003 AAPM Annual Meeting, San Diego, California, August, 2003.

[Johnston, 1990] R. F. Johnston, S. C. Pickett, D. L. Barker, "Autoradiography using storage phosphor technology," *Electrophoresis*, vol. 11(5), pp. 355–360, 1990.

[Nishikawa and Yaffe, 1990] R. M. Nishikawa, M. J. Yaffe, "Effect of various noise sources on the detective quantum of phosphor screens," *Medical Physics*, vol. 17(5), pp. 887–893, 1990.

[Palmer and Wollmer, 1990] J. Palmer, P. Wollmer, "Pinhole emission computed tomography: method and experimental evaluation," *Phys. Med. Biol.*, vol. 35(3), pp. 339–350, 1990.

[Prior, 1993] J. O. Prior, P. P. Antich, J. Fernando, J. A. Anderson, P. V. Kulkarni, R. W. Parkey, "Imaging stategies with scintillating fibers detectors: issues and preliminary results," In *Scintillating Fiber Technology and Applications. SPIE.*, vol. 2007, pp. 116–124, 1993.

[Reader, 2002] A. J. Reader, S. Ally, F. Bakatselos, R. Manavaki, R. J. Walledge, A. P. Jeavons, P. J. Julyan, S. Zhao, D. L. Hastings, J. Zweik, "One-pass list-mode em algorithm for high resolution 3D pet image reconstruction into large arrays," *IEEE Trans. Nucl. Sci.*, vol. 49, pp. 693–699, 2002.

[Rowlands, 2002] J. A. Rowlands, "The physics of computed radiography," *Phys. Med. Biol.*, vol. 47(23), pp. R123–R166, 2002.

[Schellingerhout, 2002] D. Schellingerhout, R. Accorsi, U. Mahmood, J. Idoine, R. C. Lanza, R. Weissleder, "Coded aperture nuclear scintigraphy: A novel small animal imaging technique," *Molecular Imaging*, vol. 1(4), pp. 344–352, 2002.

[Schramm, 2001] N. Schramm, A. Wirrwar, H. Halling, "Development of a multi-pinhole detector for high-sensitivity SPECT imaging," In *IEEE Nuclear Science Symposium*, vol. 3, pp. 1585–1586, 2001.

[Sonoda, 1983] M. Sonoda, M. Takano, J. Miyahara, H. Kato, "Computed radiography utilizing scanning laser stimulated luminescence," *Radiology*, vol. 148(3), pp. 833–888, 1983.

[Tenney, 2002] C. R. Tenney, "On the use of an energy-integrating detector for small-animal pinhole emission computed tomography," Presented at 2002 Annual Conference of the Academy of Molecular Imaging, San Diego, CA, October 2002.

[von Seggern, 1999] H. von Seggern, "Photostimulable x-ray storage phosphors: a review of present understanding," *Brazilian Journal of Physics*, vol. 29(2), pp. 254–268, 1999.

[Zinchenko, 2003] A. Zinchenko, E. N. Tsyganov, N. V. Slavine, P. V. Kulkarni, M. A. Lewis, R. P. Mason, O. K. Oz, R. W. Parkey, P. P. Antich, "Expectation maximization algorithm with resolution deconvolution for 3-D image reconstruction in a small animal PET imager," *Journal of Nuclear Medicine*, vol. 44(5 (Supplement)), pp.161P, No. 528. Presented at 2003 SNM Annual Meeting, New Orleans, LA, June 2003.

Chapter 25

Cardiac Pinhole-Gated SPECT in Small Animals

Tony Lahoutte, Chris Vanhove, and Philippe R. Franken*

1. Introduction

Electrocardiographically gated myocardial perfusion single-photon emission computed tomography (gated-SPECT) is a non-invasive and valuable tool for simultaneous assessment of myocardial perfusion and cardiac function in man. The use of this technique in rats is challenging because of the small size of the heart and the heart rate.

Conventional clinical imaging systems do not provide adequate spatial resolution when operated with parallel-hole collimators. The use of a pinhole collimator can improve the trade-off between sensitivity and resolution for small organs located in close proximity to the pinhole aperture.

The purpose of this work was to demonstrate the feasibility and the reproducibility of pinhole gated-SPECT to measure global and regional left ventricular function in the normal rat. The method was further evaluated to determine its ability to detect inotropic changes induced by halothane (an anaesthetic gas with known negative inotropic effects) or by dobutamine (a drug with known positive inotropic effects).

2. Animal preparation and handling

Studies were performed on male Wistar rats (Harlan Netherlands; age range, 14-18 weeks). They were allowed free access to water and food before imaging. The housing conditions were kept constant throughout the study in order to minimize variations due to physiological parameters.

The animals were anaesthetized by intraperitoneal injection of 60 mg/kg pentobarbital 15 to 20 minutes before imaging. They were then placed in a stationary supine position and instrumented with ECG electrodes connected to a standard ECG monitor (AccuSync, Medical Research Corporation, Milford, CT). Heart rate ranged from 250 to 360 beats per minutes.

The principles of the National Institutes of Health for laboratory animal care (NIH publication 86-23, revised 1985) were followed. The study protocol was approved by the Ethical Committee for Animal Studies of the University of Brussels.

*Department of Nuclear Medicine, University of Brussels, Brussels, Belgium

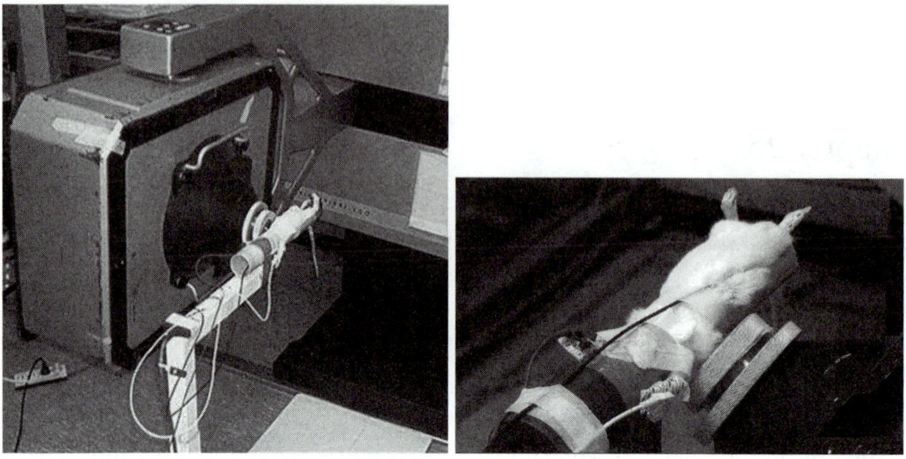

(a) (b)

Figure 25.1. Standard gamma camera (Sopha DSX) equipped with a pinhole collimator to performed gated SPECT acquisitions. The rat is studied in supine position and instrumented with ECG electrodes connected to a standard ECG monitor.

3. Radiopharmaceuticals

Technetium-99m sestamibi (440 $\pm$ 50 MBq in 0.3-ml saline) was injected intravenously 60 minutes before imaging.

4. Pinhole-gated SPECT imaging

Imaging was performed using a standard clinical single-head gamma camera (Sopha DSX) equipped with a pinhole collimator (opening: 3 mm; opening angle: 64°; focal length: 165 mm). The radius of rotation was 44 mm for all acquisitions (Fig. 25.1). The cardiac cycle was divided into 16 frames using the triggering device of the camera computer (beat acceptance window $\pm 50\%$ of average RR interval). Data were acquired over 360° using a circular orbit (64 steps; 20 seconds per step) during 22 minutes and stored in 64×64 matrices.

5. Data reconstruction

Data were reconstructed using a four-dimensional reconstruction algorithm based on OSEM (five iterations, four subsets) which takes into account the pinhole geometry, the mechanical shift, and the angular variation of the pinhole sensitivity [Vanhove, 2000]. In addition, a temporal filter based on the Fourier series is incorporated to reduce noise in the gated images [Vanhove, 2002]. No attenuation or scatter corrections were applied.

The voxel size in the reconstructed volume was 0.6 mm. Left ventricular short axis slices were obtained by manual reorientation of the reconstructed volumes along

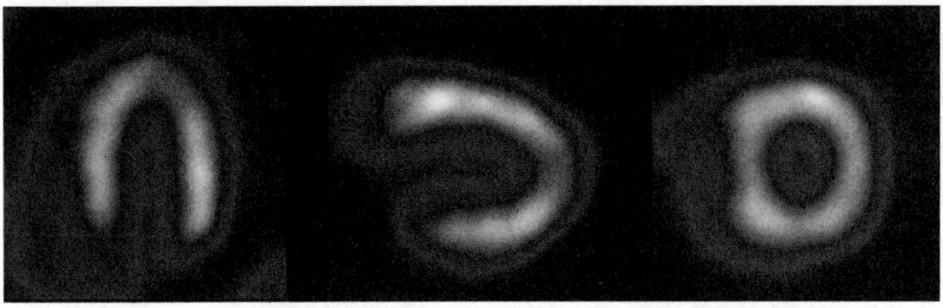

Figure 25.2. Myocardial perfusion (sestamibi) short axis, horizontal and vertical short axis slices obtained in a normal rat with pinhole SPECT(summed images).

the left ventricular long axis. No post-reconstruction filter was used. Reconstruction time was approximately 25 minutes on a Sun Ultra 5 workstation (128 MB memory installed).

6. Data analysis

High-quality images of myocardial perfusion were obtained in all animals by summing up the 16 gated frames (Fig. 25.2).

Left ventricular volumes and ejection fraction were calculated on the gated frames using the Stanford method (Mirage Processing Application, Segami Corporation, Paris, France). The method is based on statistical analysis of the activity profiles of the myocardial walls sampled in 3D from the center of the cavity. The first moment of the count distribution gives an estimate of the average position of the wall, while the second moment provides an estimate of the wall thickness [Goris, 1994]. These measurements were used to estimate the cavity volume at end-diastole (ED) and end-systole (ES). Left ventricular ejection fraction (LVEF) was calculated as (ED Ð ES) / ED.

7. Reproducibility study

Eight rats were investigated two times at 8-day interval. Images were of high quality in all animals. No significant differences were observed between the paired acquisitions. The root mean square differences between repeated measurements of ED volumes, ES volumes, and LVEF were 0.047 ml (6.9%), 0.022 ml (12%), and 0.036 (4.9%), respectively.

8. Monitoring the negative effect of halothane gas

Halothane is an anaesthetic gas with negative inotropic effect due to interactions with calcium metabolism (decreased calcium content in the sarcoplasmic reticulum and decreased myofilaments sensitivity to calcium). Six rats were investigated. For baseline measurements, the animals were anesthetized with pentobarbital. One week later, the same rats were imaged, first using the lowest halothane dosage to keep the animals asleep (1 - 1.5 vol% in 0.5 L/min oxygen) and then using high dose halothane (4 - 4.5 vol% in 0.5 L/min oxygen).

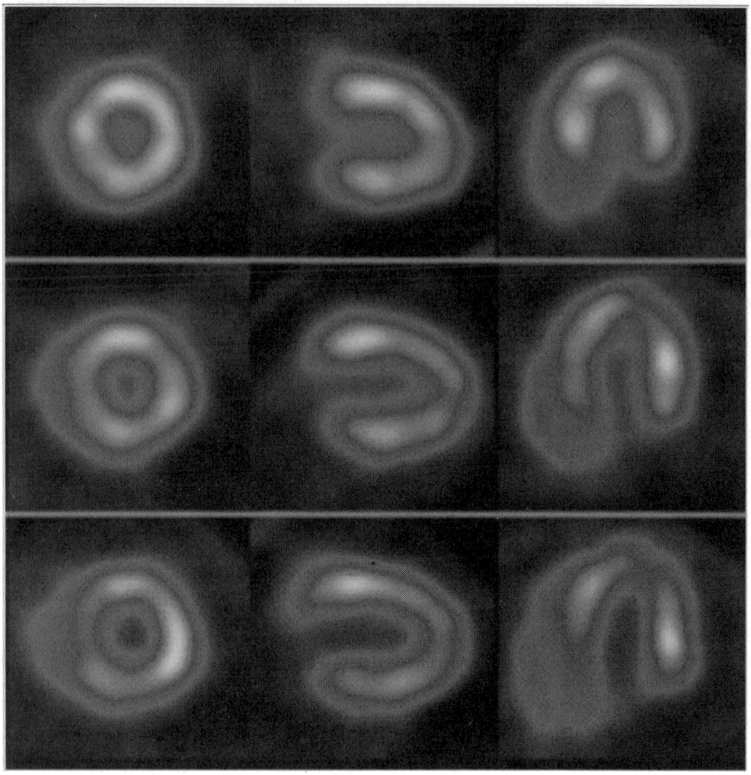

Figure 25.3. Negative inotropic effect of halothane anaesthetic gas demonstrated by serial gated SPECT end-systolic images obtained in a rat in baseline conditions (top), low-dose halothane (middle) and high-dose halothane (bottom). There is a dose dependent increase of the systolic volume reflecting reduced left ventricular contractility.

End systolic images obtained in a rat at baseline, low dose and high dose halothane are shown on Figure 25.3. An increase in ES volumes was already significant with the lowest dosage of halothane. ED volumes increased slightly. LVEF decreased from 71% at baseline to 60% during low-dose halothane ($p < 0.05$) and further decreased to 36% during high-dose halothane ($p < 0.001$). Significant decreases in wall motion and wall thickening were quantitatively measured during high-dose halothane.

9. Monitoring the positive inotropic effect of dobutamine

Dobutamine at low dose has a positive inotropic effect by direct stimulation of the beta-1 adrenergic receptors. Six rats were investigated. Serial-gated SPECT acquisitions were obtained in baseline conditions during continuous low-dose dobutamine (5 mcg/kg/min) and during higher-dose dobutamine administration (10 mcg/kg/min).

End-systolic images obtained in a rat at baseline, low-dose, and high-dose dobutamine are shown in Fig. 25.4. Decreases in ES and ED volumes were already

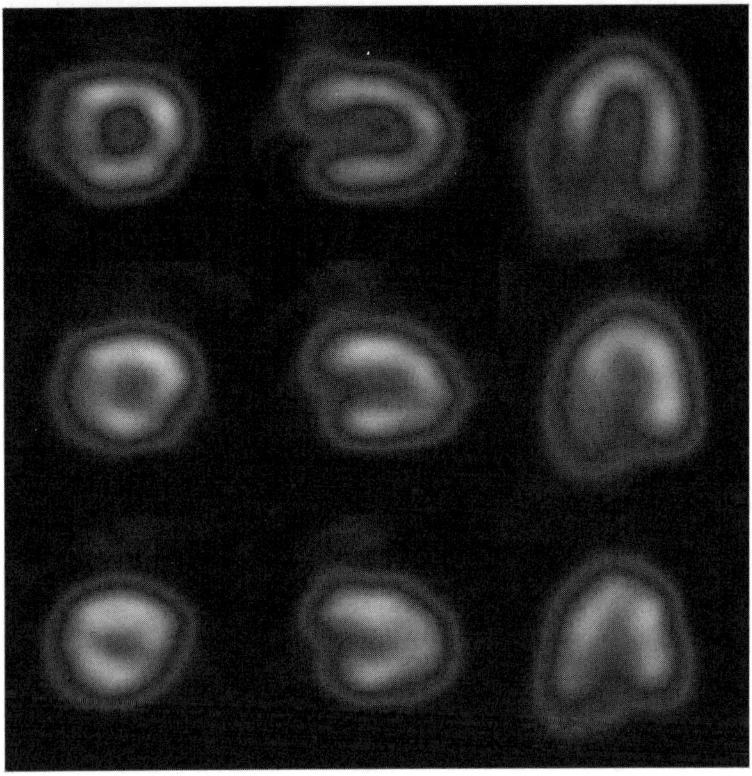

Figure 25.4. Positive inotropic effect of dobutamine demonstrated by serial gated SPECT end-systolic images obtained in a rat in baseline conditions (top), low-dose dobutamine (middle) and high-dose dobutamine (bottom). There is a dose-dependent decrease of the systolic volume reflecting increased left ventricular contractility.

significant with the lowest dosage of dobutamine. LVEF increased from 71% to 74% with low dose ($p < 0.05$) and to 78% with a higher dose of dobutamine. Significant increases in regional wall motion and wall thickening were also measured.

10. Conclusion

Besides myocardial perfusion, pinhole-gated SPECT allows objective measurements of left ventricular volumes and ejection fraction in living rats. The method is reproducible (high image quality, no operator interaction), repeatable (follow-up studies), rapid (less than 30 minutes) and inexpensive (using conventional gamma camera). The method is therefore ideally suited for investigating several cardiac rat models, new cardiovascular drugs, the cardiotoxicity of new drugs, and to evaluate the effect of new experimental treatments including gene and cell therapies.

References

[Goris, 1994] M. L. Goris, C. Thompson, L. J. Malone, P. R. Franken, "Modelling the integration of myocardial regional perfusion and function," *Nucl Med Commun.* vol. 15, pp. 9-20, 1994.

[Vanhove, 2000] C. Vanhove, M. Defrise, P. R. Franken, H. Everaert, F. Deconinck, A. Bossuyt. "Interest of the ordered subsets expectation maximization (OS-EM) algorithm in pinhole SPECT reconstruction: A phantom study," *Eur. J. Nucl. Med.* vol. 27, pp. 140-146, 2000.

[Vanhove, 2002] C. Vanhove, P. R. Franken, M. Defrise, F. Deconinck, A. Bossuyt. "Reconstruction of gated myocardial perfusion SPECT incorporating temporal information during iterative reconstruction," *Eur. J. Nucl. Med.*, vol. 29, pp. 465-472, 2002.

Index